D1473200

IMMEDIATE HYPERSENSITIVITY

The Molecular Basis of the Allergic Response

NORTH-HOLLAND RESEARCH MONOGRAPHS

FRONTIERS OF BIOLOGY

VOLUME 28

Under the General Editorship of

A. NEUBERGER

London

and

E. L. TATUM

New York

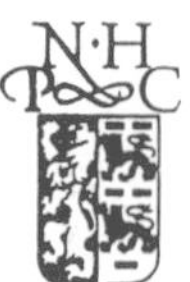

NORTH-HOLLAND PUBLISHING COMPANY
AMSTERDAM · LONDON

IMMEDIATE HYPERSENSITIVITY

The Molecular Basis of the Allergic Response

D. R. STANWORTH

Reader in Experimental Pathology
University of Birmingham

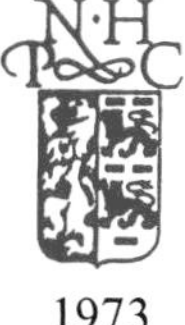

1973

NORTH-HOLLAND PUBLISHING COMPANY – AMSTERDAM • LONDON
AMERICAN ELSEVIER PUBLISHING COMPANY, INC. – NEW YORK

Library of Congress Catalog Card Number: 72-88579
ISBN North-Holland for this Series: 0 7204 7100 1
ISBN North-Holland for this Volume: 0 7204 7128 1
ISBN American Elsevier: 0 444 10444 5

Publishers:

NORTH-HOLLAND PUBLISHING COMPANY – AMSTERDAM
NORTH-HOLLAND PUBLISHING COMPANY, LTD. – LONDON

Sole distributors for the U.S.A. and Canada:

AMERICAN ELSEVIER PUBLISHING COMPANY, INC.
52 VANDERBILT AVENUE
NEW YORK, N.Y. 10017

PRINTED IN THE NETHERLANDS

Editors' preface

The aim of the publication of this series of monographs, known under the collective title of '*Frontiers of Biology*', is to present coherent and up-to-date views of the fundamental concepts which dominate modern biology.

Biology in its widest sense has made very great advances during the past decade, and the rate of progress has been steadily accelerating. Undoubtedly important factors in this acceleration have been the effective use by biologists of new techniques, including electron microscopy, isotopic labels, and a great variety of physical and chemical techniques, especially those with varying degrees of automation. In addition, scientists with partly physical or chemical backgrounds have become interested in the great variety of problems presented by living organisms. Most significant, however, increasing interest in and understanding of the biology of the cell, especially in regard to the molecular events involved in genetic phenomena and in metabolism and its control, have led to the recognition of patterns common to all forms of life from bacteria to man. These factors and unifying concepts have led to a situation in which the sharp boundaries between the various classical biological disciplines are rapidly disappearing.

Thus, while scientists are becoming increasingly specialized in their techniques, to an increasing extent they need an intellectual and conceptual approach on a wide and non-specialized basis. It is with these considerations and needs in mind that this series of monographs, '*Frontiers of Biology*' has been conceived.

The advances in various areas of biology, including microbiology, biochemistry, genetics, cytology, and cell structure and function in general will be presented by authors who have themselves contributed significantly to these developments. They will have, in this series, the opportunity of bringing together, from diverse sources, theories and experimental data, and of integrating these into a more general conceptual framework. It is unavoidable, and probably even desirable, that the special bias of the individual authors will become evident in their contributions. Scope will also be given for presentation of new and challenging ideas and hypotheses for which complete evidence is at present lacking. However, the main emphasis will be on fairly complete and objective presentation of the more important and more rapidly advancing aspects of biology. The level will be advanced, directed primarily to the needs of the graduate student and research worker.

Most monographs in this series will be in the range of 200–300 pages, but on occasion a collective work of major importance may be included somewhat exceeding this figure. The intent of the publishers is to bring out these books promptly and in fairly quick succession.

It is on the basis of all these various considerations that we welcome the opportunity of supporting the publication of the series *'Frontiers of Biology'* by North-Holland Publishing Company.

E.L. TATUM
A. NEUBERGER, General Editors

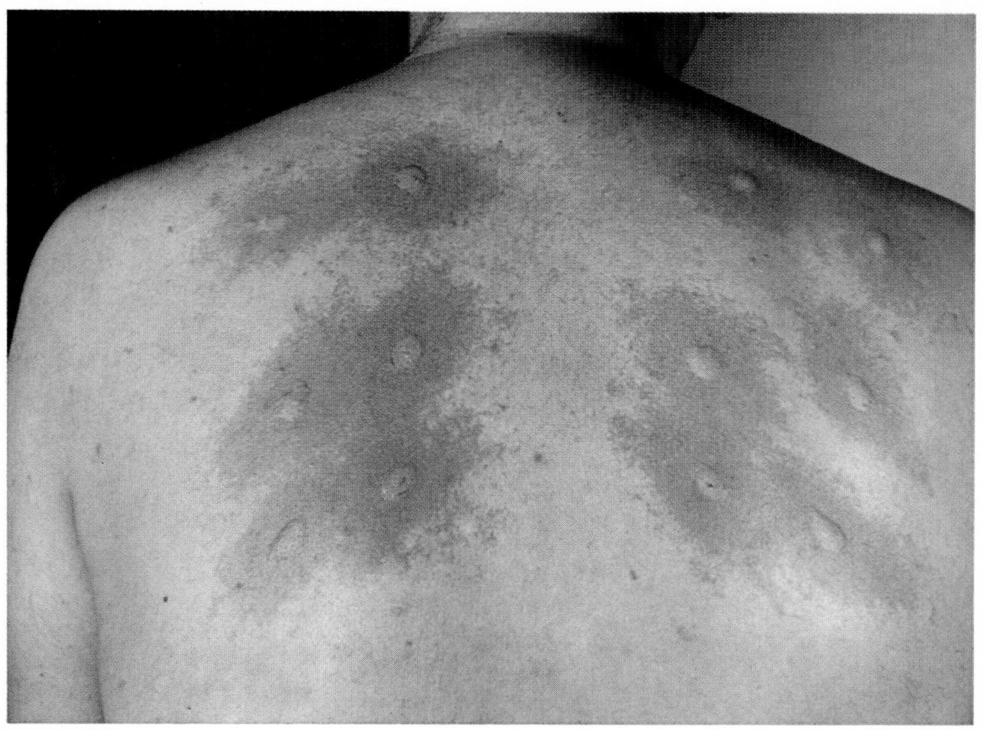

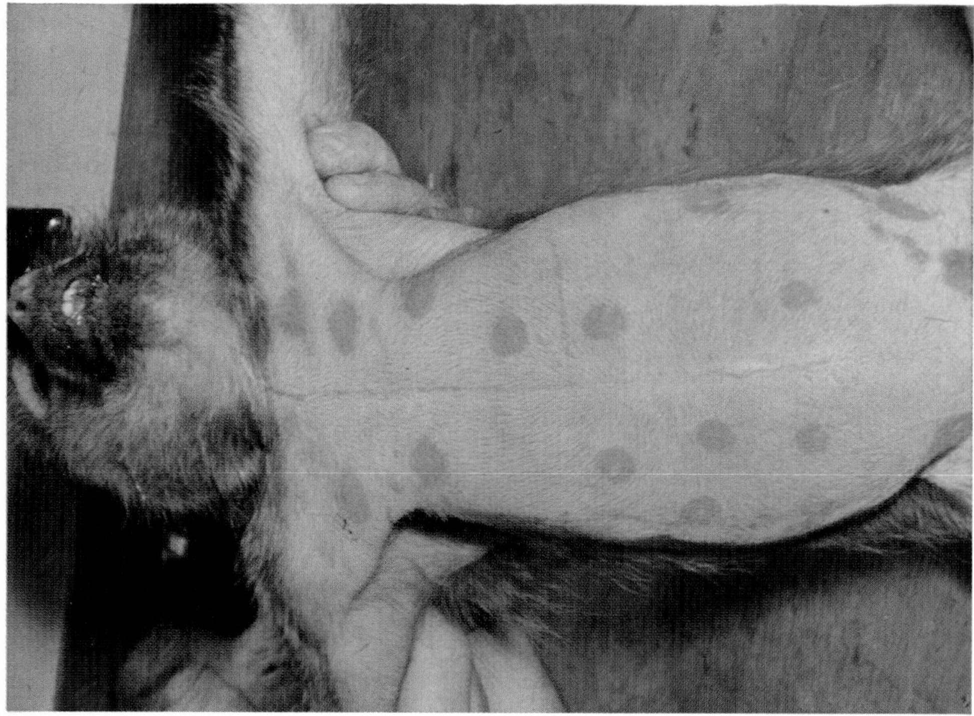

Demonstration of the passive transfer of immediate human hypersensitivity to local skin sites on a baboon.

Author's preface

Occasionally in some area of scientific endeavour the various parts begin falling into place after many years of patient, and often unconnected, observation by investigators of diverse disciplines. This applies particularly to the investigation of immediate hypersensitivity; which for many years has been hampered by the lack of adequate laboratory techniques, but which is now rapidly becoming recognised as one of the most fascinating and clinically important areas of immunology.

Like many of my former associates, I was fortunate to be inspired by The Prof: (the late John R. Squire); who, with his customary foresight, introduced me at an early stage to the challenging problems facing the immunochemist in this field of human allergy. Consequently over the last 23 years I have been in a crucial position to witness the growth of the subject, and to play an active part in its development at both the cellular and molecular levels. I am writing, therefore, with a fairly considerable experience of most of the experimental approaches discussed. The concept of the mechanism of the immediate hypersensitivity response which I have developed is, unashamedly, that of an immunochemist; for ultimately, of course, it will be necessary to explain all immunological phenomena in chemical and physical terms.

I am most grateful to the many people, throughout the years, who have made it possible for me to pursue my studies. I am referring particularly to: the many clinicians (including John Morrison Smith and Gunter Holti), who have helped me with skin testing and the provision of suitable specimens; to my friends in industry (such as Frank Milner, Head of the Bencard Allergy Unit) who have met all my requests for allergenic materials; my overseas collaborators (such as Bill Kuhns and John Willard in the U.S.A., and Hans Bennich and Gunnar Johansson in Sweden); my own technical assistants and research associates (particularly Pauline Jones, Carol Phillips, Ann Graetz, Ann Smith and Penny McLaughlan) and to the many allergic and normal blood donors in particular Pat Crockson, née Ratcliff, whose serum has found its way into many laboratories across the world). I must also mention the generous financial support which I have received from the Medical Research Council, The Wellcome Trust and the Asthma Research Council; and financial assistance from Fisons Ltd. in the reproduction of the colour plate. The human skin reactions shown there were obtained by courtesy of Peter Wolf.

Finally, I want to acknowledge much help in the preparation of this monograph. I am grateful to my young research students (such as Bharat Jasani) for many stimulating discussions; to Ray Stuckey and Dave Roberts for preparing the illustrations; and to Eileen Bishop, amongst others, for help with the typing.

I shall be forever indebted to my family (Barbara, Deborah and Sarah Jane) for their support and encouragement.

Immunoglobulin nomenclature

Since this monograph was written there has been a recommendation (Immunochem. 1972, *9*, 597), by the Sub-committee for Human Immunoglobulins of the IUIS Nomenclature Committee, that the existing dual terminology (i.e. Ig and γ) should be discontinued and that in future the usage of γ should be restricted to the designation of the heavy polypeptide chains of IgG. The recommended nomenclature has been adopted in the subject index.

Contents

CHAPTER 1

Introduction

The experimental investigation of immediate hypersensitivity started about a hundred years ago with the studies of Blackley (1873) *, a medical practitioner who was himself a hayfever sufferer. Besides demonstrating that attacks could be provoked in himself and other patients by the deliberate inhalation of grass pollen, he showed that it was possible to elicit localised reactions in the skin of the forearms by application of pollen grains to abraded areas; and in the conjunctiva following contact with an aqueous extract of pollen. This led to the practice of skin and conjunctival provocation testing with extracts of pollens and other common inhalants, such as animal danders and house dust, in order to identify the offending agents (now usually referred to as 'allergens').

The weal (edema) and flare (erythema) reactions thus elicited in hypersensitive individuals, by intradermal injection of allergen appeared within a few minutes, in contrast to the much slower development of cell-mediated hypersensitivity reactions of the delayed type. Furthermore, the involvement of circulating antibodies in a mediatory role distinguishes immediate from delayed hypersensitivity responses.

This was first suggested by the classical studies of Prausnitz

* For a fascinating description of these early investigations read 'Experimental Researches on the Causes and Nature of Catarrhus Aestivus (Hayfever or Hay-Asthma)' by C.H. Blackley. Reprinted (1959) by Dawsons of Pall Mall.

(1921), who demonstrated that local sites in his forearms could be passively sensitised by the intradermal injection of serum from a fish-sensitive donor (Küstner). The subsequent injection of the same sites (24 hr later) with fish extract evoked immediate weal and erythema reactions (see colour plate), similar to those elicited directly by intradermal injection of fish extract into Küstner's forearms. This important observation, which was confirmed accidentally on one occasion when Prausnitz inadvertently partook of a fish breakfast on the day after injecting himself with a fish-sensitive individual's serum, was soon followed by the successful passive transfer of hypersensitivity to other materials such as horse serum (De Besche 1923) and grass pollen (Freeman 1924).

Besides providing the first evidence of involvement of a circulating factor in the mediation of immediate hypersensitivity reactions, these fundamental experiments pointed to a more objective method of studying such reactions, in isolation from any influence of the hypersensitive individual. Coca and Grove (1925) went on to employ the Prausnitz–Küstner (P–K) test in an extensive study of the nature of the skin sensitising substance passively transferable in the sera of pollen-sensitive individuals. It appeared to become firmly and rapidly fixed to normal human skin, being detectable at least four weeks after transfer; and yet its activity was markedly reduced by heating the serum at 56° for 30 min. In contrast, heat stable antisera raised in rabbits against ragweed pollen and egg protein failed to sensitise passively normal human skin; although such rabbit antisera, unlike the sera of hypersensitive humans, were capable of passively sensitising guinea pig skin (in vivo) and uterus (in vitro). The human skin sensitising factor resembled precipitating antibodies in its specificity for 'antigen', by which it appeared to be neutralised in vitro as well as in vivo. Yet it failed to produce a visible precipitate, nor did it fix complement when mixed with specific allergen extract. Moreover, in its successive fractional neutralisation behaviour, it did not conform to the quantitative laws governing the fractional neutralisation of precipitating antibodies.

There appeared, therefore, to be insufficient evidence to conclude that the skin sensitising factor appeared in the circulation of hypersensitive individuals as the result of an immunological stimulus, despite the belief expressed earlier by Von Pirquet (1906) that an antigen-antibody reaction formed the basis of allergic phenomena. Consequently, Coca and Grove (1925) referred to the sensitising factor by the non-commital term 'atopic reagin', by analogy with the usage of reagin to denote the serum factor responsible for the Wassermann reaction. The term 'atopy' had already been proposed by Coca and Cooke (1923) to denote a form of human hypersensitivity associated with a hereditary predisposition, the sensitising substances being referred to as 'atopens'.

This, then, was the position fifty years ago in the field of immediate hypersensitivity. Individuals showing symptoms of the hayfever-urticaria-asthma type were known to contain substances in their circulations which possessed some of the characteristics of antibodies produced by artificial immunisation of normal humans and animals, but which demonstrated other properties which distinguished them from conventional precipitating antibodies. Foremost amongst the latter characteristics was their persistence at the site of injection of isologous skin for several weeks, in contrast to injected precipitating antibodies which diffuse away rapidly. It was thought likely that the skin sensitising factors were produced as a result of stimulus by antigenic substances within inhaled materials (pollens, animal danders etc.), particularly as immunisation of animals with extracts of these materials was shown to produce precipitating antibodies possessing anaphylactic properties. But there was no evidence that those immunogenic constituents responsible for antibody formation in animals were also involved in the induction of immediate hypersensitivity in humans.

One of the first major problems to be tackled has been, therefore, the identification and isolation of those antigens (allergens) and antibodies (reagins) involved specifically in immediate hypersensitivity reactions. Yet, despite the development of many refined protein fractionation and characterisation techniques over the last thirty years, progress has been – until recently – disappointingly slow. One of the main reasons for this has been a lack of suitable and more convenient alternatives to direct and passive skin testing, for the measurement of immediate hypersensitivity reactions in the laboratory. The last decade has seen, however, the development of several in vitro methods of assay, as well as in vivo alternatives to P–K testing in humans.

It seemed appropriate, therefore, to undertake a critical appraisal of the efficacy and reliability of the wide range of assay procedures now available, before going on to consider the fruits of their application. This has been attempted in ch. 2, which is written in the light of considerable personal experience of most of the techniques discussed; including the quantitation of the classical P–K test, which has been taken as a yard-stick. The important question of establishing a suitable allergic serum as reference standard, for circulation between laboratories, is also considered.

The complexity in composition of aqueous extracts of common inhalants has presented a formidable task to those attempting to isolate allergenic constituents in pure form. My own experiences in this direction have been concerned with the characterisation of those substances responsible for human hypersensitivity to horse dandruff; which, I believe it is fair to state, represented the first systematic chemical study of an allergenic extract. I have, therefore, outlined in some detail in ch. 3 the approach which I evolved for the isolation and characterisation of horse dander allergen in the hope that it will serve as a guide to future investigators of other allergen systems; quite apart from the light it throws on allergen structure in general. The significance of the principal studies undertaken on the other major allergen systems (ragweed and grass pollens, house dust, foods, drugs etc.) is also considered in ch. 3; leading to a discussion of the fundamental question of the structural basis of allergenic activity. It seemed appropriate to consider also in this chapter the nature of those substances responsible for the initiation of a hypersensitive state in pre-disposed individuals. Although it has been customary to refer to these substances as allergens, too, it is suggested that 'sensitogen' would be a more appropriate term; by analogy with usage of the term 'immunogen', as opposed to antigen, when referring to those substances responsible for inducing immunity states.

The isolation and characterisation of the antibodies (reagins) involved in immediate hypersensitivity responses is outlined in ch. 4. This work has been handicapped by the extremely low levels of reaginic antibodies in the sera of even the most hypersensitive of individuals; as will become apparent from the back-ground studies, reviewed at the beginning of the chapter from a historical stand-point. It was only with the emergence of zone-fractionation procedures, and sensitive immunodiffusion techniques for the characterisation of the resultant fractions, that any real progress was made with reagin characterisation. Even then, as will be noted, the many attempts to assign sensitising antibodies to one or other of the major immunoglobulin classes were clouded by considerable controversy.

The whole picture was clarified dramatically in 1967 with the unexpected discovery, in Sweden, of an unique form of myeloma gamma globulin; which has proved to be a pathological counterpart of reaginic antibody and thus provided convincing evidence that reagins belonged to a new immunoglobulin class (IgE or γE). Furthermore this paraprotein, which has since been found in a few other cases of this rare form of myelomatosis, offers the key to the complete structural characterisation of reaginic antibodies besides proving an invaluable reagent in the investigation of their various functional roles; as will be apparent from ch. 5, in which the crucial role of the antibody in the mediation of immediate hypersensitivity reactions is discussed in structural terms.

Hence it is now possible for the first time to begin to place my subject on a firm immunochemical basis. Nevertheless, despite the obvious advantages of myeloma γE globulin in this respect, there are other areas where different approaches are beginning to bear fruit. Indeed, as has been mentioned on more than one occasion, it seems likely that some forms of immediate hypersensitivity are mediated by non-γE types of antibody. For this reason, particular attention has been paid (in ch. 4) to claims of isolation of such antibodies from human allergic sera. This possibility is also raised by the demonstration of γG-type isologous tissue sensitising antibodies in artificially-sensitised animals. This and many other important conclusions about the mechanism of anaphylactic reactions, to be drawn from studies in experimental animals, are considered in a separate chapter (6). It is encouraging that recent evidence suggests that such systems are more plausible models for immediate hypersensitivity in humans than was originally suspected; even where heterologous tissue sensitising antibodies are employed in passive sensitisation studies. Moreover, it now seems reasonable to conclude that the reagin-like antibodies (sometimes referred to as 'homocytotropic') whose production can be induced by artificial means in most mammalian species investigated (e.g. rat, rabbit, mouse, dog etc.) belong, like human reagins, to a unique immunoglobulin class (i.e. IgE). Consequently the use of such species besides others like the dog, in which reaginic antibodies also occur spontaneously, is proving invaluable in defining the many factors which influence the induction of hypersensitive (as opposed to hyperimmune) states.

Studies of experimentally induced anaphylaxis are also providing important new information about the control of reagin synthesis, as well as the manner of its disappearance; both aspects which are not readily investigated in humans. Although, with the availability now of specific anti-human IgE antiserum, it is becoming possible to identify those cells involved in both the formation and subsequent uptake of reaginic antibodies. These, and certain other questions relating to reagin-cell interaction, are discussed in ch. 7; as are recent claims of the involvement of γE antibodies in processes which can be beneficial to the host.

Hence, with the identification of the principal reactants now well advanced, and reliable in vitro assay systems as well as experimental animal models now available, it is possible to consider seriously the mode of interaction between reaginic antibody and allergen at the target cell surface. This is, of course, the critical event which (as is depicted schematically in fig. 1.1) triggers the chain of reactions culminating in the release of vasoactive amines responsible for the familiar clinical manifestations of immediate hypersensitivity. A separate chapter (8) has been devoted to this important aspect of my subject; in which I have attempted to bring together not only current knowledge about the mode of action of γE (and γG) sensitising antibodies, but also recent pertinent observations on the many and varied artificial (both immunological and non-immunological) means of inducing the release of

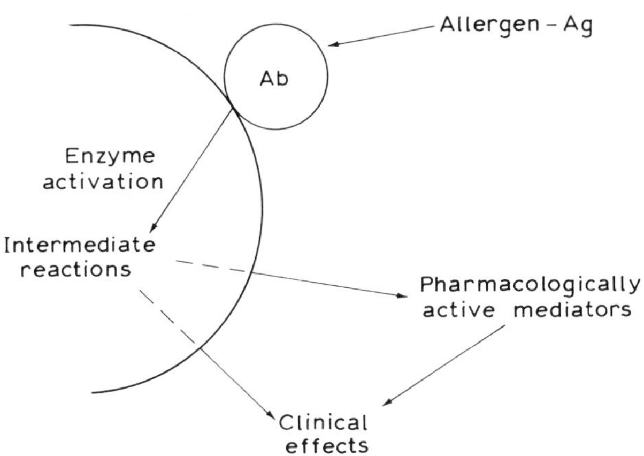

Fig. 1.1. The immediate hypersensitivity system – terms of reference.

mediators of immediate hypersensitivity responses from mast cells and basophils. Other types of release processes, involving different target cells, have also been considered for comparison; including the supposed mechanism of action of hormones which, it is felt, could have more than a little relevance to the nature and outcome of the trigger process effected by reagin–allergen interaction on mast cell surfaces. Throughout ch. 8 arguments have been developed to support the view that, despite their apparent diversity, many artificial methods of effecting release of vasoactive amines possess important features in common with reagin-mediated anaphylactic release; which should become explicable with improved knowledge about the structure and function of cell membranes and the enzyme systems which they incorporate.

An effort has been made throughout this monograph to assess the practical, as well as the theoretical, significance of the many studies cited. For it is hoped that, besides their bearing on the understanding of the mechanism of immediate-type hypersensitivity, they will lead eventually to improved methods of diagnosis and even therapy. Consequently, the principles underlying various methods employed in the experimental inhibition of immediate sensitivity responses have been discussed in ch. 9 with the clinical reader particularly in mind.

A final, short, chapter (10) is concerned with my personal speculations about future approaches, in areas yet to be chartered in this fascinating field of biological science.

CHAPTER 2

Measurement of immediate hypersensitivity reactions

2.1 *Introduction*

The need for accurate measurement of immediate hypersensitivity phenomena is two-fold: to facilitate laboratory investigation, and to provide a reliable means of clinical diagnosis. Yet, although it is now fifty years since Prausnitz's classical demonstration of the local passive sensitisation of normal recipients, it is only recently that satisfactory alternative methods of assaying reaginic antibodies have been developed.

The aim in this chapter has been an overall appraisal of the various assay procedures now available. The principles on which they are based are outlined, and their relative efficacies are discussed, but no attempt has been made to provide complete technical details (which can be readily obtained from the key sources cited in the References).

The methods now in use can be conveniently divided, on practical grounds, into in vivo and in vitro procedures. As will be noted from the master diagram in fig. 2.1, test systems in both categories exploit the tissue (cell) binding property of reaginic antibody, relying upon the direct or indirect measurement of the histamine released as a result of subsequent reaction with specific antigen (i.e. allergen).

In contrast, other methods have now been developed which are based upon the in vitro binding of allergen by reaginic (γE) antibodies. One of these (the direct leucocyte test) involves deter-

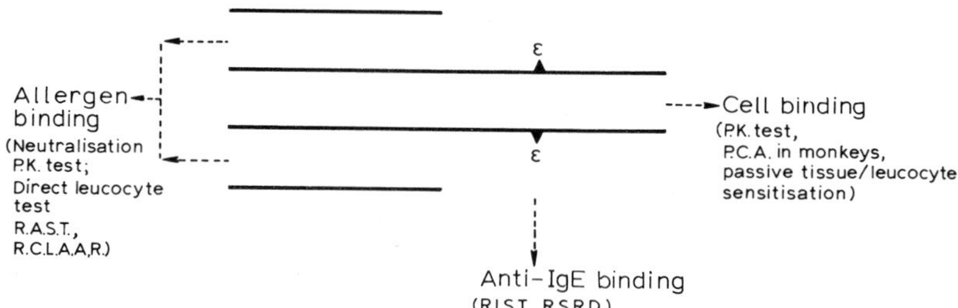

Fig. 2.1 Master diagram, illustrating the different principles on which the major methods of assaying reaginic antibodies are based.

mining the amount of allergen needed to effect the release of a standard amount of histamine (from the leucocytes of allergic donors); whilst others (such as R.A.S.T.; R.C.L.A.A.R) are based upon a quite different principle, relying upon the use of specific anti-IgE antiserum to measure the extent of reagin–allergen interaction. Specific anti-IgE antiserum is also used in other radioimmunoassay procedures (i.e. R.I.S.T.; R.S.R.D), but these provide a measure of the *total* amount of IgE (in serum or other body fluids) estimated as antigen.

It is important to recognise that none of the techniques mentioned in the previous paragraph provide a measure of the sensitising activity of reaginic (γE) antibody. In this sense, therefore, they differ from the procedures (in vitro as well as in vivo) which have evolved from the classical Prausnitz–Küstner test (fig. 2.1); and which, consequently, might be considered to provide an estimate of greater clinical significance.

2.2 In vivo passive transfer systems

2.2.1 Passive skin sensitisation in humans

Since Prausnitz passively sensitised sites on his forearm by injection of the fish-sensitive Küstner's serum (Prausnitz and Küstner 1921), the P–K test has been looked upon as the classical method of measuring immediate hypersensitivity reactions. It has become the yard-stick against which newly developed methods of assaying reaginic antibodies are assessed; and will, therefore, be considered in some depth.

Despite the early studies of Levine and Coca (1926), which indicated ways in which the accuracy of the P–K test could be improved, there has often been a tendency to perform it merely in a semi-quantitative manner. The dilution and neutralisation titration procedures originating from the work of these investigators suffer from the same disadvantage of relying upon an end-point corresponding to a weal response of minimal size where (as will be seen later) excessive variability is encountered. Nevertheless, the neutralisation procedure has the advantage that its end-point can be expressed in terms of accurately determined allergen (preferably pure) concentration, i.e. as the minimum amount of allergen protein, or protein N, needed to inhibit completely the P–K activity of a measured volume of allergic serum (with which it has been pre-incubated in vitro for 24 hr at 37°, or at lower temperatures).

Patterson and Correa (1959) have used this approach to demonstrate a constant quantitative relationship between reagin and allergen. Thus, it was shown that if an extract (of ragweed pollen) contains sufficient antigen to neutralise the reagin in an allergic serum (from an untreated patient) any dilution of the extract will neutralise an equivalent dilution of the serum. This quantitative relationship, at equivalence, is interpreted as evidence that reagin and allergen react in a similar manner to precipitating (γG) antibody and its homologous antigen. This is also suggested by more recent in vitro passive sensitisation studies (§ 2.3), which indicate that reagin–allergen interaction is suppressed by excess allergen (i.e. antigen).

It is assumed that this reaction, in neutralisation test systems, takes place in free solution in vitro (i.e. before the allergic serum–allergen mixture is injected into the normal recipient prior to subsequent challenge with allergen 24–48 hr later). It is difficult to exclude the possibility, however, that reagin–allergen interaction takes place on the cell surface, after the 'neutralisation mixture' has been injected. Indeed, immediate skin reactions have been observed in such circumstances (e.g. Patterson and Correa 1959); in view of the findings of Bowman and Walzer (1953), these premature reactions could contribute to the hypo-responsiveness of the transfer sites on subsequent challenge with allergen.

More recent findings, of Ishizaka and Ishizaka (1968A), would seem to suggest, however, that these initial skin reactions produced by reagin–allergen mixtures are effected by pre-formed complexes, and this is borne out by later observations of the same group (Ishizaka et al. 1967) which have revealed that reagin and allergen (radio-labelled ragweed antigen E) are capable of combining in vitro in the absence of cells. Thus, my earlier suggestion (Stanworth 1963) that possibly only cell-bound reaginic antibody is capable of combining with antigen appears to have no firm foundation.

2.2.1.1 Influence of blocking antibody. The neutralisation method of assaying reaginic antibodies will, of course, be particularly influenced by the presence of other types of antibody possessing anti-allergen activity (irrespective of whether they possess any capacity for binding isologous tissue). This first became apparent from tests performed by Cooke and associates (1935) on sera from ragweed sensitive patients taken before and after hyposensitisation. Thus, in contrast to the substantial weal and erythema reactions produced by mixtures of pre-treatment serum and allergen, post-treatment serum and an equivalent amount of allergen elicited negative (or relatively small) responses which were attributable to the presence of a non-sensitising, inhibitory antibody. Later studies (Cooke et al. 1937) showed that a blocking antibody possessing similar properties could be produced as a result of the injection of non-allergic individuals with a course of ragweed pollen extract.

Convincing evidence has since been obtained (Sehon et al. 1957; Connell and Sherman 1969) to suggest that blocking antibodies belong to a different immunoglobulin class to that of reaginic antibodies, being usually of the γG-type. As such they are responsible for the demonstrable ability of the sera of hyposensitised individuals to agglutinate allergen-coated erythrocytes (Rose et al. 1964) and to evoke typical PCA reactions in guinea pigs (Fisher and Connell 1962). The clinical significance of blocking antibodies will be considered later, in ch. 9.

The important point to recognise here is that the presence of blocking antibody in an allergic serum will complicate any assay procedure based on the allergen-binding capacity of the reaginic antibody. Thus, for example, in the leucocyte histamine release test (§ 2.3.3), it has been shown that competition by blocking antibody results in an increase in the amount of allergen required to effect a standard amount of histamine release. This finding can be interpreted as indicative of a greater avidity of blocking antibody, than that of reagin, for allergen. Moreover, this difference might be anticipated to be greater in the case of γM-type blocking antibody.

Obviously, therefore, the results of some modes of assay of an allergic serum could be influenced more than those of others by the previous treatment of the donor and, in particular, whether he has been subjected to injection with the offending antigen(s). Fortunately, in this connection, it has been observed that the product of reaction of blocking antibody (contained in heated post-treatment allergic serum) and allergen failed to induce immediate skin reactions of the type observed when reagin–allergen mixtures are injected into normal recipient's skin (Loveless 1940). In other words, complexes of blocking (γG) antibody and allergen (unlike γE antibody–allergen complexes) appear to be incapable of evoking such immediate reactions in vivo, and presumably of effecting immediate histamine release from human leucocytes in vitro. Obviously this is a prerequisite for the successful application of any assay procedure which involves neutralisation by the initial premixing of allergic serum with allergen in vitro.

The interference of blocking antibody with the accurate measurement of reaginic antibody activity by P–K testing has been avoided by some investigators by resort to a dilution titration procedure, involving the use of a sufficient excess of challenging allergen to meet the demands of any blocking antibody present in the allergic serum. This method suffers, however, from the difficulty of obtaining clear-cut end-points and requires the performance of a large number of tests (when there is often available only a limited area of the recipient's skin).

2.2.1.2 Quantitation of the P–K test. It is surprising that the types of P–K test to which I have referred so far have been practised for many years without any attempt being made to assess critically the accuracy of passive skin testing under carefully controlled conditions. A year's visit to New York University provided me with an opportunity to look into this question. In collaboration with W.J. Kuhns, I was able to undertake a detailed study of the various factors which can influence the accuracy of the P–K test. Our main findings (Stanworth and Kuhns 1965) are outlined below, to serve as a guide to the quantitative measurement of reaginic antibodies by this basic procedure.

Several quantitative studies had been previously undertaken of direct skin testing in allergic individuals (e.g. Becker and Rappaport 1948), and in the response of normal subjects to intradermal injections of histamine (Swain and Becker 1952); and, of course, some of their findings are also applicable to passive skin testing. As might be expected, however, extra technical problems are encountered in the transfer of allergic serum to normal skin sites, prior to subsequent challenge with allergen (as in the direct test). These include the variability in reactivity of the normal recipients available, the difficulty of accurately injecting small volumes (e.g. 0.1 ml) of serum intradermally and the problem of achieving optimal timing and siting of the allergen challenge. Any influence of blocking antibody present in the allergic serum can be avoided by using a sufficient excess of challenging allergen.

In our preliminary quantitative studies, involving the transfer of serum (0.1 ml aliquots) from a horse dandruff-sensitive individual (P.R.) into 36 sites arranged approximately 4 cm apart on the backs of three normal young male recipients, the position of the site was found not to contribute significantly to the variance of the areas of weals observed in two of the recipients (S.W. and M.D.). This is in contrast with the results of quantitative studies of direct skin testing, which indicated that the responsiveness of hypersensitive individuals to injected ragweed allergen (Becker and Rappaport 1948) and to histamine (Swain and Becker 1952) decreases as the forearm is descended and on passing from the ulnar to the radial side.

Hence, if site variance is to be avoided in human skin testing, the back of the recipient should be used in preference to his forearms. Moreover, this has the advantage of providing many more test sites in any one recipient; the maximum number which can be accomodated, with adequate spacing, on the back of an adult male of average size being of the order of 36. Even so, this number of sites is soon occupied if accurate results are to be obtained, as it is essential to perform all comparative tests in the same recipient.

This point was demonstrated by a combined analysis of variance of the areas of weals evoked in the two recipients (S.W. and M.D.) employed in our quantitative study referred to above. The variation between the results of the P–K tests in these two recipients was significantly greater ($0.05 > p > 0.01$) than the variation of the areas of weals elicited in a single individual, despite the mean areas of the weals in the two recipients being of similar magnitude (i.e. 73 ± 18 mm^2 in S.W. and 65 ± 21 mm^2 in M.D.). In contrast, P–K tests performed in the third normal (i.e. non-allergic) recipient (S.K.) used in the study revealed a considerable site to site (vertical) variation ($0.005 > p > 0.01$). He also proved unsuitable on account of his unusually low reactivity (i.e. a mean weal area of 22 ± 18 mm^2) which could possibly be attributed to his back being covered with a copious growth of hair, which had to be removed (by shaving) prior to passive sensitisation. This recipient would probably fall into the class of 'poor reactors' which, according to Coca and Grove (1925), comprise 5 per cent of normal individuals; another 11 per cent being classified as 'non-receptive' to local passive sensitisation.

A summary of the responses of various normal recipients to P–K testing on different occasions, with samples of the same diluted (1/4) serum from a horse dandruff-sensitive individual (P.R.) is given in table 2.1 (which includes the data referred to above). It will be noticed that the recipient S.K., who showed the

TABLE 2.1
Summary of responses of various recipients to P–K testing with diluted (1/5) horse dandruff allergic serum on different occasions.

Date of challenge (1961)	Recip-ient	No. of tests with 1/5 dilut-ed serum	Total no. of tests in series (excluding controls)	Mean weal area (mm^2)	Coeffi-cient of variation (%)	Noticeable features of recipient's skin
7 April	S.K.	4	48	55	35	Very hairy (re-quired shaving)
	R.D.	4	48	71	11	
9 May	R.D.	5	25	99	11	
		5 *	25 *	80	22	
26 July	J.F.	6	36	71	19	Sun-tanned
	H.S.	6	36	98	17	
	G.W.	6	36	91	20	
6 September	G.W.	36	36	73	25	
	M.D.	36	36	66	32	
	S.K.	36	36	22	85	(see above)
9 November	G.W.	6 †	36 †	73	22	
	I.P.	6 †	36 †	51	17	Readily showed flaring

* Sensitising serum diluted with 6 per cent human serum albumin solution.
† Sensitising serum diluted with recipient's serum.

marked site variance, also showed the greatest day to day variation in response. Even good reactors (e.g. R.D. and S.W.), however, showed significant day to day variation (of the order of 20 per cent). On the other hand, such reactors tested on the same day (e.g. H.S. and S.W. on 26th July; or S.W. and M.D. on 26th September), showed remarkably similary responses to the same sensitising dose of allergic serum.

Another point which emerges from the data given in table 2.1 is the apparent paradox that the greater the number of duplicate tests performed with any particular solution, the greater the variation in the area of weal elicited. This is most likely due to an increase in experimental error incurred in carrying out the much larger number of intradermal injections (e.g. 36 as compared to 6), as it is difficult to inject accurately under the epidermis a constant volume of sensitising serum at a constant depth (particularly when using 1 ml disposable tuberculin syringes). This was underlined by a quantitative study of direct skin testing by Rappaport and Becker (1949), who demonstrated the difficulty of injecting a constant volume of allergen solution to a constant depth into the dermis; even when using a specially designed stainless steel syringe, with barrel and plunger accurately machined to fit with a tolerance of 10^{-5} inches. One, unavoidable, cause of this is leakage of a variable amount of transferred fluid from the intradermal puncture hole on withdrawal of the needle. This source of variance can be minimised, however, by measuring the size of the initial injection blebs and then selecting for subsequent allergen challenge only those sites into which the standard volume of sensitising serum had been introduced. If such an approach is adopted, it is possible to restrict the variability in P–K response (as measured in weal area) to the order of 10–20 per cent in suitable recipients. This compares favourably with the degree of accuracy achieved in other types of biological assay.

If, however, the P–K test is to provide a satisfactory quantitative measure of skin sensitising antibody activity, it is essential to demonstrate (as was done in direct skin testing) that the size of weal produced is related linearly to the logarithm of antibody concentration, and that the variability in response is independent of this concentration. We (Stanworth and Kuhns 1965) showed that such conditions were fulfilled, by sensitising three normal recipients with various dilutions of serum from the horse dander-sensitive individual (P.R.) – at sites arranged randomly on their backs – followed by challenge 24 hr later by pricking in allergic solution. Typical log(dose)–response curves were obtained (an example of which is reproduced in fig. 2.2), by plotting mean weal area against serum dilution. In most cases, an approximately linear relationship was found to obtain up to a limiting dose corresponding to a 1/5 dilution of sensitising serum, whereupon the curves showed a tendency to flatten out (even when recipient's serum or 6 per cent human serum albumin solution, rather than buffered saline, were used as diluent). No evidence was obtained to suggest that this effect was due to lack of sufficient allergen for inter-

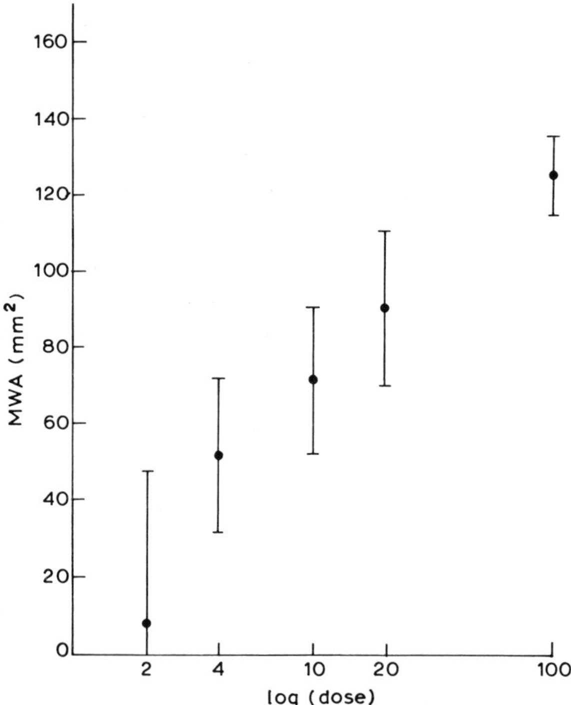

Fig. 2.2. A typical P–K test log(dose)–response curve (Stanworth and Kuhns 1965)..

action with the reagin available at sites injected with undiluted allergic serum. It could possibly be attributed, however, to an overloading of the skin sites with sensitising antibody, the excess being lost by diffusion from the transfer site.

The variability of the P–K response was found to be independent of dose, for weals of about 50 mm^2 or greater. Below this area, however, the variability increases and becomes excessive for weals of 10 mm^2 or less. This exposes a limitation of the dilution and neutralisation test procedures (discussed earlier), which rely on the accurate detection of minimal responses, corresponding to weals of this order of size. At the other end of the scale, weals larger than about 160 mm^2 are difficult to measure accurately, owing to their tendency to develop pseudopodia.

Hence, the assay of reagin activity by P–K testing is limited by the relatively narrow range over which weal responses can be quantitated accurately. Over this range a tenfold increase in dose leads to only a three- to fourfold increase in weal area. Nevertheless, the dose-response curve has a steeper slope than that revealed by measurement of response to the direct injection of histamine solutions into the forearm of individuals (allergic and non-allergic over the age of 10). In these tests, Swain and Becker (1952) showed that a 1000-fold increase in wealing agent concentration produced only a twofold increase in weal diameter. According to the calculations of Rappaport and Becker (1949), however, the measurement of weal area rather than diameter would double the slope of the dose-response curve.

In considering the various factors likely to influence the accuracy of P–K testing, attention has been paid, so far, only to the passive transfer stage. It is important to recognise, however, that other sources of error can arise at the time of allergen challenge of the sensitised skin sites. Throughout our quantitative studies (Stanworth and Kuhns 1965), allergen was injected by pricking in a concentrated solution of horse dandruff protein (in excess of the amount required to exhaust – by a single prick – sites passively sensitised with the undiluted allergen serum). Apart from the obvious advantages of prick testing, this method of introduction permits a study of the influence of allergen siting on the magnitude of P–K response. It is also possible to obtain some measure of the rate of outward diffusion of reagin from the transfer site.

For instance, we compared the sizes of weals evoked in a number of normal skin sites, each passively sensitised with 0.1 ml serum (diluted 1/1.5) from our regular horse dander-sensitive donor (P.R.), after pricking in allergen centrally (position 1), in the periphery of the injection bleb (position 2) or 5 mm outside the periphery (position 3) as is indicated in fig. 2.3a. The mean areas of weals evoked by peripheral challenge, 2 hr after transfer, were almost 25 per cent smaller than the mean areas of weals evoked by central challenge; whereas challenge at the point (position 3) selected arbitrarily 5 mm outside the periphery failed to evoke any response. Repeat challenge at the same outer site (position 3) 7–8 hr after transfer, produced weals of appreciable size

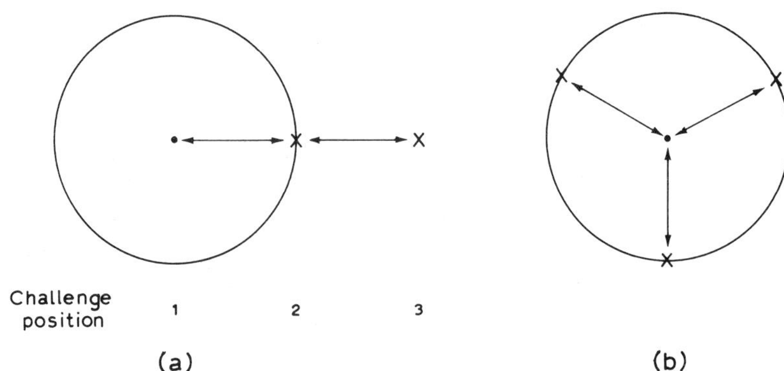

Fig. 2.3. Siting of various positions of allergen challenge (prick marked with an X) in relation to the outline of the transfer injection bleb in P–K testing.

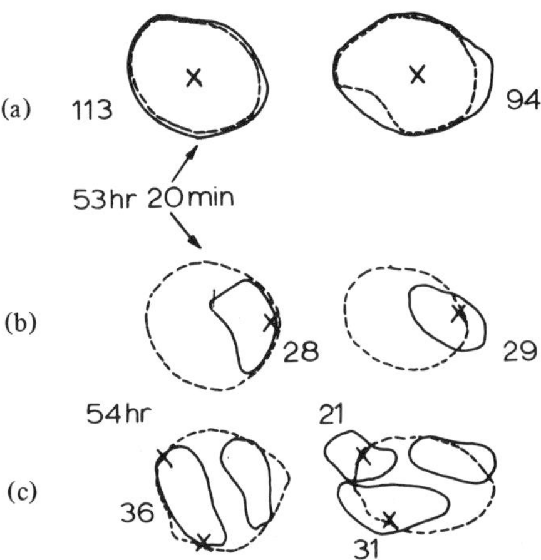

Fig. 2.4. Tracings of outlines of weals evoked by: (a) single central challenge; (b) single peripheral challenge, (c) multiple peripheral challenge of P–K test sites. (The values quoted refer to weal area in mm^2; the outlines of the initial injection blebs are shown by a dotted line.)

(i.e. 25 per cent of the area of weals elicited by central challenge) in two recipients; but a third recipient failed to respond to challenge at the outer position until 28 hr after sensitisation.

In other tests, an initial allergen challenge at a peripheral site 53 hr after transfer was followed 40 min later by challenge at two other points on the periphery as indicated in fig. 2.3b. This resulted in the elicitation of two further weals, also of appreciably smaller size than that evoked by central challenge (as is seen from fig. 2.4), but the accumulative areas of the three peripheral weals approximated to the area of the single weals resulting from the central challenge of other sensitised sites.

The results obtained from this type of investigation provide quantitative substantiation of the early observations of Coca and Grove (1925), that reagins transferred to normal individuals become attached firmly and rapidly to the fixed tissue elements. They also support the findings of Vaughan and Black (1954), that the point of inoculation of sensitising serum is surrounded by a passively sensitised zone of skin (1 inch or more in diameter) with highest sensitisation at its centre. Moreover, they indicate that the rate of outward diffusion of transferred reagin into such a zone differs in different normal recipients (which is another factor to be considered in selecting such recipients). Finally, from a practical standpoint, the results of the quantitative tests described emphasise the importance of accurate positioning of the allergen challenge in routine prick testing (which should be sited preferably at the needle mark left by the initial sensitisation injection).

The other principal factor influencing the magnitude of the response achieved in P–K testing is the timing of the allergen challenge. In other quantitative tests, we (Stanworth and Kuhns 1965) demonstrated (fig. 2.5) that maximal wealing occurred by challenging sites (in two recipients, S.W. and I.P.) at 50 hr after passive sensitisation, although weals of appreciable size were elicited at only 1–2 hr after sensitisation, i.e. soon after the initial injection blebs had subsided. A third recipient (R.D.), in whose skin transferred reagin had been found to diffuse outwards at a slower rate (as described above), showed maximal response after a 30-hr sensitisation period. Obviously the optimum period for sen-

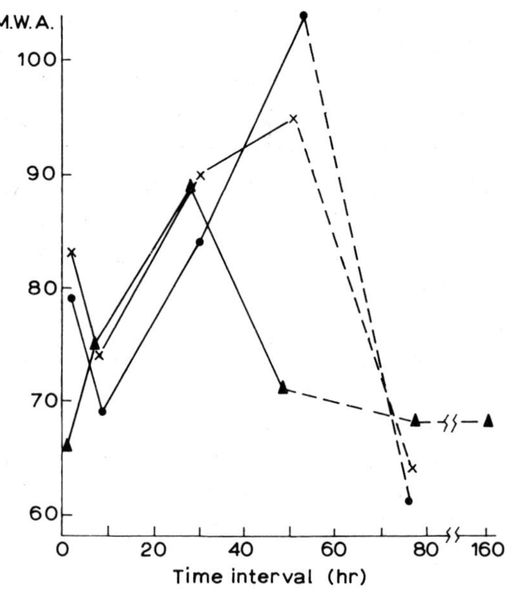

Fig. 2.5. Variation in P–K response of three different recipients (mean weal area: M.W.A.) with time period between passive sensitisation and challenge.

sitisation could be defined more precisely, by challenging many more sensitised sites after time intervals intermediate between those plotted in fig. 2.5. Similarly, quantitative evidence could be obtained to substantiate the early observations of Coca and Grove (1925), that reagins can be detected in isologous skin as long as four weeks after transfer. By determining dilution end-points at varying times after passive sensitisation with allergic serum (? from a grass pollen-sensitive individual), Augustin (1967) was able to assign a 'half-life' of about 13 days to reagins, and to demonstrate that activity was still detectable as long as 75 days after transfer. In contrast, blocking (γG) antibodies were found to disappear from an isologous skin site in less than 24 hr after transfer (Loveless 1940).

Their strong affinity for isologous tissues, and relatively strong affinity for the tissues of closely related heterologous (monkey) species (§ 2.2.2), distinguish reagins from other experimentally-induced antibodies. For instance (ch. 6), guinea pig γ_1-type anti-DNP antibodies were found to sensitise isologous skin sites for only 2–4 days, whilst a similar dose (0.25 μg) of rabbit or monkey γ_2-type anti-DNP antibodies sensitised heterologous (guinea pig) skin for about one day (Ovary et al. 1964).

Turning, finally, to the rate of development of the weal after allergen challenge in P–K testing, the response has been found to reach a maximum in 20–30 min. In our quantitative studies (Stanworth and Kuhns 1965) it was observed that weals approximately doubled in size during the 10–20 min period after challenge. Statistical analysis showed, however, that measurement of the larger weals, produced after the longer time interval, did not lead to greater accuracy in the assay of P–K activity.

These, then, are the main factors to be considered in the estimation of reaginic antibodies by the classical Prausnitz–Küstner technique. As a routine assay it is handicapped, of course, by the need for suitable human recipients and the danger of transmitting hepatitis virus in the sensitising serum.[1*] Consequently, it has never proved a practical proposition for clinical diagnosis. Nevertheless, the method possesses some important advantages as a research tool. Foremost amongst these is its exquisite sensitivity; the minimum dose of reaginic (γE) antibody needed for obtaining a positive P–K response having been estimated to be of the order of 10^{-6}–10^{-5} μg antibody N (Ishizaka and Ishizaka 1968).

2.2.1.3 Direct skin testing. At this point, it should be mentioned that direct skin testing – although admittedly more sensitive – is by no means as informative as the passive transfer system just described for the measurement of immediate hypersensitivity. As it takes place within the allergic individual's own tissues it is obviously subject to influences which are avoidable (or, at least, controllable) in the indirect approach. Moreover, it fails to provide a clear-cut measure of the reaginic antibody involvement; indeed, it is difficult to exclude the possibility of a contribution of more than one type of sensitising antibody (ch. 4) in some direct reactions. On the other hand, it seems probable that these could be

* See notes at end of chapter.

distinguished on the basis of their different optimum time periods for passive sensitisation.

Despite these limitations, quantitative direct skin testing has been frequently relied upon for the assay of allergen activity (ch. 3); and, as already mentioned, the careful studies of Becker and Rappaport (1948) have indicated the means of achieving greatest accuracy from this technique.

2.2.2 Passive sensitisation of sub-human primates

The inability of reaginic antibody to sensitise passively the skin of guinea pigs, and other suitable laboratory animals, has always been a severe handicap in the measurement of the immediate hypersensitivity response. Consequently any method which offers a satisfactory alternative to the use of human recipients deserves serious appraisal.

Early investigators (Grove 1928; Caulfield et al. 1936; Straus 1937) found that the skin reactions evoked in monkeys, by sensitisation with human allergic serum followed some hours later by challenge with specific allergen, were not as easy to measure as the characteristic weal and erythema responses evoked in normal isologous tissue. Owing to a difference in skin texture, and a tendency of the injected fluid to spread out, the response observed in monkeys is manifested as an ill-defined oedema with no surrounding flare. The difficulty of measuring this accurately, compared with the button-like weal produced in P–K testing in humans, was no doubt a major factor in the lack of interest shown initially in the use of monkey skin testing as an alternative system. In the last ten years, however, this problem has been overcome by the use of intravenously injected dye to reveal the extent of antigen-induced extravasation (Layton et al. 1961, 1962, 1963); in a similar manner to the method used in PCA testing in guinea pigs (see colour plate).

Tests carried out by Layton and his associates in a variety of species have indicated that the higher primates (monkeys and apes) are the most readily sensitised with human allergic serum; whereas primate-like species, such as the tree shrew, proved unreceptive. Other primate species, such as catarrhine, platyrrhine and prosimian monkeys, showed marked local reactions. In my own experience both rhesus monkeys (*Macaca mulatta*) and baboons (*Papio cynocephalus* and *P. anubus*), with body weights in the range of 3–6 kg, have proved suitable recipients. The latter appear to be potentially safer to handle, however, as no case of B. virus has been reported in this species; nor do they appear to carry hepatitis virus, in contrast to other primate species such as marmosets and chimpanzees.

The suitability and reliability of the monkey PCA test, as an alternative to P–K testing, in the assay of reaginic antibodies has been assessed in various laboratories (e.g. Rose et al. 1964; Buckley and Metzgar 1965). Of the various methods of effecting allergen challenge which were tried by Rose and his associates that involving the simultaneous intravenous injection of a mixture of dye (e.g. 2 ml 1 per cent Evans Blue solution) and allergen (e.g. 2 ml 5 per cent w/v ragweed pollen extract) – following the prior (24 hr) intradermal injection (0.1 ml) of the skin sites – proved the most satisfactory. The intravenous administration of dye followed by allergen was found to be technically less convenient; whilst the direct intradermal injection of antigen into each sensitised site proved more laborious and usually produced smaller reactions. It would be preferable to adopt this approach, if responses to different allergens are to be compared in the same animal; and it is obviously much more economical in the use of allergen.

There is need for caution, however, when challenging by direct intradermal injection into sensitised sites, because in my own experience such a practice can lead to the 'firing off' of remote sites. Consequently, in my laboratory we prefer to effect challenge by the sub-cutaneous injection of allergen solution into the animal's arm, i.e. into an area remote from the passively sensitised sites on the shaved chest and abdomen. Furthermore, we find that a much smaller dose (e.g. 2–4 mg) of allergen than that used by many investigators is sufficient to evoke blueing reactions when the dye is administered immediately before, by intravenous injection. Typical blueing reactions produced in a passively sensitised baboon by this procedure are shown in the colour plate. We have found Evans Blue (10 ml, 0.5 per cent soln) to be the most satisfactory indicator dye. It is very stable and ideal, therefore, for lengthy experiments; although its persistence in the animal's skin can sometimes be troublesome. In an attempt to avoid this problem we have also tried using Coomassie Blue, but we found this most unsatisfactory (contrary to the experience of Augustin 1967). Other investigators prefer to use Pontamine Sky Blue.

Reagin-mediated skin reactions in monkeys show certain characteristics which distinguish them from isologous skin responses, noticeably piloerection at the transfer site. According to Layton et al. (1963) this effect – together with blanching and wealing – might be expected to occur prior to extravasation; since allergen may come into contact with, and begin to react with, reagin in extra vascular tissue before it can reach and penetrate the capillary walls. Vasoactive amines liberated by reagin–allergen interaction within the extravascular tissue supposedly act, subsequently, directly upon the capillary walls to elicit the observed extravasation phenomenon.

The time course of development of the skin reaction in passively sensitised monkeys, after allergen challenge, has been shown to resemble closely that seen in P–K testing in humans' skin. For instance, Rose and his associates (1964) observed that 3–5 min following the intravenous injection of allergen-dye mixtures circular areas of blue colour appeared at sites sensitised with human allergic serum. The reactions became more intense over a 5–10 min period, reaching a maximum after 30 min. The time of development of reactions effected by our allergen challenge procedure, outlined above, is somewhat longer. The optimal sensitisation period (i.e. interval between sensitisation and challenge) was found to be between 24 and 48 hr. It will be noted, by reference to the previous section, that this is less than the optimum time for passive sensitisation of human skin by reagins. Positive reactions were observed, however, from 4–96 hr after passive sensitisation of monkeys; and other investigators (Layton 1965; Augustin 1967) have shown that passively transferred reagins are detectable in monkey skin sites as long as 10–14 days after sensitisation.

As in human P–K testing, the magnitude of the response in monkeys can be assessed by measurement of the area of the skin

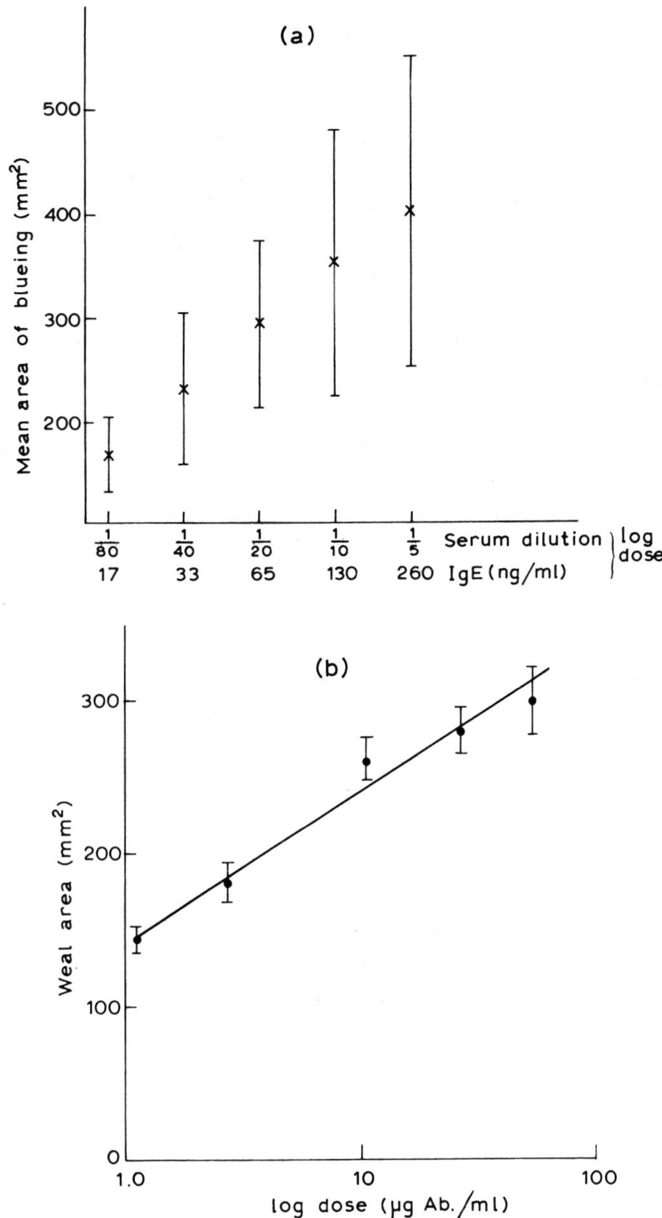

Fig. 2.6. Log (dose)–response relationships revealed by PCA testing varying dilutions of: (a) a grass pollen-sensitive individual's serum in a baboon; (b) a rabbit anti-*p*-azobenzene-arsonate antiserum in a guinea pig (Keogh 1970). (Diluent in a: buffered saline containing 10 per cent normal human serum.)

reaction (here manifested as a blueing, of course, rather than an oedema with surrounding flare). Moreover, in addition, the relative intensity of the blueing provides an arbitrary means of grading the response. A thorough quantitative assessment of the accuracy of this procedure, along the lines which we (Stanworth and Kuhns 1965) adopted in the study of the accuracy of the P–K test, has not been reported; most investigators tending to rely upon a dilution titration procedure despite its drawbacks. Nevertheless, it is possible to demonstrate a linear relationship between the log (sensitising human serum dose) and the response in baboons, expressed as mean area of blueing (fig. 2.6a). From that plot it will be seen that a ten-fold increase in reaginic antibody concentration produces about a two-fold increase in blueing area; a relationship which is comparable to that shown by isolated rabbit γG antibodies in guinea pig PCA testing, as is also indicated in fig. 2.6b. It will also be noticed from fig. 2.6a, perhaps surprisingly, that a greater degree of variance between duplicate test results was found with higher doses of antibody. This can possibly be attributed to a greater susceptibility of the responses to higher doses to site variation, the abdominal area of the recipient proving more reactive than the chest. It should be mentioned in contrast, however, that Rose and associates (1964) found that potent allergic sera (from untreated ragweed-sensitive individuals) produced approximately the same reactivity at different sites in cynomologus (*Macaca irus*) and rhesus monkeys; although the delicate skin of the eyelids and anterior trunks gave slightly larger blueing reactions than did the skin of the thighs when weaker sensitising sera were used. Obviously these factors become more important when it is necessary to use the maximum number of test sites in one animal (e.g. as many as 54 have been passively sensitised).

Most investigators have found the monkey PCA test to be less sensitive than the P–K test in the detection of reaginic antibodies. For example, Buckley and Metzgar (1965), in a direct comparison of the dilution titration end-points of three allergic sera (from untreated patients, sensitive to ragweed or orchard grass), observed that a serum which gave a maximal reciprocal P–K titre of 5000 in human recipients showed a dilution end-point of only 160 in rhesus monkeys. Likewise, Patterson (1969) and his associates found that approximately ten times the concentration of human reaginic serum was required to sensitise monkey skin as was required to sensitise human skin. Rose and his associates (1964), on the other hand, observed that sera from untreated ragweed sensitive individuals gave end-point titres in rhesus monkeys comparable to those shown in P–K tests in human recipients.

There are several factors which could influence such comparative tests. For instance, the receptivity of monkeys of the same species to passive sensitisation varies widely; being related, quite possibly, to a pre-existing state of sensitivity to *Ascaris* (which can be ascertained by prior direct skin testing with *Ascaris* extract). Another factor which can influence the outcome of dilution P–K and PCA titrations is the composition of the diluent employed. Patterson (1969) has found that dilution of human allergic serum with normal human serum, or normal monkey serum, resulted in significant reduction of the monkey PCA titre compared with that shown by sensitising serum diluted with physiological saline. This he attributed to competitive inhibition, as a result of the normal serum proteins binding to reagin-receptor sites; but it could be related to the frequently observed non-specific skin irritative property of undiluted sera. In my experience, the inclusion of 10 per cent normal serum in physiological saline diluent produces no reduction in PCA titre; but it can be expected to afford some protection to the labile reagin molecules which become more vulnerable in dilute solution. The buffering of the diluent does not appear to be very critical in passive transfer tests in vivo, presumably because there is adequate time for equilibration during the relatively long sensitisation periods employed. But this is essential when performing passive sensitisation tests in vitro, as will become apparent from the next section.

The results of recent investigations into the stability of skin sensitising activity during storage of allergic sera are discussed in a separate section (2.6), at the end of this chapter.

Turning to the interpretation of monkey PCA test data, the specificity of the responses observed is a fundamental issue. As some human non-reaginic (i.e. precipitating) antibodies are known to evoke PCA reactions in guinea pigs, it is reasonable to suppose that similar antibodies might contribute to the PCA reactivity shown by human allergic sera in monkeys. There is, however, substantial evidence to suggest that antibodies other than those of the γE (reagin) type are not involved in the classical monkey PCA reaction evoked by allergen challenge after an appropriately long sensitisation period (i.e. 24 hr, or longer). For example, skin tests carried out with three sera from ragweed-sensitive individuals (by Rose et al. 1964) indicated that pre-heating (2–4 hr, 56°) destroyed completely both PCA activity (in monkeys) and P–K activity (in humans) without influencing the hemagglutination titres of the sera (measured by use of allergen-coated erythrocytes). Moreover, similar heat treatment had no effect on the ability of rabbit anti-bovine serum albumin antibodies (presumably of the γG type) to produce PCA reactions in monkeys or guinea pigs. There is also, less direct, evidence that the PCA reaction produced by human allergic sera in monkeys is not effected by precipitating antibodies. For instance, γG- and γM-globulin fractions isolated from allergic sera, unlike reagin-rich γA-globulin fractions, failed to show any PCA activity (Buckley and Metzgar 1965; Augustin 1964).

It might perhaps be concluded, therefore, that blocking antibodies do not contribute to the PCA activity of allergic sera in monkeys, despite their capacity to agglutinate allergen-coated erythrocytes. In this connection it is possibly significant, however, that all of the investigations mentioned above were performed on sera from untreated allergic patients, in which the level of blocking antibodies would be expected to be low. Sera from some patients who have been hyposensitised with relatively large doses of allergen in mineral oil emulsions, and which would therefore contain much higher amounts of blocking antibody, were found to produce PCA reactions in guinea pigs (Fisher and Connell 1962). In contrast, several attempts to induce PCA reactions in guinea pigs by transfer of sera from untreated allergic individuals have resulted in failure (Augustin 1955; Stanworth 1963; Rose et al. 1964).

The best chance of provoking passive skin reactions in monkeys by transfer of blocking antibodies, or indeed any other type of human γG antibody, would seem to be by the adoption of a short sensitisation period (e.g. 2–4 hr); because there is no evidence available to suggest that human γG antibodies show long lasting affinity for either isologous or heterologous tissue.[2] It is significant, therefore, that Augustin (1967) has obtained evidence of non-γE-type sensitising antibodies in the sera of horse serum-sensitive individuals by this approach; and, more recently, Parish (1970) has provided similar evidence of the presence of short-term (1–4 hr) anaphylactic antibodies in purified IgG fractions from the sera of persons showing weal and flare responses (10 min) to prick testing with milk proteins, ovalbumin or tetanus toxoid – despite the absence of any detectable γE antibody in the test solutions. There were adequate reasons for concluding that the response observed in the latter investigations were not of the Arthus type; but the heat stability (after 2 hr at 56°), and apparent complement dependence, of the antibodies concerned pointed to a fundamentally different mode of action to γE (reaginic) antibodies. Nevertheless, the reaction of the antibody with specific antigen seemed to lead to the release of histamine, and it was found to differ from human γG antibodies which evoke PCA reactions in guinea pigs after short term (i.e. 4 hr) passive sensitisation.

Human γG-type sensitising antibodies obviously deserve further study. It will be important to establish their clinical significance, which might include a contribution to the tissue changes seen in those diseases (e.g. aspergillosis) associated with the formation of precipitins. It seems of possible significance that they are seen in patients who have been exposed to allergens by injection, rather than via the respiratory tract (which would appear to favour a γE antibody response, as is discussed in ch. 7).

There is little danger of confusing monkey PCA reactions induced by this type of antibody with those mediated by the γE (reagin) type. For, even where short-term sensitisation is employed, any effect due to reaginic antibodies can be abolished by pre-heating the allergic serum at 56° for 1 hr; or by administration of an inhibitory dose of human myeloma IgE concomitantly with, or prior to, the sensitising serum (ch. 5). In the light of the latter observation it might, perhaps, be expected that γG mediated monkey PCA reactions are similarly inhibited by human γG myeloma proteins of a particular sub-class. This presupposes, however, that cell binding is a prerequisite in the mode of action of human γG type sensitising antibodies; a requirement that could perhaps be established by measuring their short term monkey PCA reactivity before and after absorption with suitable tissue (e.g. chopped normal human lung).

In view of Parish's (1970) observations on the inability of his human γG antibodies to evoke PCA reactions in guinea pigs, it might perhaps be anticipated that they would prove to be of the γG2 class (i.e. the only one of the four human γG sub-classes which has proved incapable of passively sensitising guinea pig skin). Another way of investigating this possibility, and of bringing the problem closer to the clinical situation, would be to perform passive sensitisation tests with human γG anaphylactic antibodies in myelomatosis patients with monoclonal gammopathies representative of each of the four sub-classes (if such an investigation was deemed to be ethically acceptable). This supposes, however, that such antibodies are going to behave similarly in isologous human situations to the manner in which they behave in heterologous monkey skin. The possible involvement of human anaphylactic antibodies of the γG-type in penicillin, and other drugs, sensitivities is discussed further in later chapters.

There would seem to be less likelihood that human antibodies of other (non-γE) immunoglobulin classes are capable of producing anaphylactic responses following short-term passive sensitisation of humans or monkeys, because paraproteins representative of these classes (i.e. γM, γA and γD) have been shown (Terry 1965) to be incapable of binding to heterologous (guinea pig) skin in reverse PCA testing. Such extrapolations, from one species to another, sometimes prove to be ill founded, however. In this connection, it is interesting to note that there has been a report of the in vitro sensitisation of monkey ileum by what appears to be an 11*S* heat-labile secretory γA component of human parotid secretions (Arbesman, Dolovich, Wicher, Dushenski, Reisman and Tomasi 1968). But, in view of the greater sensitivity of the monkey ileum system than even the P–K test (as mentioned earlier), it will be important to show unequivocally that this observation is not attributable to trace amounts of γE antibody in the secretory

IgA preparation tested. It should be possible, theoretically, to rule out the involvement of any particular immunoglobulin class in tissue sensitisation by pre-absorption of the sensitising serum with mono-specific anti-immunoglobulin antiserum; but, as is illustrated in ch. 4, even this approach can have its pitfalls.

Finally, having examined the grounds for concluding that skin testing in monkeys provides a satisfactory alternative to the P–K test in the measurement of reaginic antibody, it is worth considering the advantages and disadvantages of the technique in practical terms. The risks involved in human transfer experiments are, of course, avoided. Moreover, as will be discussed further in later chapters (6 and 9), the use of sub-human primates permits the study of systemic as well as local sensitisation processes. Admittedly specialised assistance is required in the housing and handling of the animals, but the use of the drug Sernylan (phencyclidine phenocylohexyl piperidine hydrochloride, produced by Parker Davies & Co.)[3] has greatly facilitated experimentation. For example, intramuscular injection (e.g. 1 mg/lb body wt) of baboons results in rapid (i.e. within 5–10 min) anesthesia; and it is possible to maintain animals in a state of sedation for long periods, without fear of undesirable side-effects (Kalter 1969; Mortelmans 1969).

The cost of purchasing, quarantining and maintaining monkeys is unavoidably high, but this problem may be alleviated to some extent by the services provided at the Primate Centres being established in several European countries (Britain not included, unfortunately). Moreover, it is possible to economise by using animals on more than one occasion for passive transfer studies, provided that one is aware of the possible complications and always includes adequate reference allergic sera in repeat test series. For instance, we have used the same baboons for local passive skin testing of human allergic serum on as many as four different occasions, with suitably long rest periods in between (i.e. at least 26 days); and Rose et al. (1964) report that they used one animal six times, allowing two weekly intervals. Too frequent use, however, runs the risk of evoking a systemic anaphylactic response to the human serum or allergen proteins; or the induction of a state of refractoriness to the sensitising serum.

Radermecker and Goodfriend (1968) have shown that the latter effect can be induced by the intravenous injection of normal human or even rabbit serum (i.e. 40 ml dose), suggesting that it is unlikely to be due to the formation of monkey anti-reagin antibody as Patterson and his associates (1965) claim. This refractory state developed 10–14 days after the systemic injection of the foreign serum and lasted for about a month. It is interesting to note that P–K test sites in humans show a similar period of unresponsiveness (Bowman and Walzer 1953), which has been attributed to an exhaustion of histamine within the sites.

It is not possible to generalise, because the minimum amount of human serum and time required for the onset of the refractory state in passively sensitised monkey's skin varies from animal to animal. Indeed certain monkeys have been found to be naturally unreceptive to local sensitisation by human reaginic antibody (Patterson 1969). Nevertheless, with care, repeated usage is a feasible proposition in many animals.

In conclusion, the development of the monkey PCA test has provided a useful and reliable alternative to human P–K testing for the measurement of reaginic (γE) antibodies.

2.3 Passive sensitisation in vitro

2.3.1 Sensitisation of contractile tissue preparations

In vitro passive sensitisation systems have only come into use relatively recently in the study of immediate human hypersensitivity. This is surprising when it is realised that Dale first demonstrated in vitro anaphylaxis in guinea pig tissue (ileum and uterus) as long ago as 1913, and that similar gut bath systems have been used regularly ever since in studies of the passive sensitisation by heterologous antibodies of the γG-type. The narrow species specificity requirements for passive sensitisation by human reaginic antibodies has, however, been one of the main stumbling blocks; as it is not always easy to obtain suitable primate tissues.

The demonstration of allergen induced histamine release in the isolated bronchial muscle of a pollen-sensitive patient (Schild et al.

1951) might have been expected to spur experimental allergists on to the development of a comparable in vitro system involving the passive sensitisation of non-allergic human bronchial preparations in an organ bath. The problem has always been, however, the acquirement of suitably fresh tissue; a need which is often difficult to meet and which is very much dependent upon what the surgeon can provide. It has been shown recently, however, that other types of human tissue such as appendix (Chopra et al. 1966), ileum and uterus (Tollackson and Frick 1966), can be passively sensitised in vitro by human reaginic antibodies. For instance, human appendix cut into four or five rings (4–5 mm thick), looped together with silk thread to form a chain, can be passively sensitised for allergen-induced histamine release by the small amounts of reagin in highly diluted (e.g. 1/10 000) sera from ragweed-sensitive individuals (Kobayashi et al. 1967). Tollackson and Frick (1966), on the other hand, have found that human smooth muscles strips, passively sensitised with sera from untreated allergic individuals, were much less responsive to subsequent challenge with grass pollen or animal dander allergen. They frequently observed a lack of response to histamine or allergen, which they suggested might be attributed to an effect on the contractility of the smooth muscle strips by the disease process of the donor and the proximity of the disease to the specimens of ileum obtained. Another point which emerged from the work of the same investigators was that human uterine strips procured from classical caesarean sections were more reactive than those from lower segment sections, and that gravid uterus was 10–100 times more sensitive than fibromatous uterus to histamine and anaphylaxis.

Some of the difficulties of using isolated human tissue can be overcome by the use of monkey tissue preparations. Moreover, it has been shown (Kobayashi et al. 1967) that these systems (e.g. ileum set up in strips in a Schultz–Dale bath) are appreciably more sensitive (i.e. by a factor of 50–500 times) in detecting allergic sera than in vivo PCA testing in monkeys; which means that they are even more sensitive even than the P–K test (which is usually reckoned to be about ten times more sensitive than the monkey PCA test). The in vitro assay procedure suffers from the disadvantage, however, of a rather large variability in sensitivity (standard deviation not quoted) between different strips of ileum from the same monkey, as well as between strips of tissue obtained from different animals of the same species.

In order to quantitate reactions, therefore, it is necessary to measure the contraction responses to histamine for each strip. Another difficulty is that certain strips of monkey ileum are found at times to have spontaneous contractions, that are too great to permit their use immediately. This problem can apparently be overcome, however, by keeping the tissue at 40° overnight or by cooling it to −1° to −2° for 10–30 min prior to testing. Furthermore it is suggested (by Arbesman et al. 1964) that the variability in responsiveness of different ileum preparations could be minimised by performing quantitative tests with several strips; a task which is simplified these days by the use of automated assay equipment, such as that developed by Boura et al. (1954).

A typical dose-response curve, obtained by tests on isolated strips of monkey ileum, sensitised with varying concentrations of serum from a ragweed-sensitive individual is shown in fig. 2.7. As might have been anticipated perhaps from the similarity of the PCA responses observed in monkeys and guinea pigs, a similar

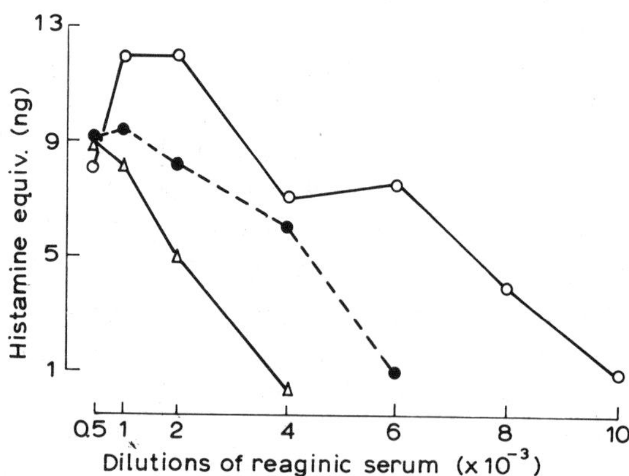

Fig. 2.7. Typical dose–response curves obtained by testing varying dilutions of human allergic serum in the monkey ileum system. (Reproduced from Kobayashi et al. 1967, by permission of the authors.)

relationship to that shown in fig. 2.7 was revealed by the studies of Mongar (1965) of the in vitro sensitisation of guinea pig ileum by non-reaginic (precipitating) antibodies. He considers this to be indicative of two (or three) point attachment of antibody molecules which become singly attached at high antibody concentrations. As Kobayashi and his associates (1967) have pointed out, however, it is difficult to explain on the basis of this hypothesis why histamine release from sensitised ileum is inhibited by excess antigen (allergen); an effect which has been observed in in vitro passive cell and tissue sensitisation systems, including passive leucocyte sensitisation (as will be seen from the next section).

As in other in vitro assays of reagin activity, therefore, it is important to work at optimal allergen concentration if maximum release of histamine from monkey ileum strips is to be effected. Other practical points worth noting from the studies of Kobayashi et al. (1967) are that the in vitro sensitisation of monkey ileum can be enhanced (2–10 times) when the sensitising allergic serum is diluted with isotonic buffered glucose solution rather than Tyrode solution (the optimum time for sensitisation being 10–15 min); and that an approximately threefold enhancement can be achieved by challenging with allergen containing added maleic acid (0.05 mM) or succinic acid (0.05 mM). A similar enhancing effect was observed when these dibasic acids were added just prior to allergen challenge, but not if they were added to the serum at the time of sensitisation. This observation is in agreement with findings from a study of the mechanism of passive anaphylaxis in isolated guinea pig lung tissue, undertaken by Austen and Brocklehurst (1961). They suggested that the enhancement of the muscle response is due to potentiation of some step activated by antigen–antibody combination, which is common to both the release of histamine and slow reacting substance. Incidentally, comparative studies (Kobayashi et al. 1967) have shown that monkey and guinea pig ileum preparations react equally to histamine and bradykinin; whereas the monkey ileum is more responsive to SRS-A and the guinea pig ileum shows a greater response to serotonin. Neither heparin (1.4 U/ml), nor EDTA (4 mM), had any effect on the passive sensitisation of monkey ileum; in contrast to their enhancing effect on the passive sensitisation of human leucocytes in vitro.

2.3.2 Sensitisation of chopped tissue

2.3.2.1 Lung systems. The in vitro assays considered so far rely upon the use of a Schultz–Dale system, in which the pharmacological response to the vasoactive amines liberated on reaction with specific allergen is manifested in situ by the contraction induced within the tissue preparation itself. This approach is not readily applicable, however, to the multiple assay of allergic sera, even where automated equipment is available. A promising development, therefore, has been the use of an alternative method (Goodfriend et al. 1966), involving the passive sensitisation of fragments (70–130 mg wet wt) of monkey lung tissue suspended in Tyrodes solution (50 ml/mg wet tissue). Portions of fragments were randomly paired to give 200 mg aliquots, which were placed in screw cap vials and passively sensitised by incubation (at 5° or 37°) with allergic serum (0.4 ml) for periods ranging from 30–12 min. After washing (× 3) with Tyrode solution, the aliquots of sensitised lung fragments were challenged with allergen (2 ml ragweed pollen extract) for 15 min at 37°. The supernatant fluids (now containing the specifically liberated histamine, and other smooth muscle spasmogens) were assayed, using an unatropinised guinea pig ileum in a jacketed organ both (10 ml) equipped with an isotonically recording physiograph. Determinations were made on duplicate (and sometimes triplicate) lung samples, aliquots (0.1 ml) of the supernatants being assayed simultaneously on two ileum preparations by reference to the responses evoked by testing histamine standards intermittently with the samples.

The results of tests performed by Goodfriend and his associates (1966) in this manner, on varying dilutions of human allergic serum (with a 1/2000 P–K titre), suggested that the in vitro chopped lung assay was less sensitive than P–K testing in humans (in contrast to the monkey ileum assay procedure discussed earlier). As will be observed from fig. 2.8, the dose response curve is

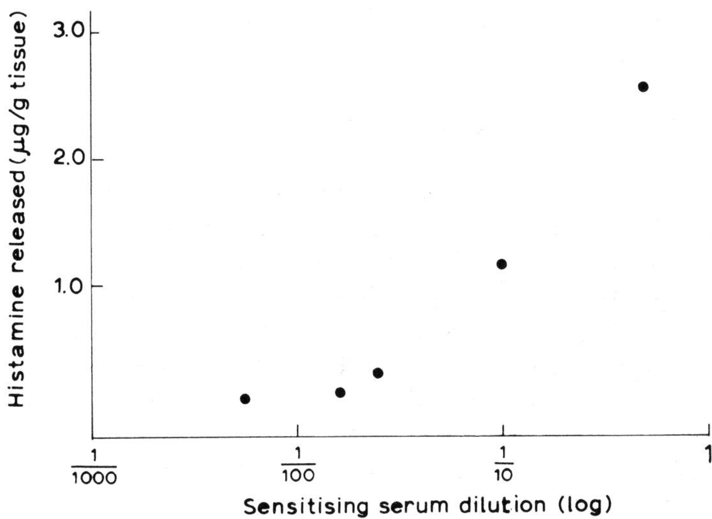

Fig. 2.8. Dose–response curve obtained by assay of varying dilutions of allergic serum in the monkey lung (chopped) system. (Plotted from the data of Goodfriend et al. 1966.)

beginning to flatten out at a serum dilution of 1/160; although even at this dose level the responses obtained were twice those produced by a non-allergic normal serum.

The procedure outlined is, of course, analogous in principle to the passive leucocyte sensitisation test (illustrated schematically in fig. 2.15b); but in that method it has been customary to assay the liberated histamine by a sensitive spectrofluorometric technique rather than by bio-assay. An analogy between the two procedures is suggested also by the results of studies (Goodfriend et al. 1966) on the effect of time and temperature of incubation of the monkey lung fragments with allergic serum; and on the influence of allergen (ragweed) concentration. The response observed (fig. 2.9a) increased with time of incubation up to 2 hr, and was greater (by approx. 2-fold) at 37° than at 5°. Furthermore, the curve obtained (fig. 2.9b) by plotting response against allergen concentration showed a similar form to that observed in passive leucocyte testing (fig. 2.25), showing a maximum at a well-defined

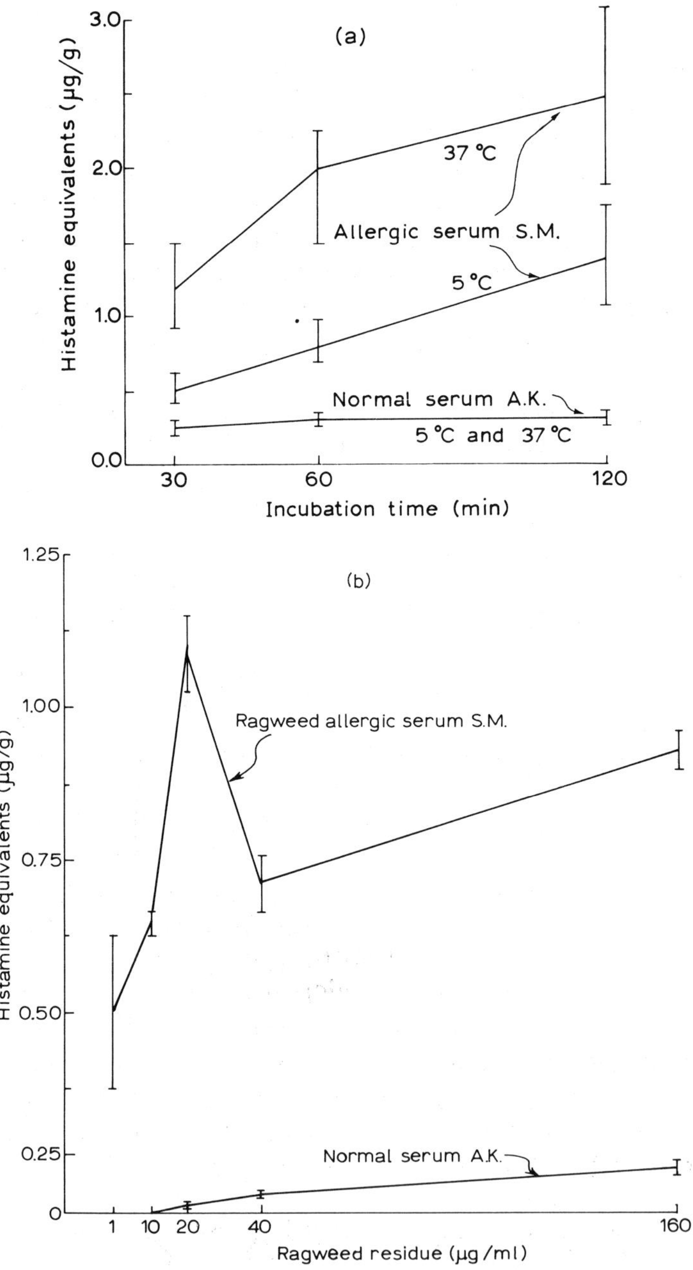

Fig. 2.9. Effect of: (a) time and temperature of incubation with ragweed allergic serum; (b) dose of challenging allergen, after 30 min incubation with sensitising serum at 5°; on the anaphylactic response of monkey lung fragments. (Reproduced from Goodfriend et al. 1966, by permission of the authors.)

allergen concentration (20 mg ragweed residue per ml) and then ultimately rising again at excessive allergen concentrations.

As has been found with the other in vitro sensitisation systems considered in this chapter, there is every indication that γE (reaginic) antibodies were being measured by the chopped monkey lung procedure. For example, the responses were shown to be: allergen specific, approximately correlative with P–K titre but unrelated to the hemagglutination titre of the allergic serum, and abolished by pre-heating the sensitising serum at 56° for one hour.

As might be expected, it has also proved possible to demonstrate allergen-induced histamine release from chopped human lung fragment which has been sensitised by prior incubation with human allergic serum. Yet the potentialities of such a system for the assay of human γE (reaginic) antibodies have only recently been investigated, although an essentially similar procedure, based on the use of chopped guinea pig lung, was first employed some time ago in studies (Mongar and Schild 1957) of the anaphylactic properties of γG antibodies.

Fresh specimens of macroscopically normal human lung, obtained at the time of surgery for carcinoma, have been used for this purpose (Sheard et al. 1967). After transport of the specimens to the laboratory in ice-cold oxygenated Tyrode solution, the primary bronchi and blood vessels were dissected out and the lung parenchyma was chopped finely with sharp scissors in a 103 Universal bottle. Some investigators (e.g. Augustin 1967) have preferred not to remove the pleura, because it is expected to contain most of the mast cells; but Bukhari (1967) has observed that the amount of histamine present in the parenchyma was surprisingly greater than that in samples containing pleura and so he has routinely dissected off the pleura before slicing the underlying tissue. We have adopted a similar procedure in my own laboratory, and have found a McIlwain chopper useful for fragmenting our material after preliminary cutting up with scissors (in contrast to Augustin's experience).

According to the procedure of Sheard and his associates (1967), the chopped tissue is mixed with about 200 ml of cold Tyrode solution, filtered through gauze, washed thoroughly and drained

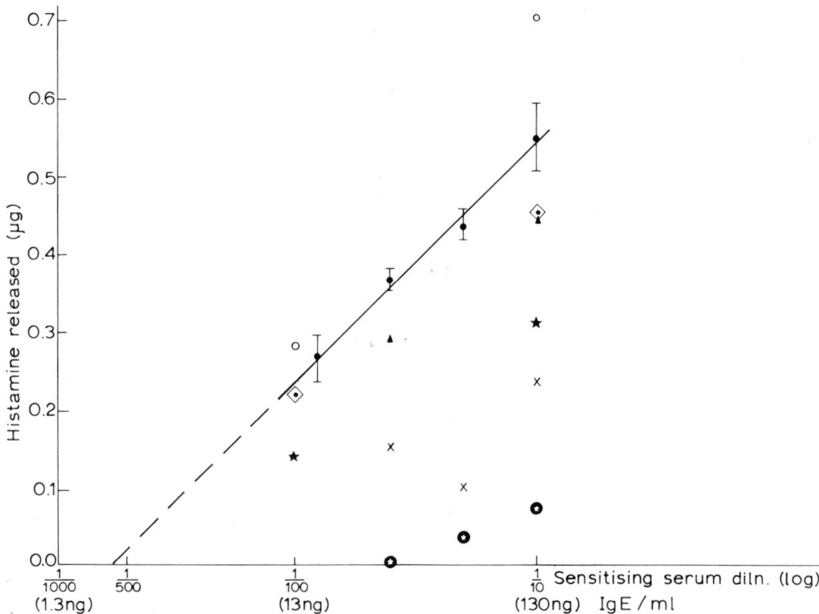

Fig. 2.10. Dose–response relationships obtained by assay of varying dilutions of the same standard allergic (pollen-sensitive) serum using different specimens of chopped human lung (distinguished by different symbols).

of excess fluid. Portions (400 mg) of the washed chopped lung (rapidly weighed on a torsion balance) are suspended in aliquots (4 ml) of allergic sera and diluted (1/10) with Tyrode solution; chlortetracycline (0.01 mg/ml) being added as bacteriostat. After incubation at room temperature overnight, and at 37° for 1 hr next day, the samples are washed thoroughly to remove excess serum proteins before incubation for 15 min at 37° with Tyrode solution (4 ml) containing allergen (e.g. cocksfoot pollen protein). Finally the supernatants are separated, placed in ice, and assayed for histamine and SRS-A on the same day using an isolated guinea pig ileum bathed with Tyrode solution containing atropine sulphate (10^{-6} M).

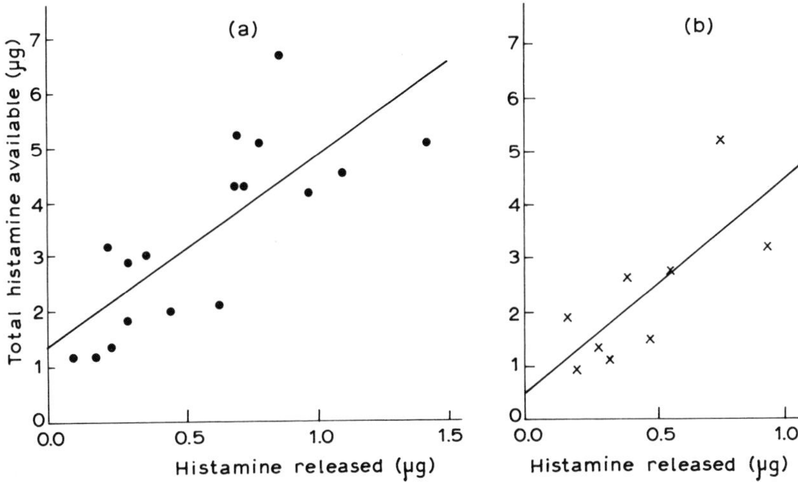

Fig. 2.11. Relationship between amount of histamine released specifically and the total available histamine in portions (400 mg) of passively sensitised human lung, following challenge with: a) cocksfoot, b) timothy pollen allergen. Each test was performed on lung from a different patient.

Other investigators (e.g. Augustin 1967) have used smaller portions (around 100 mg) of tissue, divided into uniform samples by pushing the fragments into even sized holes in a perspex tray (Mongar and Schild 1953) and then removing excess liquid by means of a nylon suction brush similar to that employed by Brocklehurst et al. (1961) in dealing with chopped guinea pig lung.

Despite the dubious physiological conditions obtaining during the relatively lengthy procedure outlined, and the markedly polluted state of many lung specimens, it is possible to obtain a reasonably accurate measure of human reaginic (γE) antibody activity by this procedure. The dose–response relationships shown in fig. 2.10 were plotted from data obtained by the technique outlined,[4] using 400 mg portions of human lung which had been fragmented by use of a McIlwain chopper. As will be noted (from the main curve) a tenfold increase in serum concentration effected an approximately fourfold increase in response; thus resembling the P–K test dose–response relationship (fig. 2.2).

TABLE

Accumulative data obtained by assaying a standard allergic serum (dil. 1/10)

Aller-gen*	Sensitising serum		Total available histamine (μg)	Allergen-induced histamine released (μg)
	Batch No.	Time (months) of storage in frozen state		
T	1	2	3.160 ± 0.435	0.925 ± 0.050
T	1	4	2.640 ± 0.218	0.380 ± 0.006
T	1	5	1.480 ± 0.263	0.470 ± 0.036
T	1	5	1.080	0.305 ± 0.040
T	1	5	0.887 ± 0.042	0.190 ± 0.012
T	1	6	X 1.300 ± 0.128	0.270 ± 0.108
T	1	7	2.720 ± 0.153	0.550 ± 0.035
T	1	7	5.200 ± 0.195	0.750 ± 0.114
T	1	7	1.400	0.153 ± 0.000
C	1	7	3.160 ± 0.076	0.205 ± 0.029
C	1	9	5.200 ± 0.733	0.700 ± 0.140
C	1	9	2.900 ± 0.013	0.288 ± 0.000
C	1	9	2.100 ± 0.039	0.630 ± 0.153
C	1	9	2.000 ± 0.008	0.445 ± 0.000
C	1	12	X 1.340 ± 0.072	0.220 ± 0.000
C	1	12	6.625 ± 1.484	0.865 ± 0.040
C	1	12	3.035 ± 0.575	0.355 ± 0.066
C	2	1 wk	# 1.803 ± 0.181	0.285 ± 0.000
C	1	12	1.172 ± 0.193	0.080 ± 0.016
	2	1 wk		0.155 ± 0.015
C	1	13	5.030 ± 0.467	0.790 ± 0.017
	2	1		1.425 ± 0.270
C	2	1	4.250 ± 0.502	0.685 ± 0.047
	2	1 +		0.725 ± 0.166
C	2	2	4.150 ± 0.029	0.975 ± 0.030
C	2	2	X 4.500 ± 0.129	1.100 ± 0.079

* C = cocksfoot, T = Timothy pollen.

† 200 mg portions of chopped lung used.

\+ Reconstituted lyophilised serum used.

x Non-specific release effected by allergen on non-sensitised lung: 14.2 per cent TAH.

X TAH determined on fresh portions of lung.

\# TAH determined on allergen-challenged portions of lung.

2.2
on specimens of chopped human lung (400 mg portions) from different donors.

% TAH	Non-specifically released histamine (μg)	% TAH	Observations on conditions of lung specimens
28.4	0.100 ± 0.050	3.1	
14.0	0.000	0.0	
30.9	0.008 ± 0.004	2.6	
28.2	0.027	8.9	
17.0	0.030	3.4	
20.8	0.000	0.0	
20.2	0.000	0.0	
14.4	0.000	0.0	
8.0	0.020 ± 0.000	3.6	very clean – min. pollution†
6.3	0.000	0.0	heavily polluted with carbon
13.4	0.000	0.0	
9.9	0.198	6.8	signs of infection
30.0	0.000	0.0	
22.3	0.000	0.0	
13.4	0.160 ± 0.003	0.6	†
13.0	0.400 ± 0.000	6.0	
11.7	0.075 ± 0.005	2.5	
15.6	0.045 ± 0.000	2.5	
6.8	0.055 ± 0.024	4.7	
13.2	0.080 ± 0.030	6.8	
15.7	0.150 ± 0.015	3.0	very clean, well aerated
28.4	0.105 ± 0.000	2.1	
16.1	0.250 ± 0.020	5.9	sooty, poorly aerated
17.1	0.300	7.1	
23.5	0.290	7.0	
24.4	0.550 ± 0.023	12.2 *x*	signs of infection †

N.B. On all other occasions the TAH was calculated by addition of amount of histamine released by TCA from control sensitised lung specimens to the amount found in the supernatant after their incubation with Tyrode solution.
IgE (RIST) level of sensitising serum: batch 1, 1100 ng/ml; batch 2, 1300 ng/ml.

Substantial amounts of histamine are usually released from sensitised chopped human lung preparations, on challenge with specific allergen, which correlate with the total amount of histamine available (fig. 2.11); and it is usually possible to achieve satisfactory agreement between duplicate assays. This will be seen from the accumulative data in table 2.2; which were obtained in my laboratory (by the same operator) using the *same* standard allergic serum (obtained from one of our grass pollen-sensitive donors) throughout. As will be noted, however, the allergen-induced histamine release rarely reached 30 per cent of the total available histamine (released by trichloroacetic acid treatment); and sometimes it is appreciably less, although still significantly higher than the amount of histamine released non-specifically on incubation of the sensitised lung with Tyrode solution.

This variability in response would seem to reflect a high degree of variation in the capacity of lung specimens from different individuals to become sensitised. For although the data from comparative tests of old and new batches of the standard allergic serum (on the same specimens of lung) suggest that some loss in sensitising capacity might have occurred during storage in the frozen state, the observed differences in response on different occasions do not appear to be related to the age of the sensitising serum. Moreover, the variability does not appear to be related to the macroscopic appearance of the lung specimen; nor, apparently, to its degree of contamination with carbon particles which would cause an error in the wet weights of the test portions. Indeed, in view of the contamination shown by many of the lung specimens used, the agreement between duplicate estimates of histamine released specifically and by trichloroacetic acid treatment is surprisingly good.

The data listed in the table emphasise the importance of always including a reference serum standard when performing chopped lung assays, against which to calibrate the particular tissue preparation being used. In this connection, it is encouraging to note that despite the obvious difference in responsiveness of the lung specimens used in the two comparisons made of the activity of the old and new batches of the standard allergic serum, the ratio of the activities measured on the two occasions showed fairly good agreement. Furthermore, samples of the same batch (1) of sensitising serum which had been stored in two different ways (i.e. frozen and in lyophilised form) showed very similar sensitising activities when tested on the same specimen of lung (table 2.2).

An allergic serum similar to that employed to obtain the data under discussion might meet the requirements for a reference standard, which could be circulated between different laboratories. The problem of storage of such serum for relatively long periods of time, without loss in activity, is under current investigation in our laboratories (and will be discussed further, § 2.6). In this connection, it should be pointed out that the observed difference in reactivity of the two batches of sensitising serum used in our study, despite a negligible difference (i.e. 200 μg/ml) in total IgE level, might well reflect a change in the level of pollen-sensitising antibody IgE over the interval of a year between the two blood donations.

It is not feasible, practically, to perform many more than about 18 chopped lung assays at any one time, which does not leave much scope for testing unknowns if a full standard curve is to be constructed on each occasion. As a compromise, therefore, in many of our own test series we have included duplicate assays on two different dilutions (e.g. 1/10; 1/40) of the standard serum; together with duplicate tests on similarly sensitised portions of lung incubated with the medium (e.g. Tyrode solution) instead of allergen, in order to determine the amount of non-specific release. Typical two- (or three-) point calibration curves obtained in this manner are included in fig. 2.10, to permit a comparison with a full standard curve. As will be noticed, the slopes of most of them approximate to that of the main calibration curve.

Incidentally, another control assay which should be included in every test series involves the addition of the allergen solution to chopped human lung which has been pre-incubated with Tyrode solution, rather than with sensitising serum. This reveals the occasionally encountered complicating situation, where lung has been inadvertently obtained from a donor who is sensitive to the allergen in question.

There seems to be little doubt that the chopped human lung assay like that employing monkey lung, is measuring reaginic (γE) antibodies; as investigations carried out on pollen-sensitive (Sheard et al. 1967) and milk-sensitive (Parish 1963) individuals' sera have indicated. Its ability to detect γG-type human antibodies, on the other hand, is questionable. This is suggested by the negative findings of Augustin (1967), from studies on γG antibodies raised by hyperimmunisation of a non-atopic individual with grass pollen, and the difficulty experienced by Assem and Schild (1968) in the detection of sensitising antibodies against penicillin by use of the lung assay. The latter workers' observations raise further, however, the possible involvement of γG-type sensitising antibodies in drug sensitivity (a question which will be returned to in ch. 4). In this event, it might be expected that the relatively long lung-sensitisation period (14–20 hr at room temperature, before bringing to 37°) employed in the analysis of sera from penicillin-sensitive individuals would be far from optimal for binding by an antibody thought (from the monkey PCA testing described earlier) to possess a weak tissue affinity. It seems, moreover, significant in this connection, that Assem and Schild (1968) found that the penicillin-sensitive individuals' sera sensitised *monkey* lung preparations more readily than human lung.

It is interesting to note that the reagin-mediated immediate hypersensitivity response evoked in the chopped human lung system shows many characteristics in common with the in vitro anaphylactic reactions demonstrable in guinea pig lung preparations following initial sensitisation with heterologous γG-type antibodies. For instance, the time course of antigen-induced histamine release in the two systems is practically identical (Bukhari 1967). Furthermore, the longer period apparently necessary for the passive sensitisation of human lung by reagin is presumably attributable to the relatively low level of γE antibody present in human allergic serum. A minimum sensitisation period of 3 hr at 37° would seem to be necessary (Augustin 1967). Although the practice of incubating the lung with allergic serum at room temperature overnight (e.g. for 17 hr) is often more convenient, it can lead to greater non-specific histamine release; because, by this time, the tissue is beginning to show signs of deterioration. In contrast, monkey skin preparations seem to be more stable, usually showing only minimal non-specific histamine release.

Other evidence of human γE antibody binding to chopped human lung is provided by the results of some preliminary absorption studies undertaken in my laboratory on the serum of a grass pollen-sensitive individual. Repeated absorption with several portions (100 mg) of fresh human lung was sufficient to remove completely the ability of the allergic serum to sensitise passively a further portion of fresh lung. Nevertheless, parallel estimations by the radio-immunosorbent test (§ 2.5.2) revealed a residual IgE level of 730 ng/ml in the absorbed serum (corresponding to approx. 28 per cent of the starting serum). Moreover, in separate tests, inclusion of myeloma IgE in the sensitising serum (at a concentration of 500 μg/ml) brought about a partial inhibition of chopped lung sensitising activity; whereas, in contrast, a comparable amount of human γG1 myeloma protein showed no measurable inhibitory effect.

Further experiments along these lines are needed, to throw more light on the mode of sensitisation of lung tissue. As Parish (1970) has pointed out, however, it will be important to avoid confusion caused by unspecific binding of non-antibody immunoglobulin. In this connection, the results of an investigation (Paul and Weir 1969) of histamine release effected from normal human lung by treatment with specific antisera against different classes of immunoglobulin are of interest. Although a (sheep) anti-human IgE antiserum proved most active, a (goat) anti-human IgG antiserum appeared to show some histamine releasing activity. In a similar type of approach it would be interesting to see whether there was any evidence of preferential uptake by human lung of human γG-globulin of a particular sub-class, by incubating chopped lung preparations with representative myeloma proteins followed by treatment with specific antiserum. There would be need for caution, however, in interpreting the findings; and in ensuring that any uptake of immunoglobulin observed had not resulted from mere non-specific adsorption.

In summary, the chopped human lung assay would seem to be of greater value in the research laboratory than as a routine method of measuring reaginic antibody activity. Although it has been found to be much more sensitive than the monkey lung system (Assem and Schild 1968), it is still appreciably less sensitive than the classical P–K test. Moreover, its dependence upon a supply of fresh human tissue puts it beyond the scope of many investigators.

2.3.2.2 Skin assays. An alternative in vitro sensitisation procedure, which avoids some of the disadvantages of the chopped lung assay, relies upon the use of monkey skin suspension (Goodfriend and Luhovyj 1968). The technique is essentially similar to that adopted in the chopped lung, and passive leucocyte sensitisation (§ 2.4) procedures, with one or two notable differences. For instance, unlike the other in vitro passive sensitisation systems, it was found that Ca^{2+} ions (2×10^{-3} M) were needed in the sensitisation as well as the challenge phase.

The skin excised from the abdomen of closely shaved animals (e.g. rhesus monkeys or baboons) is first freed of subcutaneous fat and connective tissue, before being mixed with Tyrode solution and cut into fragments of approximate dimension: $0.1 \times 0.5 \times 0.5$ cm. We found that the use of scissors was essential, but Goodfriend and Luhovyj (1968) succeeded in using a tissue chopper to obtain a uniform suspension. After being washed by centrifugation, the packed skin suspension is conveniently used in 200 mg (wet) aliquots for passive sensitisation with human allergic serum (by incubation for 1.5 hr at 37°, or at room temperature overnight). The histamine liberated into the suspending medium on subsequent reaction with specific allergen can be estimated spectrofluorometrically or by bioassay in a similar manner to that employed in the other in vitro sensitisation systems.

Of 21 ragweed sensitive individuals' sera tested in this manner, 20 were found to evoke significant in vitro anaphylactic reactions in contrast to the lack of reactivity shown by 6 non-ragweed sensitive atopic and 3 non-atopic individuals' sera; furthermore, heating at 56° for 1 hr was found to destroy the tissue sensitising activity;

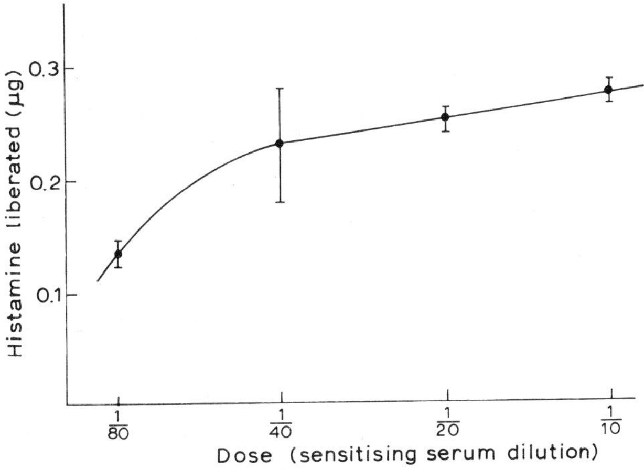

Fig. 2.12. Log dose–response curve obtained by assay of varying dilutions of an allergic (pollen-sensitive) serum by means of the monkey skin suspension technique.

and the sensitising activity of untreated allergic sera did not appear to be related to their capacity to agglutinate erythrocytes coated with ragweed allergen (Goodfriend and Luhovyj 1968). Hence, it can be concluded that γE (reaginic) antibodies are being detected by this system, too. As will be seen from fig. 2.12 (based on observations in my own laboratory), however, the dose-response curve is flatter than that obtained using the chopped human lung assay referred to earlier.

It is interesting to note that the data from which this curve was plotted were obtained by sensitisation with the same batch of allergic serum as that used to obtain the chopped lung assay data given in table 2.2. Using this same serum (from a grass-pollen sensitive individual) at a 1/10 dilution for passive sensitisation of skin suspension, the amounts of histamine released (on a tissue weight basis) on specific allergen challenge were comparable to those measured in the chopped lung assay. Moreover, it was noticeable that the amount of non-specific histamine release encountered after monkey skin suspensions had been incubated with allergic serum overnight was significantly less than that occurring in the chopped lung system; presumably because of the greater stability of the skin preparations.

The total amount of histamine released from monkey skin suspensions (200 mg aliquots) by treatment with trichloracetic acid (5 per cent) in some test series approximated to the histamine content reported (Perry 1956) for human skin (i.e. about 8 μg/g); but, on other occasions, the amount of total available histamine was found to be somewhat lower. Presumably local variations in the histamine content of monkey skin, similar to those observed in human skin (Feldberg and Miles 1953), would influence this value; as would many other factors, such as skin thickness and the distribution of mast cells. Nevertheless, skin preparations might be expected to be more uniform in composition than the average human lung preparation taken at pneumonectomy.

Some investigators will find the acquirement of monkey skin easier than that of human lung; as this can be obtained when animals which have been used for other purposes are sacrificed. In this event, however, it might be felt that the use of ileum or lung (in the type of systems already outlined) would be more rewarding. A case might ultimately be made for the use of skin, however, because of its greater stability; as this could possibly lead to the development of a procedure for its long term storage. Attempts in my laboratory to store chopped human lung by freezing in liquid nitrogen were, not surprisingly, unsuccessful. Neither glycerol nor dimethyl sulphoxide, two reagents commonly used in the preservation of mammalian cells in the frozen state, afforded any protection against non-specific histamine release. The results of preliminary attempts to preserve monkey skin in the frozen state, on the other hand, seem more promising.

It was shown some time ago (Billingham and Medawar 1952) that rabbit-skin which had been frozen slowly after impregnation with glycerol solution and stored for 4 months at $-79°$ was indistinguishable, on transplantation, from a freshly removed graft. Although it might be expected that the requirements for graft viability are not as stringent as those necessary for the maintenance of the integrity of tissue mast cells (which are notoriously vulnerable to disruption under a wide range of conditions), we have made attempts to preserve monkey skin in a similar form. For example, discs of skin were soaked in various preserving agents (such as 15 per cent, w/v glycerol), placed in round bottom centrifuge tubes, frozen slowly by immersion in solid CO_2 in acetone and later thawed rapidly. In other experiments, chopped skin suspensions in 15 per cent glycerol were similarly treated; but every process adopted led to the premature loss of a major portion of the skin histamine. On the other hand, preliminary results from experiments in which large pieces of monkey skin were wrapped in polythene sheeting and kept in a deep freeze for several days were more encouraging. For, although 50 per cent of the histamine released on allergen challenge of passively sensitised suspensions of the stored tissue was attributable to non-specific effects, measurable amounts (e.g. 0.1 μg/g wet tissue) of specific release were recorded. [5]

An interesting outcome of these preliminary studies (Graetz and Stanworth to be published in detail elsewhere) has been the demonstration that discs of monkey skin could be used as an alternative to suspensions of chopped material in the assay of tissue sensitising antibodies. After preparation of the skin in the usual way, the outlines of the discs are marked with a No. 10 cock borer (15 mm diameter) and cut out with scissors. The discs, which differed in weight by not more than ± 6 per cent, were then sensitised by incubation (at room temperature overnight) with allergic serum in stoppered glass tubes and subsequently challenged with allergen in the usual way. In table 2.3, data obtained in this manner are compared directly with those from parallel chopped skin assays using skin from the same monkey, and the same standard allergic serum as that used to obtain the chopped lung assay data provided in table 2.2. As will be noted, the proportion of histamine release effected by challenge with specific allergen is not appreciably different in the two procedures, but the overall amount released from the skin suspensions is substantially greater than that recovered from the discs; presumably because of the greater accessibility of the mast cells in the former type of preparation.

The success, albeit only partial, of the disc procedure raises the possibility (suggested by my colleague, A. Graetz) of performing the complete assay on skin discs located in wells in plastic trays

TABLE 2.3

Monkey skin assays: comparison of data obtained using skin suspensions and skin discs.

(a) Chopped skin assay

Sensitising serum dilution	Total available histamine (μg)	Weight of test aliquot (g)	Allergen-induced histamine released (μg)	% TAH	Non-specific histamine released (μg)	% TAH
1/10	0.550 ± 0.066	0.2000	0.118 ± 0.004	21.5	0.000	0.0
1/10	0.748 ± 0.059	0.2000	0.098 ± 0.009	13.1	0.016	2.1
1/20		0.2000	0.083 ± 0.004	11.1	0.015	2.0
1/40		0.2000	0.090 ± 0.001	12.0	0.010	1.3
1/80		0.2000	0.080 ± 0.006	10.7	0.010	1.3

(b) Skin disc assay

Sensitising serum dilution	Weight of disc (g)	Total available histamine (μg)	Allergen-induced histamine released (μg)	% TAH	Non-specific histamine released (μg)	% TAH
1/10	0.2170 ± 0.0272	0.170 ± 0.000	0.037 ± 0.003	21.8	0.000	0.0
1/10	0.1908 ± 0.0028	0.420 ± 0.016	0.039 ± 0.001	9.3	0.010	2.4
1/20	0.1908 ± 0.0068		0.030 ± 0.002	7.1	0.005	1.2
1/40	0.1914 ± 0.0022		0.019 ± 0.002	4.5	0.000	0.0
1/80	0.1777 ± 0.0067		0.020 ± 0.001	4.8	0.000	0.0

IgE (R.I.S.T.) level of sensitising serum = 1300 ng/ml.

(like haemagglutination trays) maintained at 37° into which the various reagents (sensitising serum, wash fluid, allergen solution etc.) are introduced and subsequently withdrawn in sequence. Such an in vitro system would seem to approximate most closely to the classical in vivo P–K system, and might ultimately be capable of automation.

In conclusion, the chopped monkey skin technique in its present form does not provide any outstanding advantages over the chopped human lung assay referred to earlier; on the other hand, human skin which, like human lung, has been shown to bind reagin (Parish 1970) has the advantage of greater availability.[6] Furthermore, it would seem to offer the best chance of long term storage of tissue; a development which would overcome the most serious handicap of in vitro passive tissue sensitisation procedures, namely the difficulty of obtaining suitably viable material at the appropriate time.

2.3.3 Peripheral leucocyte sensitisation

As I predicted in a review article nine years ago (Stanworth 1963) leucocyte sensitisation has proved to be – in many ways – the most useful in vitro alternative to P–K testing for the measurement of immediate hypersensitivity reactions. After several years practical experience of the technique, however, it is fair comment to state that it is by no means the easiest of assay procedures. Nevertheless, its application (particularly by Osler and his associates 1968) has provided important new insights into the various factors operative in reagin (γE) mediated anaphylactic reactions.

2.3.3.1 Background. As long ago as 1941, Katz and Cohen had shown that the incubation of ragweed-sensitive individuals' blood with specific allergen in vitro evoked a release of histamine into the plasma, in contrast to the negative effect produced by similar treatment of blood taken from non-allergic individuals. This important observation was later confirmed and extended by other investigators (Noah 1954; Noah and Brand 1955; Van Arsdel et al. 1958), whose work demonstrated that histamine release from leucocytes in the blood of individuals sensitive to a wide range of materials (including the common inhalants and various foods) can be induced by incubation with the appropriate allergen. For example, in the studies of Van Arsdel and his associates (1958), large aliquots (25–40 ml) of blood from 41 allergic individuals was incubated at 37° with varying amounts of allergen (in 1 ml vol); and the histamine thereby released into the plasma was determined spectrophotometrically by reaction with dinitro-fluorobenzene, after first separating the cells and precipitating the plasma proteins with trichloroacetic acid. The amount of histamine released was found to vary with allergen (i.e. ragweed pollen extract) concentration, reaching a maximum at 20 μg. protein N/l blood; whereas higher allergen concentrations suppressed histamine release, and excessive amounts (i.e. 4000 μg allergen protein N/l blood) provoked non-specific histamine release. The rate of histamine release was shown to be linear, reaching a maximum after 30 min incubation of allergic blood with allergen at 37°.

These important initial observations were later followed by the demonstration that allergen-induced histamine release could also be effected from allergic leucocytes which had been washed free of humoral sensitising antibody and resuspended in Locke–Ringer solution (at *p*H 7.4–7.8). The amount of histamine thus liberated was found to be 56–84 per cent as much as that released after resuspension of the washed allergic leucocytes in their own plasma (Middleton and Sherman 1960). Resuspension of washed allergic leucocytes in plasma from hyposensitised allergic individuals, on the other hand, brought about a depression of allergen-induced histamine release (Van Arsdel 1962) unless high allergen concentrations were employed (presumably to allow for the binding by blocking antibody present in such plasma).

The findings of Middleton and Sherman provided the first convincing evidence of the firm binding of reaginic (γE) antibodies to the leucocytes of hypersensitive individuals, besides 'paving the way' for the development of a leucocyte assay procedure. The demonstration that serious cell damage (as revealed by non-specific histamine release) was not caused by the repeated washing necessary to remove occluded allergic plasma proteins meant that the

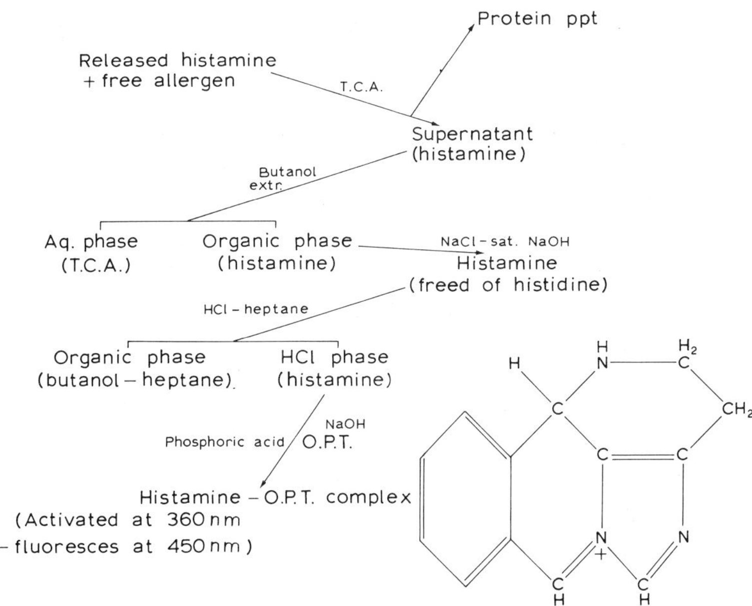

Fig. 2.13. Outline of procedure used in extraction and spectrofluorometric assay of histamine ((Abbreviations: TCA, trichloroacetic acid; OPT, orthophthaldehyde))

various factors influencing allergen-induced histamine release could now be studied using washed cells, suspended in well-defined plasma-free media. Moreover, it encouraged the later attempts to sensitise passively washed leucocytes from normal human donors, by incubation with serum from hypersensitive individuals.

Another crucial step in the development of the leucocyte assay has been the application of a sensitive spectrofluorometric procedure to the measurement of the histamine released from sensitised cells on allergen challenge (Noah and Brand 1961). This method, devised originally by Shore et al. (1959) for the assay of histamine in various tissues, and since refined by Kremzner and Wilson (1961), avoids the lengthy column adsorption procedures which are a necessary preliminary to the spectrophotometric assay. As outlined in fig. 2.13, it involves extraction of the liberated histamine from trichloroacetic acid supernatants into *n*-butanol, return

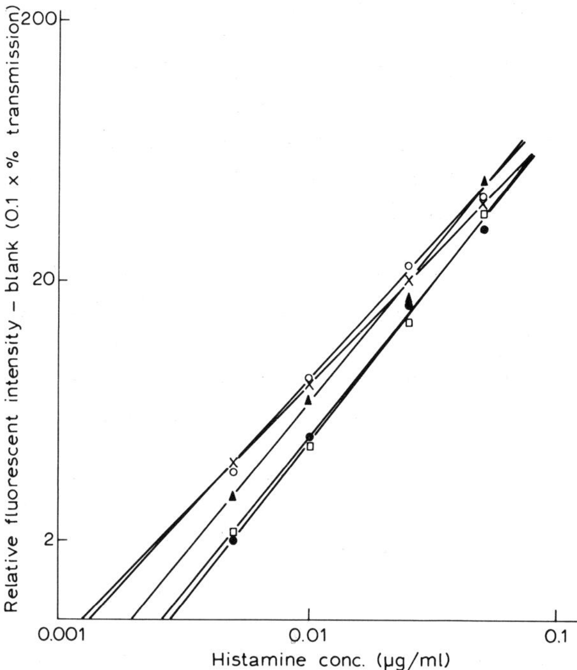

Fig. 2.14. Typical work curves (plotted on log-paper) used in the spectrofluorometric assay of histamine.

of the histamine to an aqueous solution and condensation with O.phthaldehyde (OPT) to yield a product with a strong stable fluorescence at 450 nm when activated at 360 nm. This can only be measured, however, in spectrofluorometers with sufficiently intense emission sources at 360 nm (such as the instruments manufactured by Aminco-Bowman or the Farrand Optical Co.). The fluorescence intensity of the modified histamine OPT complex is stable for at least 30 min, which means that about 20 assays (including the standards) can be conveniently coped with in one test series.[7] Moreover, it is proportional to histamine concentration over the wide range of 0.005–0.5 µg/ml (i.e. 5–500 ng/ml), as can be seen from the work curves reproduced in fig. 2.14. Hence the procedure is considerably more sensitive than the spectrophotometric assay which it superceded, comparing favourably in this respect with the standard bio-assay procedure based on the measurement of the contractile effect of histamine on guinea pig ileum in a Schultz–Dale bath. Consequently, it is possible to use appreciably smaller volumes of leucocytes per assay (e.g. cells from 2–4 ml portions of blood) than were required previously, when the released histamine was measured by the much less sensitive spectrophotometric method.

2.3.3.2 Passive sensitisation of normal leucocytes. The conditions necessary for in vitro passive sensitisation of normal human leucocytes are as might be expected more demanding; foremost amongst these being the technically difficult problem of maintaining the unstable granulocytes in a viable form for considerably longer periods than in the testing of hypersensitive individual's leucocytes, which have been pre-sensitised with reaginic (γE) antibodies in vivo. Hence, it is not altogether surprising that the first attempts to sensitise passively the leucocytes of normal human donors (Middleton 1960) met with only partial success. The technique employed involved the incubation (2 hr, 37°), with occasional mixing, of mixtures of heparinized whole normal blood (36 ml) and plasma (4 ml) from ragweed-sensitive individuals (which had been matched with respect to the major blood groups), followed by incubation (30 min, 37°) with allergen. Of 10 attempts, using 6 different sensitising plasmas and 7 normal blood donors, only 3 succeeded in effecting passive sensitisation as revealed by subsequent allergen-induced histamine release.

Later studies (Van Arsdel and Sells 1963) in which allergic serum rather than plasma was used, provided more encouraging evidence of the feasibility of in vitro passive sensitisation of normal leucocytes which had been separated by centrifugation and washed in Tyrode solution. All subsequent assay procedures have been based on this approach (illustrated schematically in fig. 2.15); where normal individuals' leucocytes are washed and incubated with allergic serum (to effect their sensitisation), followed by further washing to remove excess serum prior to challenge with specific allergen. Finally, after separating the cells and removing the protein from the supernatant by precipitation with trichloroacetic

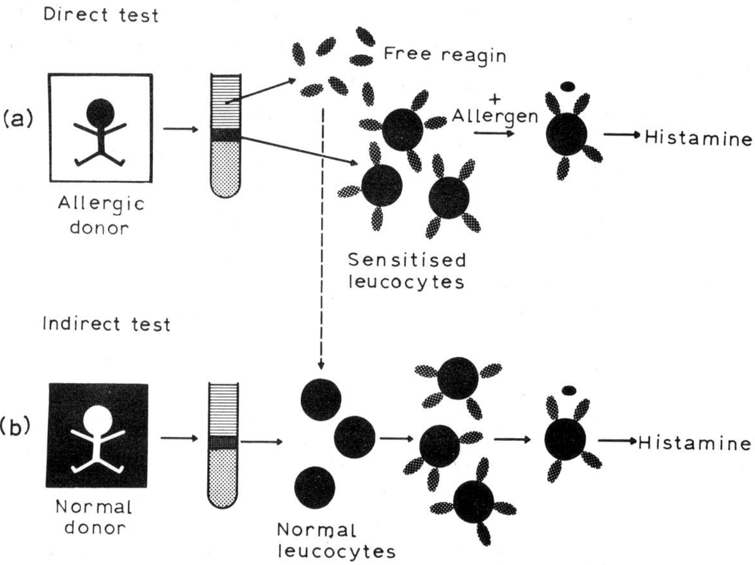

Fig. 2.15. Outline of major steps in the direct (a) and indirect (b) leucocyte assay.

acid, the liberated histamine is estimated spectrofluorometrically (fig. 2.13). The method currently in use in my own laboratory has been evolved from the procedure of Van Arsdel (communicated personally), modified according to the more recent extensive observations of Osler and his associates (Lichenstein and Osler 1964, 1966A and B; Levy and Osler 1966).

2.3.3.3 Factors influencing leucocyte sensitisation. The studies of Levy and Osler (1966) have shown that temperature, *p*H, divalent cation concentration and reagin concentration are all factors which influence the in vitro sensitisation of normal human leucocytes. The effect of temperature on the passive sensitisation of normal human leucocytes by serum from a ragweed-sensitive individual is shown in fig. 2.16. The differences in histamine release observed at 3 temperatures chosen (4°, 20° and 37°) are attributable to the temperature dependency of the sensitisation process, since the histamine releasing capacity of the allergic leucocytes

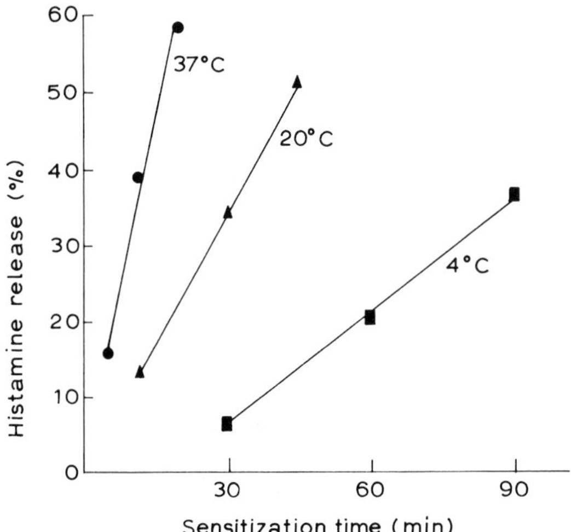

Fig. 2.16. Effect of temperature on the passive sensitisation of normal human leucocytes with serum from a ragweed-sensitive individual. (Reproduced from Levy and Osler 1966, by permission of the authors.)

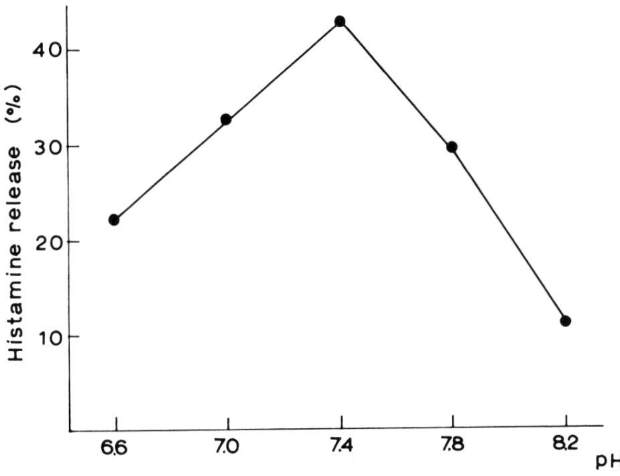

Fig. 2.17. Effect of *p*H on the passive sensitisation of normal human leucocytes. (Reproduced from Levy and Osler 1966, by permission of the authors.)

was shown to be unimpaired after 3 hr incubation in 10 per cent autologous serum with EDTA at 4° or 20°. Despite the slower rate of sensitisation at 4°, it was claimed that prolonged incubation (overnight) with allergic serum at this temperature yielded cells as reactive as those prepared at 37°. As, also, in the case of tissue sensitisation (referred to in preceding sections), prolonged treatment leads to high 'blank' values; presumably as a result of the loss of viability to which granulocytes in particular are susceptible, when maintained for relatively long periods in vitro.

The effect of *p*H on the passive sensitisation of normal leucocytes by serum of a ragweed-sensitive individual is illustrated by fig. 2.17; plotted from data obtained by diluting allergic serum with Tris-albumin buffer (*p*H 7.35 ± 0.05) containing EDTA (which is now preferred to the previous use of Tyrode solution as a suspension medium for leucocytes) and then adjusting the *p*H (at 37°) with small volumes of IN.NaOH or HCl to the required *p*H value. An aliquot (1 ml) of leucocyte suspension (at *p*H 7.5) was added to diluted (1/20) allergic serum (9 ml) thus adjusted to the required *p*H, and the mixture incubated for 60 min at 37° prior to challenge with ragweed allergen (1.5×10^{-2} μg/ml). As will be noted, a fairly sharp optimum occurred at *p*H 7.4 with the amount of histamine released falling to half the maximum value when the *p*H was increased or decreased by less than one unit. In contrast, the degree of passive sensitisation of isolated guinea pig ileum by rabbit antibodies has been shown to be the same at *p*H 5.6 and 8.2; although when carbon dioxide was used to lower the *p*H, sensitisation diminished with increasing acidity (Halpern et al. 1959).

Levy and Osler (1966) excluded the possibility that their observed effect of *p*H was due to an alteration of the histamine releasing mechanism of the suspended leucocytes, by demonstrating that release by cells from allergic donors was not altered by pre-incubation at the various *p*H values (fig. 2.17), except for a decreased response from the cells pre-incubated at the highest *p*H studied (i.e. *p*H 8.2). In our own experience, this observation is of considerable practical significance because we have found that the *p*H of allergic serum (e.g. that from our regular horse dander-sensitive donor P.R.) which has been stored in lyophilised form and reconstituted in sterile distilled water can be as high as 9.0. Moreover, the buffering capacity of the Tyrode solution originally used as a suspension medium for washed leucocytes was not sufficient to compensate for this. Presumably any potentially deleterious effect of this high *p*H would be counteracted in P–K testing, by the buffering occurring in the normal recipient's tissues during the relatively long sensitisation period; possibly through the agency of the mast cells themselves, which have been implicated in the maintenance of the homeostatic *p*H of connective tissue (Chu 1963). On the other hand, it is necessary to adjust the *p*H of the reconstituted allergic serum (to *p*H 7.35) prior to its use in the in vitro sensitisation of normal leucocytes. The use of a Tris buffer as suspension medium will adequately maintain this *p*H throughout sensitisation and subsequent allergen challenge; whilst the inclusion of human serum albumin (30 mg/100 ml) affords extra protection to the leucocytes.

The presence of EDTA in the sensitising allergic serum–leucocyte mixture at a concentration of 5 mM (i.e. in considerable excess of the amount required to bind the estimated quantity of divalent cations in a 5-fold serum dilution) was found to enhance sensitisation (Levy and Osler 1966). By performing passive leucocyte sensitisations test with and without EDTA present during the separation and washing of the normal leucocytes, and during their subsequent incubation with allergic serum, it was established that allergen-induced histamine release was doubled when EDTA was present during sensitisation. But, the presence of the chelating agent in the fluid (Tris-albumin buffer) used for washing the cells, prior to sensitisation, had little effect. Consequently, EDTA (4 mM) has been incorporated in all sensitisation reaction mixtures (in addition to the 1×10^{-2} M EDTA contained within the syringe used to take the blood from the leucocyte donor). In our experience there are also good practical grounds for using EDTA in all suspending fluids during the isolation and sensitisation of the leucocytes, as this discourages the agglutination which is more likely to occur when heparin has been used as anticoagulant (particularly when the removal of platelets has been incomplete).

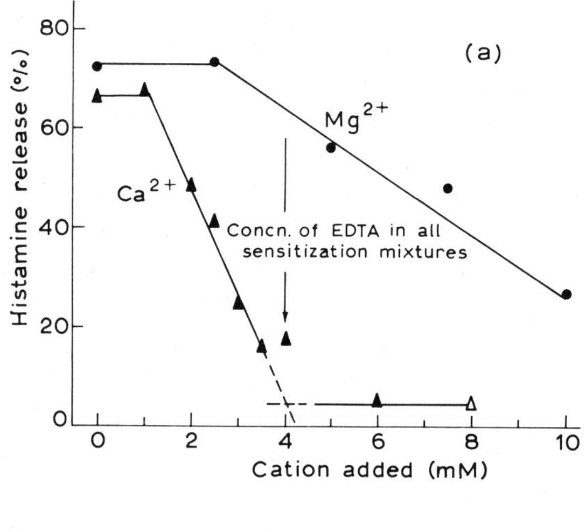

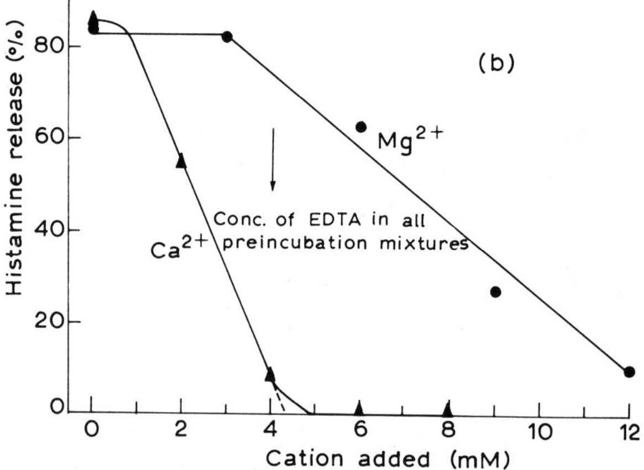

Fig. 2.18. Effect of Ca^{2+} and Mg^{2+} ions on the in vitro (a) and in vivo (b) sensitisation of human leucocytes (Reproduced from Levy and Osler, 1966 by permission of the authors.)

Contrary to its effect during the sensitisation stage, however, EDTA has been shown to inhibit antigen-induced histamine release from sensitised cells by removing the divalent cations, Ca^{2+} and Mg^{2+} (Lichenstein and Osler 1964).

As might be anticipated from such observations, it was shown

(Levy and Osler 1966) that passive leucocyte sensitisation in vitro – as judged by histamine release – is highly sensitive to calcium, but somewhat less sensitive to magnesium ions (fig. 2.18a). The virtually complete suppresion of histamine release was effected by a Ca^{2+} ion concentration of 4.1 × 10^{-3} M, whilst twice this concentration of Mg^{2+} ions produced a 50 per cent inhibition. It is interesting to note, however, (fig. 2.18b) that Ca^{2+} and Mg^{2+} ions exerted similar inhibitory effects on allergen-induced histamine release from leucocytes 'sensitised in vivo', when these cells were pre-incubated in autologous allergic serum containing 4M EDTA to which the divalent cations had been added. Furthermore, the unresponsiveness of leucocytes following such treatment with Ca^{2+} ions could not be restored by incubation with allergic serum containing EDTA in excess.

It is interesting, therefore, that there is indirect evidence that calcium ions act directly upon the cell surface, in the sensitisation of leucocytes for allergen-induced histamine release. The possible significance of this observation to the understanding of the mechanism of immediate hypersensitivity reactions will be considered further in ch. 8. If, however, the precise involvement of Ca^{2+} ions in leucocyte sensitisation is to be established it will obviously be important to employ much more homogeneous cell preparations in future studies; a refinement which should also lead to a technical improvement in the routine assay of reaginic antibodies by this procedure.

2.3.3.4 Cellular requirements for allergen-induced histamine release. This would seem to be an opportune time to consider, briefly, the cellular requirements of the passive leucocyte sensitisation assay. As the method is employed at present, it is customary to use concentrated suspensions of total leucocytes, containing approximately 1.0 × 10^7 cells per ml suspension. The volume of blood yielding this number of leucocytes varies from donor to donor, as is indicated by our data plotted in fig. 2.19. Furthermore, the total available histamine (TAH) content also varies; even from cell suspension to cell suspension obtained from the same donor on different occasions. This will be seen from the examples

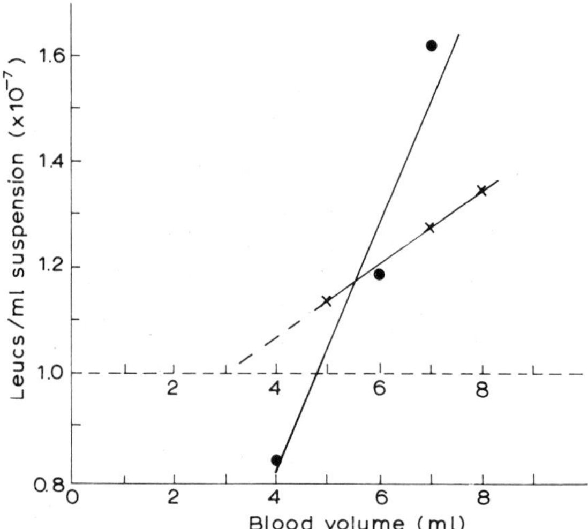

Fig. 2.19. Variation of total leucocyte yield with volumes of blood taken from 2 different donors.

taken from our accumulative data (fig. 2.20), obtained from repeated tests on leucocytes from three of our regular donor panel. The lack of correlation between the total histamine available in a standard cell suspension (derived from 4 ml blood), and the total leucocyte content, presumably reflects differences in the number of viable basophils recovered on the different occasions; because the amount of specifically released histamine showed no correlation with the total available histamine (as is also apparent from fig. 2.20). This is, of course, one of the main factors limiting the sensitivity of the passive leucocyte assay; as is illustrated in fig. 2.21, where the absolute amount of histamine released on allergen-challenge of sensitised cells is plotted against the volume of blood yielding the leucocyte suspension employed and the non-specific (base-line) release resulting from the treatment of non-sensitised leucocytes with allergen is included for comparison. This finding is typical of those obtained using cells from other members of our normal leucocyte donor panel, with the sensitising serum in question (from the horse dander-sensitive individual P.R.); indicating that the absolute minimal blood test volume is around 2.5 ml.

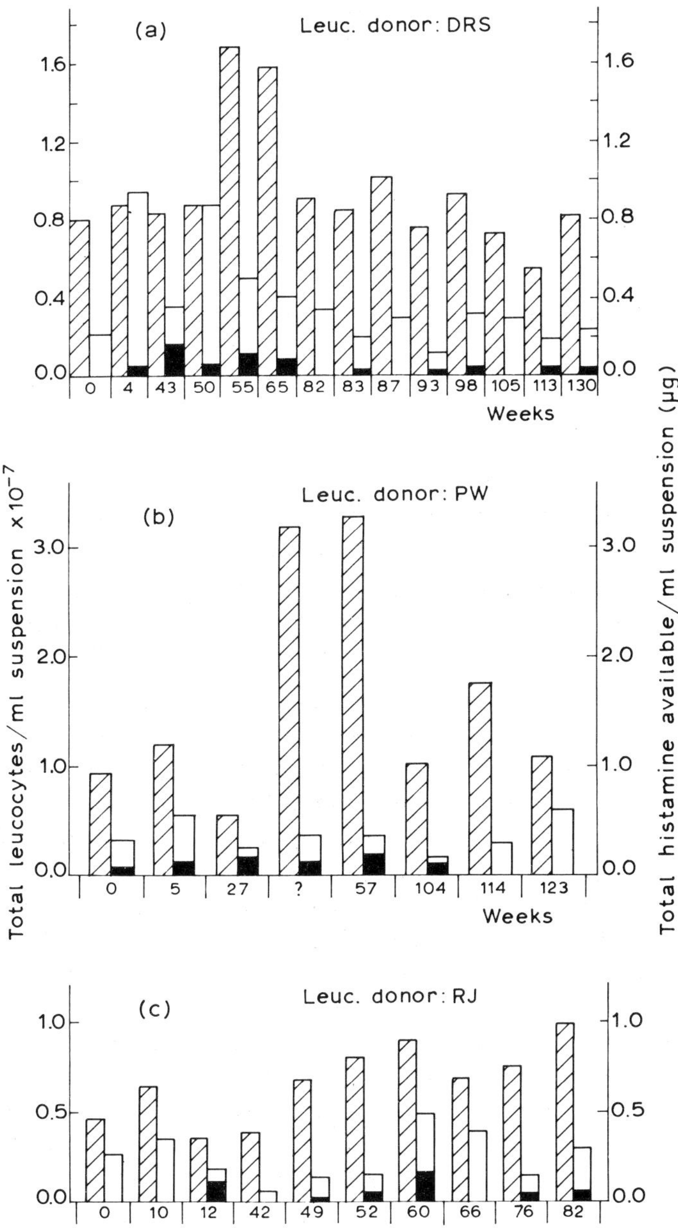

Fig. 2.20. Comparison of total leucocyte yields (▨) and total available histamine (□) from standard aliquots (4 ml) of blood taken on different occasions from 3 of our regular normal leucocyte donors. The black areas indicate the proportion of histamine released specifically on allergen challenge, following passive sensitisation with the same standard allergic (horse dander-sensitive) serum.

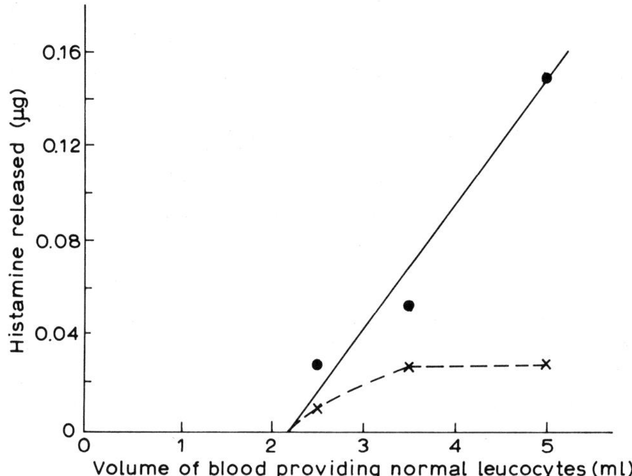

Fig. 2.21. Variation in allergen (horse dandruff)-induced histamine release with the total leucocyte content of the test aliquot used for passive sensitisation with allergic serum. (The dotted line refers to non-specific histamine release effected by buffer alone.)

But, in practical terms, it is usually necessary to use leucocyte suspensions from somewhat greater volumes of blood (i.e. 3–5 ml) if a measurable yield of histamine above the base-line is to be obtained.

It is possible to obtain satisfactory results using smaller volumes of blood from atopic individuals themselves; which, of course, precludes the need for in vitro sensitisation prior to allergen challenge. For instance, aliquots of leucocytes from 2.0 ml volumes are usually then quite adequate; and there has been a recent report (May et al. 1970) of the performance of ten such tests on as little as a total blood volume of 10 ml (from children) by the adoption of technical modifications which included the combining of protein precipitation and histamine extraction into one operation.

At the other end of the scale, the effect of using relatively large concentrations of total leucocytes (i.e. 120, 240 and 480 $\times$ 10^6 in 20 ml volumes) for passive sensitisation has been investigated (Levy and Osler 1966), using aliquots of serum (diluted 1/20) from the same ragweed-sensitive donor. After incubation (at 37° for 60 min), followed by centrifugation in the cold, the cells were resuspended in Tris-albumin buffer (containing calcium and magnesium ions) at a concentration of 1.6 × 10^7 leucocytes per ml. Measurement of the histamine released on challenge with specific allergen revealed a relative insensitivity of the passive sensitisation process to fourfold changes in total leucocyte concentration. We have made similar observations, in studies of the passive sensitisation of normal human leucocytes (in suspension containing up to 1.7 × 10^7 cells/ml) by serum from our regular horse-dander-sensitive donor (P.R.). The use of suspensions containing more than 2.4 × 10^7 leucocytes per ml for in vitro sensitisation is prevented, however, by their agglutination (Levy and Osler 1966).

Leucocyte agglutination is thought to be discouraged in washed cell suspensions by the presence of contaminating erythrocytes (Van Arsdel 1964), but it is possible that they adsorb reaginic antibody non-specifically. For this reason, it is preferable to layer the freshly taken blood on to dextran solution (e.g. 8 per cent w/v 'Dextraven 110') as an initial separation procedure; a practice which (in our experience) reduces the contamination by erythrocytes by at least tenfold that occurring in suspensions of cells isolated merely by centrifugation. Even so, the ratio of erythrocytes to total leucocytes in the suspensions is still of the order of 4 to 10 times; and the use of dextran precludes subsequent basophil counting by conventional techniques.

2.3.3.5 Cells involved in histamine release. It is assumed, of course, that the circulating basophils – which bear a close morphological and histochemical resemblance to tissue mast cells – are primarily involved in the passive sensitisation of normal human leucocytes by reaginic antibodies. Merely on the basis of a statistical analysis of histamine contents and total and differential leucocyte counts, of blood samples, Graham et al. (1955) have concluded that the basophils contain more than half of the total histamine of normal blood despite their scarcity (i.e. comprising less than 1 per cent of the total leucocytes). More direct evidence of basophil involvement would seem to be provided by the demonstration of Shelley and Juhlin (1961) that it is possible to induce the basophils of hypersensitive individuals to degranulate in vitro on reaction with specific allergen. The system employed differs, however, in certain important respects from that involving reagin-mediated histamine release; and, as will be discussed further in § 2.4.1, it has yet to be demonstrated unequivocally that it measures reagin–allergen interaction. Nevertheless, recent findings from immunofluorescent studies with labelled anti-IgE antibody (Ishizaka et al. 1970) and from a rosette-forming procedure (Wilson et al. 1971) have provided evidence of the presence of γE molecules on the basophil surface.

In preliminary studies in my laboratory, employing the improved method of Cooper and Cruickshank (1966) for the direct counting of basophils, there was no significant decrease in the number of cells detectable following reaction of blood from a grass pollen-sensitive donor with the specific allergen in vitro; but 48 per cent of the basophils counted showed evidence of granular depletion. Similarly Greaves (1968) found that incubation of basophils from artificially-sensitised rabbits, with specific antigen (ovalbumin), had no significant effect on the number of cells detectable by metachromatic staining with Toluidine Blue. When, however, these experiments were repeated using living (unstained) rabbit basophil preparations, it was observed by phase contrast microscopy that addition of specific antigen (at 37°) caused immobilisation of the basophils, accompanied by the rapid oscillation of the granules. The granular material coalesced around the periphery of the cell; and, in some cells, vacuolation appeared and the cell membrane developed blister-like protrusions and ultimately the cell became inert and moribund. It seems significant that Hastie (1971) has observed similar types of morphological changes in basophils from grass-pollen sensitive individuals, on presentation of the specific allergen in a chamber designed to ensure maintenance of cell viability during microscopic examination.

It is possible, of course, that other types of peripheral leucocyte, such as eosinophils and neutrophils, are also involved in allergen-induced histamine release; but Greaves (1968) found no evidence of eosinophil involvement in experiments employing enriched fractions of leucocytes from artificially sensitised rabbits, separated by differential sedimentation. Similar fractionation procedures are being employed in attempts to isolate the less robust human basophils, in a high state of purity. The various steps per-

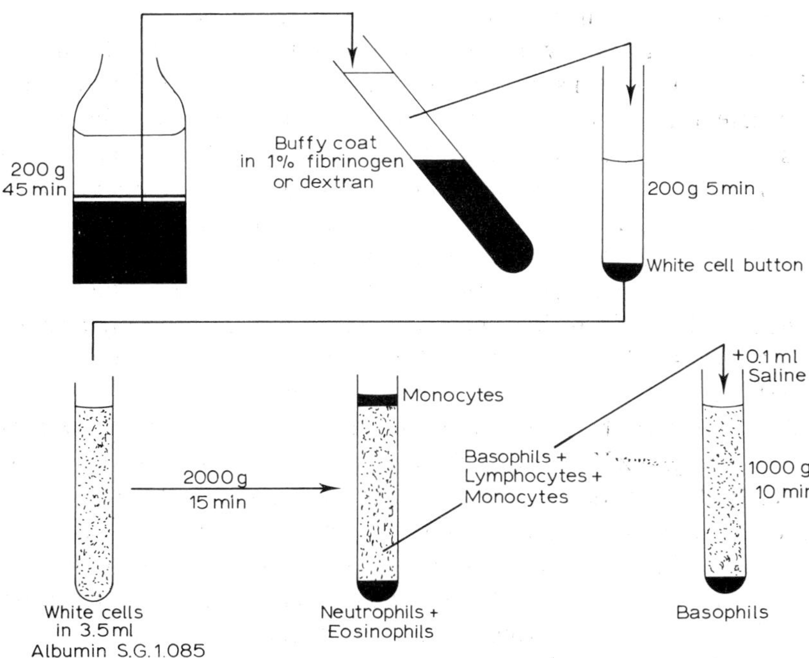

Fig. 2.22. Schematic outline of procedure used in differential sedimentation of human leucocytes. (Reproduced from Sampson and Archer 1967, by permission of the authors.)

formed in one such procedure (Sampson and Archer 1967), based on the differential sedimentation of a total leucocyte suspension obtained by an initial separation in 1 per cent fibrinogen or dextran, are outlined in fig. 2.22. Preparations thus obtained, however, comprised only 5–20 per cent basophils: which were shown to contain $2.4 \pm 0.6\ \mu g$ histamine per 10^6 basophils. This confirmed the calculations of Graham and his associates (1955), suggesting that the basophils contained a significant amount of total leucocyte histamine. Unlike the earlier investigators, however, Sampson and Archer (1967) failed to obtain evidence of any histamine in eosinophils or neutrophils. By assuming that human mast cells contain a similar amount of histamine to rat mast cells, they have concluded that only a small proportion of the total body histamine is contained in the circulating human basophil; mast cells being far more numerous in the body than basophils (Archer 1959). Unfortunately it is not possible to use human mast cells for in vitro passive sensitisation testing; nor is it practicable to compensate for the scarcity of basophils in normal human blood by using leucocytes from patients with chronic leukemia, for instance, because their basophils have been found to contain significantly less histamine than normal (Sampson and Archer 1967).

Against the advantage of using enriched leucocyte preparations, obtained by relatively long fractionation procedures, has to be weighed the risk of damaging the cells by the extra manipulations involved. As already mentioned, granulocytes are particularly susceptible to loss of viability under in vitro conditions. Human basophils prepared by the differential sedimentation procedure outlined in fig. 2.22 were found, however, to retain their capacity for specific histamine release; besides proving capable of active movement and phagacytosis of sensitised group A erythrocytes. The fragility of the granulocytes is an obstacle to attempts to preserve large batches of human leucocytes (for later passive sensitisation testing, by deep freezing in liquid nitrogen in the presence of glycerol or dimethyl sulphoxide), as has been accomplished with lymphocytes; and as was attempted in the preliminary studies on the preservation of human lung and monkey skin referred to in the previous section. The development of a satisfactory procedure would obviate the present need for maintaining a panel of normal leucocyte donors. The fragility of basophils would also seem to preclude their separation by the types of column procedure in current use for the fractionation of lymphocytes. In this connection, it would seem significant that Pruzansky and Patterson (1970) have observed that allergen-induced histamine release from allergic individuals' basophils which have been separated by passage through glass beads appears to be a cytotoxic process; contrary to the findings of studies on non-fractionated sensitised human leucocytes (Lichenstein and Osler 1964), which suggested that the allergen triggers an active secretion of histamine. It will obviously be essential, however, to establish that this form of fractionation treatment has not rendered the basophils more labile and susceptible to cytotoxic changes.

2.3.3.6 Variability in behaviour of normal leucocytes towards passive sensitisation. Finally, whilst dealing with cellular aspects of the passive leucocyte sensitisation system, it is worth noting that some normal donors' leucocytes appear to be more readily sensitised in vitro than others; whilst yet others are relatively unreceptive to reaginic (γE) antibody.

For instance, Levy and Osler (1966) have confirmed the earlier observations of Van Arsdel and Sells (1963), that the speed of sensitisation of normal leucocytes varies with their source as well as the concentration of the sensitising allergic serum. It was found that maximal histamine release (on allergen challenge) was usually obtained within the second hour of sensitisation (at 37°), whilst sensitisation beyond this period (e.g. for 4 hr, with 10-fold dilutions of relatively potent allergic sera) sometimes leads to diminished release (e.g. 67.1 per cent at 4 hr, as compared to 87.2 per cent at 2 hr).

Furthermore, it has been shown (Levy and Osler 1966) that the allergen dose–release relationship for leucocytes sensitised (to ragweed) in vitro varies markedly with cells from different non-allergic donors. For instance, of 84 non-allergic cell donors, whose leucocytes were incubated with numerous and potent allergic sera, only 16 provided cells which released more than 40 per cent of their available histamine on reaction with allergen; but cells from these donors were readily sensitised (for maximum response) by the sera of many different-allergic individuals. As Levy and Osler have pointed out, however, these findings seem to conflict with the early in vivo studies of Coca and Grove (1925), confirmed later by Stanworth and Kuhns (1965); which indicated that over 80 per cent of normal individuals were satisfactory recipients for P–K testing. It is possible, however, that this apparent discrepancy between the in vitro and in vivo findings can be attributed to a difference in the rate of sensitisation of different individuals' tissues compared to their leucocytes. Such a difference would not be apparent from P–K testing, as challenge is made after a relatively prolonged sensitisation period. In contrast, in their in vitro studies, Levy and Osler (1966) passively sensitised the normal leucocytes from various donors by incubation for only 60 min with allergic

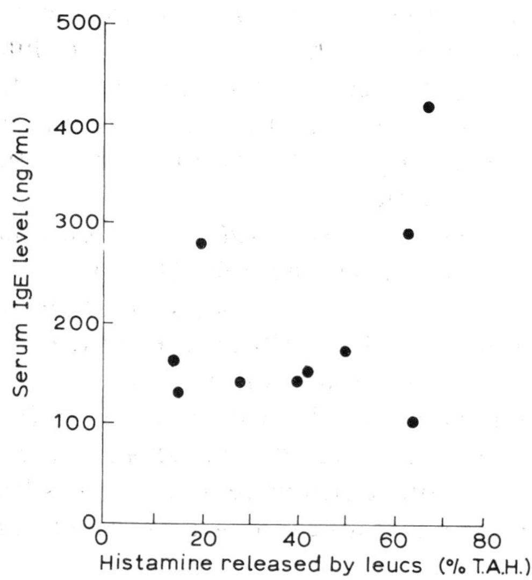

Fig. 2.23. Comparison of maximal specific (i.e. allergen-induced) histamine release shown by the passively sensitised leucocytes of regular normal donors with their serum IgE (total) levels determined by R.I.S.T.

serum; and yet, as already mentioned, the speed of sensitisation over this limited time period, was observed to vary considerably between the leucocytes from different donors. Is it perhaps possible, therefore, that cells which were apparently unreceptive after 60 min required longer incubation times for optimal sensitisation?

In this connection it is possibly significant that in our studies of the passive sensitisation of leucocytes from a smaller number of normal donors, we find that a greater percentage appear to be receptive (on some occasions) to reaginic antibody binding after 3 hr incubation with allergic serum. Cells of 6 of the 10 individuals on our leucocyte donor panel have on occasions released 40 per cent or more of their total available histamine, following sensitisation with serum from our horse dander-sensitive blood donor (P.R.) followed by allergen challenge. On other occassions, however, even the cells from these donors appeared to be much less receptive (see fig. 2.20); an observation which cannot be attributed entirely to experimental variation, but which would seem to suggest perhaps some day-to-day variation in the receptivity of an individual's leucocytes or – more likely – in the yields of viable basophils obtained.

There are, no doubt, many factors which could influence the capacity of an individual's basophils to bind reaginic antibody. For instance, if recent findings from experimental animal systems can be taken as a guide, it is conceivable that there might be interference from the binding of unrelated γE antibodies (directed against other allergens) or even from that of other classes of immunoglobulin. In this connection, the interesting suggestion has been made that the receptivity of a normal donor's basophils will be governed by the γE-globulin already on their surface; which is proportional to that found (in low levels) in their circulation. The data presented in fig. 2.23 would seem to refute the latter possibility, however; assuming that the total serum IgE level (as estimated by R.I.S.T.) gives a true reflection of basophil-bound IgE, and that the latter remains relatively constant. For, as will be seen, there was no obvious relationship between the serum IgE level of the leucocyte donor and the maximum allergen-induced histamine release shown (after sensitisation with serum from our horse dander-sensitive donor, P.R.)[8].

As will be discussed further later, however, the decisive factors controlling basophil sensitisation might prove to be more subtle than this.

2.3.3.7 Effect of allergen concentration. As has been found in the other sensitisation systems already considered, the concentration of challenging allergen influences the extent of histamine released specifically from sensitised leucocytes. This is observed both in the direct test, using cells from allergic donors, and also with leucocytes which have been sensitised by in vitro incubation with allergic serum under the conditions already outlined.

Representative allergen dose–response relationships observed by Lichenstein and Osler (1964), in studies on leucocyte suspensions from 3 of their ragweed-sensitive donors, are reproduced in fig. 2.24. Apparently the upper 2 responses are the more typical, the third being characteristic of about 20 per cent of donors

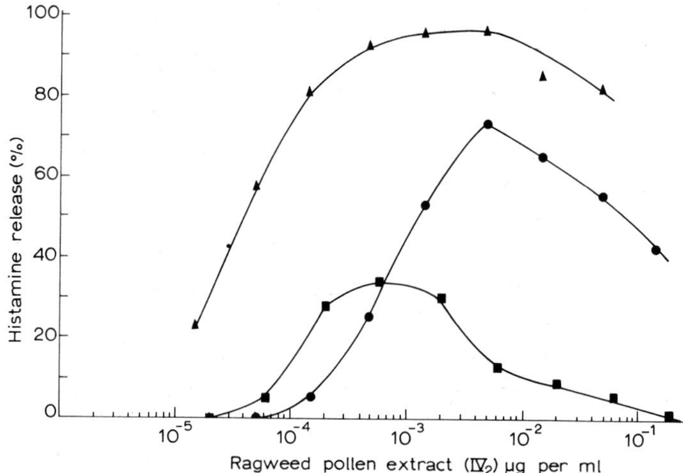

Fig. 2.24. Allergen dose–response relationships shown by leucocytes from 3 ragweed-sensitive donors. (Reproduced from Lichenstein and Osler 1964, by permission of the authors.)

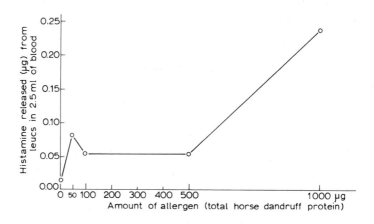

Fig. 2.25. Allergen dose–response relationship shown by a normal human's leucocytes passively sensitised by treatment with serum from horse dander-sensitive individual.

whose leucocytes release only a small proportion of the total available histamine on allergen challenge. From studies on several hundred different cell populations, threshold allergen levels have been found to range from 10^{-7} to 10^{-3} μg/ml; whilst about 10–30-fold greater amounts of allergen evoke maximal histamine releases (70–100 per cent of the total available). Excessive amounts of allergen, on the other hand, suppress the response; as is the case in other allergic reactions. We have observed a similar dependence upon allergen concentration in passive leucocyte sensitisation systems, as will be seen from the curves in fig. 2.25 plotted from data obtained from sensitisation with the serum of a horse dander-sensitive individual. Here, too, excessive amounts of allergen suppress the response. Hence, it is obviously important in any application of the passive leucocyte sensitisation assay to first establish the optimal allergen concentration for maximum specific histamine release in the system in question.

The amount of allergen needed to evoke a 50 per cent response from the leucocytes of allergic individuals has been employed as a measure of their degree of sensitivity, and has been shown to be inversely related to the severity of symptoms recorded by the patients or their physicians (Osler et al. 1968). This has the advantage that reactivity can be expressed in terms of an accurately measurable protein (allergen) concentration. As will be apparent from the master fig. 2.1, however, this parameter provides a measure of the allergen-binding capacity of cell-bound reaginic (γE) antibody; in contrast to the tissue sensitising activity of humoral antibody determined in the indirect systems, where it is usual to maintain the allergen concentration at a constant optimal value.

2.3.3.8 Performance of the passive leucocyte sensitisation technique. Having considered the major theoretical aspects of the passive leucocyte sensitisation technique, it is important finally to attempt an assessment of its practical potential (in keeping with the approach already adopted in previous sections of this chapter).

As already indicated, there can be little doubt that the procedure is measuring reaginic antibodies. This is illustrated rather neatly by the data in fig. 2.26, where the P–K activity of varying

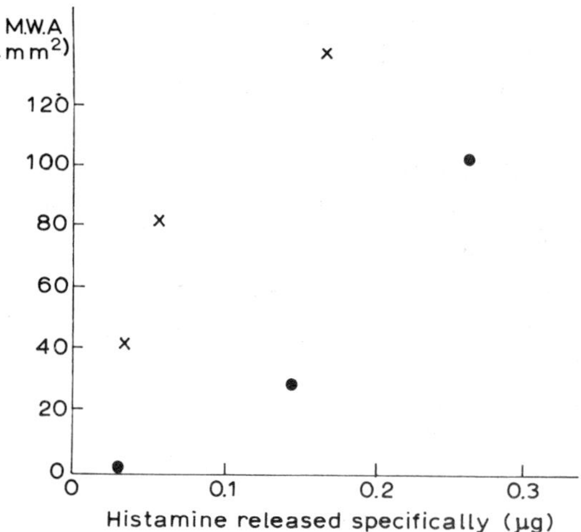

Fig. 2.26. Comparison of P–K activity (expressed as mean weal area: M.W.A.) of varying dilutions of serum from a horse dander-sensitive individual (P.R.) with their capacity to sensitise the leucocytes of the skin test recipient for histamine release on allergen challenge (10 and 20 min weal areas plotted).

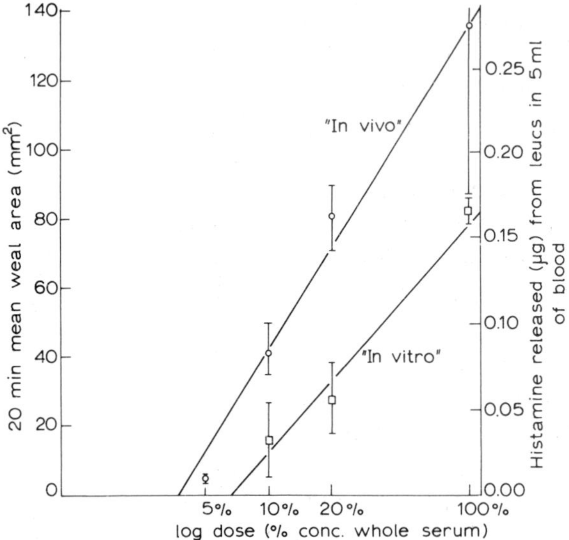

Fig. 2.27. Separate dose–response curves obtained from the quantitative P–K testing and passive leucocyte sensitisation assay referred to in fig. 2.26.

TABLE 2.4A

Effect of heat treatment on the passive sensitising activity of human allergic sera as measured by the leucocyte test (Stanworth, unpublished data).

Normal leucocyte donor	Allergic serum donor	State of serum	Allergen	Total available histamine (from leucocytes from 4 ml blood) (μg)	Specifically released histamine (from leucocytes from 4 ml blood) (μg)	% total
D.R.S.	P.R.	untreated	horse dander	0.32	0.15 (0.14)	47
		heated (56°C/30′)			0.03 (0.05)	9
R.J.	M.D.	untreated	Timothy grass	0.16	0.10	63
		heated (56°C/30′)	pollen		0.00	0

TABLE 2.4B

Effect of heat treatment on the passive sensitising activity of human allergic sera as measured by P–K testing (Stanworth and Kuhns, unpublished data).

Allergen	Time of heating allergic serum at 56° (min)	Recipient H.S.				Recipient J.F.			
		20 min weal area (mm^2) 1	2	Mean	% untreated serum M.W.A.	20 min weal area (mm^2) 1	2	Mean	% untreated serum M.W.A.
Horse dandruff	0	115	89	102	100	104	64	84	100
	15	133	124	129	129	59	84	72	86
	30	26	23	25	25	10	10	10	12
	60	0	0	0	0	0	0	0	0
	120	0	0	0	0	0	0	0	0
	240	0	0	0	0	0	0	0	0
Diphtheria toxoid	0	31	48	40	100	43	35	39	100
	15	18	13	16	40	13	15	14	36
	30	0	11	6	15	0	0	0	0
	60	0	12	6	15	0	0	0	0
	120	0	0	0	0	0	0	0	0
	240	0	0	0	0	0	0	0	0

dilutions of an allergic serum (expressed as mean weal area) is compared with their capacity to sensitive passively leucocytes from the recipient of the passive skin tests. Furthermore, heating at 56° for 30 min destroyed a major part of the leucocyte-sensitising activity; as is indicated by the data in table 2.4A; thereby paralleling its effect on P–K activity (table 2.4B).

There is a linear relationship between the logarithm of the sensitising serum concentration and the amount of allergen-induced histamine released from passively sensitised leucocytes. Moreover, the coefficient of variation of a single in vitro assay in our experience is comparable to that observed in the P–K test (fig. 2.27, comprising separate plots of the data compared directly in the previous figure). But the passive leucocyte sensitisation assay appears to be about 5 times less sensitive than the in vivo procedure, and its log (dose)–response curve is flatter. On the other hand, the direct leucocyte test – on cells from ragweed-sensitive individuals – has been shown to be more accurate than the P–K testing of the same individuals' sera (Lichenstein et al. 1967).

Lack of reproducibility [9] of assays performed on successive occasions is another difficulty encountered particularly with the passive leucocyte sensitisation system (fig. 2.20). In our experience this problem is difficult to avoid, even where the same leucocyte donor's cells are used (with the same sensitising serum); on some occasions only negligible amounts of histamine release being recorded on specific allergen challenge, in contrast to the appreciably larger amounts released more consistently from passively sensitised human lung (table 2.2). At the other end of the scale, maximum specific release rarely exceeds 65 per cent of the total available histamine (released by trichloroacetic acid treatment); whereas non-specific release, brought about by the addition of buffer alone to the sensitised leucocytes, can sometimes be as high as 30 per cent of the total available histamine. Yet in our experience, using total leucocyte numbers of around 1×10^7 for passive sensitisation, it is not possible to measure accurately specific responses of less than 10 per cent by the spectrofluorometric procedure.

One of the main problems is the poor yield of basophils often achieved by the leucocyte separation procedures available[10] Admittedly, this could be compensated for by using suspensions of cells from larger aliquots of blood; but only at the expense of reducing the already limited number of tests possible with cells from any one leucocyte donor. Another difficulty would seem to be the achievement of efficient sensitisation of those basophils obtained, which form only a minor proportion of the total cells (leucocytes and erythrocytes) within the test suspension. As has already been indicated, many factors can thwart this aim; the conditions for optimum sensitisation varying with the source and concentration of the sensitising serum. Allergen-induced histamine release is more readily demonstrated, on the other hand, from leucocytes of allergic donors; presumably because the in vivo sensitisation process is more efficient.

The passive leucocyte sensitisation technique shares many of the drawbacks of the other in vitro sensitisation procedures already discussed, although it is usually easier to obtain fresh normal human blood than human or monkey tissue. It is a laborious and time-consuming procedure, demanding a high degree of technical skill and access to a suitable spectrofluorometer (or, alternatively, a facility for bioassay of the released histamine). As practised in my own laboratory, the 50 ml (approx.) of blood taken from each normal leucocyte donor provides sufficient cells for only 3 duplicate test and 3 duplicate control assays, in addition to cells used for the separate determination of total available histamine.

It is questionable, therefore, whether it will ever become established as a routine method of assaying reaginic (γE) antibodies. Nevertheless, it seems probable that passive leucocyte sensitisation will form the basis of many future investigations of the mechanism of immediate hypersensitivity reactions; particularly when it becomes possible to employ highly pure human basophil preparations[11] with homogeneous antibody and allergen reactants.

2.3.3.9 Attempted development of modified leucocyte assay system. In an attempt to devise a simpler routine test, preliminary investigations have been made in my laboratory into the possibility of adapting the leucocyte assay into a rapid passive in vivo procedure. The idea was to use a convenient experimental animal's skin as a live 'cell reaction chamber', from which the histamine released by the interaction of allergen with passively transferred sensitised human leucocytes would initiate an extravasation response in the host animal's tissue (revealed by pre-injected indicator dye). As the combination of human reaginic antibody on the recipient animal's tissue would not theoretically be a prerequisite for allergen-induced histamine release in this situation, the narrow species range over which it is possible to effect a P–K-type reaction (discussed in § 2.3.3.3) would not be expected to offer any limitation. We chose, therefore, guinea pigs as recipients for the intradermal injection of aliquots (0.1 ml) of suspensions (containing approx. 2.1×10^7 total leucocytes per ml) of leucocytes from a grass-pollen-sensitive individual. Allergen challenge was effected 10 and 30 min later by either intravenous or local injection (into the site), Evan's Blue being used as indicator. In no test, however, was the extent of blueing effected significantly greater than that produced by the use of a comparable number of leucocytes from a non-allergic individual.

It is possible, that these negative findings are attributable to the use of an insufficient number of basophils, because an approximately 10-fold larger volume of allergic leucocyte suspension has been required for the allergen-induced release of sufficient amounts of histamine for in vitro measurement. In this case, the value of the method would be questionable on the grounds of a relative lack of sensitivity compared with that of the in vitro leucocyte assays discussed earlier. There could, however, be other complicating factors because even in the case of the transfer of allergic human leucocytes to isologous skin, the weal reactions induced on subsequent allergen challenge were often relatively small; and prolonged inflammatory responses, lasting for at least 6 days after transfer of the leucocyte suspensions, were observed (Walzer and Bowman 1960).

2.4 Alternative in vitro cell systems

Histamine release is, of course, not necessarily the only measurable indicator of cell bound reagin–allergen interaction. Alternative 'end-points' to have been considered include basophil degranulation and leucocyte agglutination. There have also been innumerable attempts to employ erythrocytes as allergen carriers in agglutination systems.

2.4.1 Indirect basophil or mast cell degranulation

Despite extensive efforts to demonstrate its applicability there is serious doubt as to whether the basophil degranulation test devised by Shelley and Juhlin (1961, 1962) is capable of detecting reaginic (γE) antibody activity; moreover its reliability and accuracy compare unfavourably with those of the in vitro systems already discussed in this chapter.

In the indirect system (Shelley 1962) the more abundant (i.e. 10 times) rabbit basophils are used in preference to normal human basophils, in a microscope slide test requiring only minute amounts of reactants (e.g. 0.005 ml allergic serum; 0.005 ml allergen solution). The buffy coat, separated from a drop of rabbit's blood by centrifugation in narrow polythene tubing, is mixed with the serum and allergen solution on a slide covered with a thin film of supravital stain (e.g. 0.05 ml ethanolic solution of Neutral Red). In a microscopic examination made under oil (after covering the reaction mixture with a vaseline edged cover slip), by scanning the living field at varying time intervals from 5–30 min later, the basophil granules are seen stained a brick red colour in contrast to the yellow neutrophils and light-brown eosinophils. According to Shelley (1962) the reaction can be assumed to be positive when 'the majority of basophils show loss of sphericity, cell distortion, swelling granulosis, granular swelling, less staining, rapid oscillation or dancing of granules, loss of granules, appearance of a clear nucleus, cell wall bleb formation and streaming of granules from cells'. Furthermore, cells treated with sera from strongly sensitive individuals were seen to 'degranulate explosively'.

Other investigators have employed Toluidine Blue to stain the mucopolysaccharides in the basophil granules, together with detergent (e.g. saponin) to lyse the erythrocytes present, thus permitting their direct counting (in a Fuchs-Rossenthal hemocytometer). But, in the experience of Cooper and Cruickshank (1966), the staining of basophils by aqueous Toluidine Blue is often confused, because the water solubility of the polysaccharides makes identification difficult and counting time consuming. Moreover, the clotting and aggregation of platelets which occurs renders counting inaccurate, because aggregates associate with degranulated basophils in their vicinity thereby producing spuriously low counts. Attempts have been made, however, to overcome these difficulties by the inclusion of acetyl pyridinium chloride in the toluidine solution to lyse the erythrocytes and at the same time render the granular mucopolysaccharides insoluble; and, in addition, aluminium sulphate is included to mordant the dye. Thus, the basophils are stained purple-red in contrast to the other leucocytes, platelets and erythrocytes (which all remain unstained); and, as staining is fast, counts may be made some time (e.g. up to a week) after taking the sample. In a similar type of improved staining technique (Levin 1967), relying upon a non-aqueous fixative (absolute ethanol-glacial acetic acid–chloroform 6/2/2), 30 per cent degranulation of the rabbit basophils is taken as a base-line above which the reaction is considered to be positive.

It is essential to exercise caution, however, in the interpretation of results obtained using these staining techniques, because Greaves (1968) has found that anaphylactic histamine release from the basophils of actively sensitised rabbits is not accompanied by a change in the number of metachromatically staining cells when a non-fixative stain is used (such as 0.08 per cent Toluidine Blue in aqueous phosphate buffer, *p*H 7.6). If, on the other hand the basophils are collected in the presence of saponin-alcohol fixative a fall in the number of metachromatically stained cells is seen in the antigen-treated cell suspension; but not in a Tyrode-treated suspension, nor in antigen-treated normal cell suspensions. A detailed study of the cytological changes occurring in washed rabbit basophils during anaphylaxis confirmed that histamine release from actively sensitised cells can occur without loss of the ability of the basophils to stain with basic dyes, and in the absence of degranulation; although the process is accompanied by characteristic morphological changes. It seems likely, therefore, that the basophil degranulation observed when Toluidine Blue stain is employed in Shelley's technique can be attributed to an effect of the fixative on the antigen-treated cells and not to a direct manifestation of the antibody–antigen reaction. Nevertheless, it is still possible that the effect observed is mediated indirectly by antibody; for, as Greaves (1968) has suggested, it is conceivable that the detergent exerts a destructive action on basophil cell membranes which have already been rendered susceptible by anaphylactic antibody.

It seems most unlikely, however, that reaginic (γE) antibodies are responsible for such an effect on basophils. Indeed, there is every indication that the basophil reaction has nothing to do with reagin (cell-bound)-allergen interaction, as it occurs under conditions which differ markedly from those known to be optimal from allergen-induced histamine release from passively or actively sensitised skin in vivo and from leucocytes, tissues or lung in vitro. For instance, as was indicated in the previous section (2.3.3), reagin-mediated histamine release from normal human leucocytes occurs optimally at 37° (after a sensitisation period of 90 min) in the presence of precisely defined amounts of divalent action (Ca^{2+} and Mg^{2+}). In contrast, human basophil degranulation has been shown (Haye 1965) to occur, within a few minutes, at 20° in the presence of EDTA. Moreover, reagin-mediated reactions have been found to be independent of complement, and γE antibodies (as opposed to aggregated IgE) have proved incapable of fixing complement in vitro; whereas the capacity of allergic sera (from penicillin-sensitive individuals) to evoke rabbit basophil degranulation was destroyed by heating at 56° for 30 min (Schwartz et al. 1965A), but was restored by the addition of fresh complement (or several individual components, of which C1 and C2 proved indispensable).

Similar doubts about the involvement of reaginic (γE) antibodies have been cast on the results of attempts to detect human hypersensitivity by indirect rat mast cell degranulation (Schwartz et al. 1965B); which has been employed as an alternative to the indirect rabbit basophil test because of the superiority of rat peritoneal mast cells (in terms of greater in vitro stability, absence of degranulation and the suitability of any donor animal's cells). On the other hand, it is not inconceivable that some other (non-γE) type of human antibody is capable of evoking the degranulation effects observed in rabbit basophils and mast cells. In this connection, it is perhaps significant that the effect appears to have been achieved most readily with sera of patients showing sensitivity to antibiotics and other drugs (e.g. insulin, horse serum), where there are suspicions that non-γE antibodies are implicated. Furthermore, direct evidence has been reported (Goodfriend et al. 1969) of a lack of correlation between the rabbit basophil degranulating activities and P–K titres of DEAE sephadex fractions of serum from a (treated) ragweed-sensitive individual. There also appears to be a lack of correlation between direct basophil degranulation and the direct skin activity of allergic (grass-pollen sensitive) donors, if the small number of preliminary data (Stanworth and Haye, unpublished) in table 2.5 can be considered as representative; nor, as will be observed from the table, is there apparently any correlation with the amount of histamine released specifically from the same

TABLE 2.5

Comparison of the direct degranulating activity of grass pollen-sensitive individuals basophils, with their direct skin activity and allergen-induced histamine release from their leucocytes (Stanworth and Haye, unpublished data).

	Direct skin reaction (M.W.A. in mm^2) to Timothy ext. (10 mg prot./ml)		Histamine released (μg/l plasma) by Timothy ext. (10 mg prot./ml)		Basophil degranulation (% degranulated)		
					Timothy ext.		NaCl
	1/100	1/1000	1/100	1/1000	1/100	1/1000	(control)
W	146	38	77	91	34	47	13
B	106	67	139	139	48	44	32
F	61	28	81	32	14	10	20
Wi	15	6	113	65	2	4	5
L	45	28	146	129			10
K	33	22	97	58	20	40	10

donors' leucocytes following in vitro incubation of whole blood samples with specific allergen. It is possible that the presence of γG-type blocking antibodies are influencing such findings, but the results of indirect basophil degranulation tests performed on the sera of ragweed-sensitive patients (Kravis et al. 1965) suggest that this is unlikely.

The manner in which indirect basophil (or mast cell) degranulation tests are conducted suggests that the reaction responsible for the morphological effects observed is fundamentally different from the γE-mediated reactions measured in the in vitro systems discussed previously. For instance, it seems highly significant that despite the claims of Perelmutter and Khera (1970) of cell-bound γE antibody involvement in the induction of morphological changes, it is not possible (Jasani 1971) to effect allergen (e.g. cocksfoot pollen) induced histamine release from rat mast cells which have been adequately washed prior to incubation with sensitising serum in the manner adopted in the passive leucocyte (human) sensitisation test. This raises, therefore, the possibility that antigen–antibody complex formed in the fluid (i.e. serum) phase can (possibly with the aid of complement components) effect the changes seen in rat mast cells or rabbit basophils; in a manner analogous to the antigen–antibody mediated reaction in rabbit platelets, to be referred to later.

Admittedly recent reports of an antigenic relationship between human γE-globulin and the γE-globulins of the rat and rabbit raises the possibility that human reaginic antibodies might possess some binding activity for the mast cells and basophils of these animal species; but it seems more likely that any morphological changes mediated by γE antibodies under the test conditions usually employed would be initiated *subsequent to* their prior complexing with specific allergen whilst in the medium rather than on the target cell. This possibility is quite consistent with the picture which is beginning to form of the supposed role of γE antibodies in the triggering of immediate sensitivity responses (ch. 5 and 8); for, according to the mechanism which I have proposed there, reagin–allergen interaction on the mast cell (or basophil) surface results in the formation of an activating site (within the Fc region of the antibody) whose action would not necessarily be restricted to the triggering of target cells of the species of origin of the γE antibody. Moreover, this could account for a recent report (Korotzer et al. 1971) that rat mast cells which have been 'passively sensitised' with pollen-sensitive individuals' sera can be caused to degranulate by subsequent treatment with monospecific rabbit anti-human myeloma IgE antiserum; as human IgE-anti-IgE complexes (like aggregated human IgE) would be expected to possess mast cell-reactive sites which had been revealed in the γE antibody as a result of its cross-linking by anti-γE antibody. On the other hand, it is quite conceivable that the structural requirements for mast cell binding by γE antibodies are more stringent; and, therefore, incapable of transcending the human–rat species barrier.

Technically, the indirect basophil test also poses problems owing to the tendency of cells to degranulate non-specifically (even in the absence of antigen or sensitising antibody) and owing to the lack of reproducibility of results; and the toxicity of many human allergic sera (Haye 1965) presents another difficulty. Furthermore, even if these problems are surmounted by the use of very fresh (not more than an hour old) allergic serum and the blood of healthy donor rabbits possessing basophil counts between 150–400/mm^3 as suggested by Shelley (1965) it has still to be recognised that the indirect basophil degranulation test relies essentially on a subjective assessment of the extent of reactivity. In the words of Shelley himself: 'without an individual who has an eye for cytology, a good visual memory and attention for detail' the test cannot proceed; always assuming, of course, that it is possible to solve the problem of recognising a basophil which has already degranulated. Nevertheless, if the difficulties could be overcome a simple test of this type has obvious attractions to the clinician anxious to screen for drug sensitivity, for example, without subjecting the patient to the risks involved in in vivo testing.

It is possible that a more reliable method of measuring cell alteration could be developed, such as the release of a radioisotope marker from suitably labelled basophils or mast cells. Release of ^{51}Cr has been used, for instance, to provide a very sensitive index of the damage to antigenic target cells effected by lymphoid cells (Perlman and Holm 1970). But this, like cell-mediated lysis in tissue culture suspensions or the destruction of erythrocytes in hemolytic disease (other situations where the method has been applied), is a cytotoxic process; unlike the changes induced in reagin-sensitised mast cells and basophils on challenge with specific allergen.

A promising new method of studying cell bound reagin–allergen interaction, which is under active consideration in my own laboratory, involves the application of micro-calorimetry to the measurement of the small heat-changes induced (Stanworth et al. 1972). The results obtained so far are encouraging, and are beginning to provide new information about the mechanism of immediate hypersensitivity reactions. But the procedure is unlikely to prove suitable for the routine assay of reaginic antibody activity.

2.4.2 Indirect agglutination systems

The failure to demonstrate reagin–allergen interaction by conventional precipitin techniques has stimulated many attempts to develop a more sensitive agglutination assay system, based on the use of antigen (allergen)-coated particles. Understandably red cells have featured prominently as carriers, but attempts have been made to use many other types of particles; including leucocytes, platelets, collodion particles and even pollen grains themselves (as was discussed in a review article some years ago; Stanworth 1963).

2.4.2.1 Erythrocyte agglutination. In early studies allergen was linked directly to erythrocytes by means of bis diazotised benzidene or indirectly through incomplete antibody to which the diazotised allergen had been coupled (Coombs 1955; Britton and Coombs 1955). The latter approach avoids the risk of chemical alteration of the erythrocyte surface by coupling reagent, which can lead to the non-specific adsorption of γ-globulin from the test serum.

There was no evidence, however, that reaginic (γE) antibodies

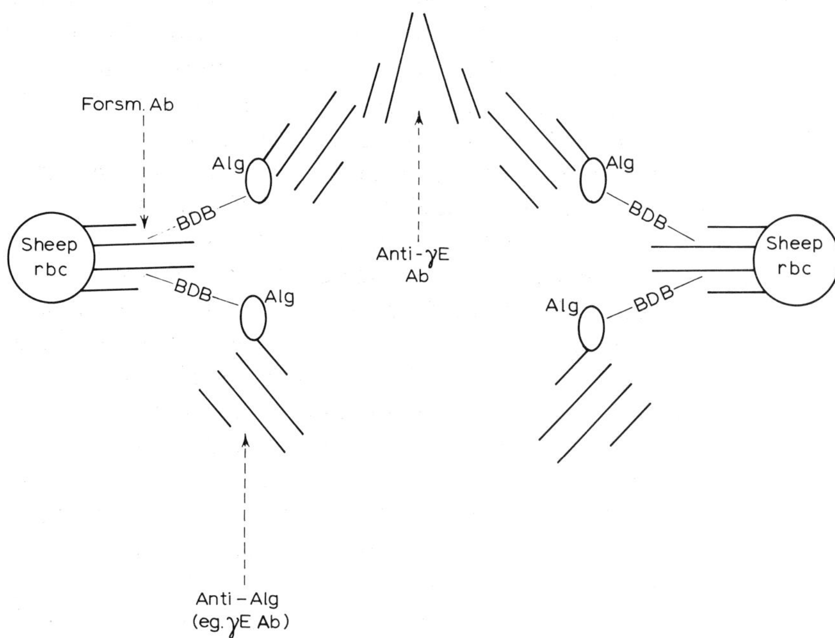

Fig. 2.28. Schematic illustration of the basic principle of the red cell linked antigen-antibody reaction (RCLAAR). Alg: allergen (antigen).

were being measured specifically in these systems. On the other hand, the high agglutination titres shown by the sera of hayfever patients after specific hyposensitisation (Britton and Coombs 1955) suggested that 'blocking' (γG) antibodies were being detected. This conclusion was also apparent from the measurement of hemagglutinating antibody levels in the sera of treated and untreated hypersensitive individuals by means of the tanned cell technique of Boyden (1951).

As might have been anticipated, antigen-linked red cells are agglutinated by any complete antibody with specificity for that antigen, irrespective of its immunoglobulin class. This has been demonstrated by the more recent studies of Coombs and his associates, by means of a modified red cell linked antigen system (Steele and Coombs 1964) in which specific anti-globulin antisera are used to identify the reactive antibodies. The basic principle of this 'red cell linked antigen–antiglobulin reaction (RCLAAR) system, as it is termed, is illustrated schematically in fig. 2.28 (see also master fig. 2.1). First rabbit anti-Forssman antibody is photo-oxidised to render it non-agglutinable yet still capable of reacting with rbc antigenic determinants. This photo-oxidised anti-erythrocyte antibody is linked to antigen (allergen) by means of bis diazotised benzidine, and the resulting conjugate used to sensitise sheep erythrocytes. Washed cells which have been sensitised in this manner are then mixed with the serum to be tested. Agglutination at this stage indicates the presence of agglutinating antibodies against the red cell linked antigen; for example, γG blocking antibodies resulting from hypo-sensitisation treatment would be demonstrable in this manner. If no agglutination occurs the cells are washed again, and aliquots are treated with specific rabbit antiserum directed against human immunoglobulins of the different major classes.

Coombs and his associates (1965) have used this method to demonstrate IgA antibodies, together with those of the IgG class, in infant sera which are reactive with casein, α-lactalbumin and β-lactoglobulin. IgA antibodies were demonstrated more frequently in sera from suspected allergic subjects and from suspected cot death cases. On the assumption that reagins were associated with γA-globulins, and despite the observation that the γA antibody titres were not affected by heating the infants' sera at 56° for 4 hr, it was concluded that reagin-mediated anaphylaxis was a possible cause of cot death. It should be mentioned, however, that in a later study (Hunter, Feinstein and Coombs 1968) it was shown that sera obtained at post-mortem after cot death failed to produce a PCA reaction in baboons, in contrast to two sera from a child clinically sensitive to milk and from another with Aldrich's syndrome.

As it has now been established that reaginic antibody activity is associated with a distinctive class of immunoglobulin (IgE), as will be considered in detail in ch. 4 and 5, it has become necessary to reappraise the red cell linked antigen–antiglobulin reaction as a means of detecting reagins. This has been done by Coombs and his associates (1968), who have employed an anti-IgE (myeloma) antiserum as well an antisera directed specifically against the other four major immunoglobulin classes. Tests were performed on sera from patients with allergic asthma to castor bean, using red cells to which the allergen had been coupled through a photo-oxidised anti-Forssman antibody in the usual way. A comparison of the IgE antibody level of the sera thus examined with the patient's clinical histories, and with the PCA activity in baboons (of some of the sera), suggested that reagins were probably being measured. Moreover, it proved impossible to demonstrate by this method γE antibody in the sera of individuals who showed no signs of clinical sensitivity to castor allergen although possessing high serum total IgE levels (Bennich and Johansson 1971). It was also significant that heating two of the castor bean sensitive individuals' sera at 56° (one for only 30 min, and the other for 4 hr) destroyed the detectable combining activity of the γE antibody without affecting the γG antibody titre.

Despite its apparent complexity, the red cell linked antigen–antiglobulin assay would seem to be the most promising agglutination yet devised for the measurement of reaginic antibodies. It will be important, therefore, to assess critically its ability to measure γE antibodies in the sera of patients showing the more common type of inhalant sensitivities, which have been assayed independently by in vivo P–K testing and by the in vitro passive sensitisation procedures already described. In this connection, it should be recognised that (like the R.A.S.T. procedure, to be considered in the next section) the technique is measuring antigen (i.e. allergen) binding rather than tissue-sensitising activity. Unfortunately, pollen allergens are apparently not easily coupled to rabbit anti-Forsmann antibody; and other allergens (e.g. from *Ascaris* preparations) seem to be damaged during the coupling process (Bennich and Johansson 1971).

As far as can be established from the data published so far, the sensitivity of the R.C.L.A.A.R. is comparable to that of PCA testing in baboons. It is difficult not to suspect, however, that the technical expertise of a Coombs is required for its successful execution!

2.4.2.2 Leucocyte agglutination. The demonstration that washed cells recovered from the buffy coats of normal donors' blood, following sedimentation, can be passively sensitised for allergen-induced histamine release by incubation with serum from a hypersensitive individual (§ 2.3.3) suggested that reaginic (γE) antibodies have the capacity to bind at least to some types of human leucocyte. This raised the possibility that a leucocyte agglutination procedure might be evolved as a method of assaying reagin activity.

Fitzpatrick and his associates (1967) have attempted this in the development of their so-called double layer leucocyte agglutination (DLLA) test, which involves reacting passively sensitised cells with specific allergen (e.g. grass pollen) followed by incubation with rabbit anti-allergen antiserum. According to Augustin (1967) the test is 'tedious and difficult to perform' (involving 18 washings and a number of incubations with sera etc., and the taking of at least 3 counts in each test) and, moreover, it is not specific for reagin-type antibodies. It is probable, therefore, that any blocking antibodies present in the test sera, which have the capacity to agglutinate allergen-coated red cells (as mentioned in the previous sub-section), would interfere with the agglutination of allergen-coated sensitised leucocytes by the rabbit anti-allergen antiserum. Another complicating factor is non-specific adsorption of allergen by the normal donors' leucocytes. Studies carried out by Pruzansky and Patterson (1966), using ^{125}I-labelled ragweed allergen, indicate that this can be relatively large and comparable to the amount of allergen taken up by leucocytes from ragweed-sensitive individuals.

Nevertheless, it is interesting to note that whereas the lymphocytes in the system employed by Fitzpatrick et al. (1967) failed to take up reagins, the agglutinates seemed to be composed primarily of neutrophils. Obviously it would be an advantage if a test system could be devised involving reagin–allergen reaction with this type of cell, which is very much more abundant in human blood than is the histamine-containing basophil.

2.4.3 Other possible indirect methods of assaying reaginic antibodies

2.4.3.1 Phage inactivation. An interesting and original approach, which has been applied by Haimovich et al. (1967) to the measurement of anti-penicilloyl antibodies, is based on the very sensitive phage neutralisation technique used by Mäkelä (1966) and Haimovich and Sela (1966) for the measurement of extremely low concentrations of antibodies to well defined determinants. The haptens are coupled chemically to bacteriophage and the highest antiserum dilution giving at least 50 per cent inactivation of the phage, on incubation at 37°, is determined. When incubation periods of 5 hr were adopted, penicilloylated T4 phage was neutralised by dilutions of rabbit anti-penicilloyl antiserum as low as 10^6–10^7-fold (corresponding to antibody concentrations of 1.0–0.1 mg/ml); no effect being observed with unmodified phage.

Haimovich et al. (1967) have measured the anti-penicilloyl antibodies in the sera of a group of allergic and non-allergic individuals in this manner, before and after heat treatment (of the diluted sera) at 56° for 5 hr. The capacity of the sera to evoke PCA reactions in baboons was also determined, but only two proved to be reactive in this system. Solely, therefore, on the basis of the observation that some of the allergic sera examined lost their phage inactivating capacity as a result of the somewhat prolonged heat treatment adopted, it was concluded that the procedure was capable of detecting reaginic antibodies. Moreover, the failure to evoke PCA reactions with most of the sera, in contrast to phage-inactivation titres which ranged from 10^{-4}–10^{-1}, was taken to indicate that the phage neutralisation technique possessed a significantly greater sensitivity in reagin assay.

In view of the growing evidence which suggests that antibodies other than those of the γE-type might be involved in immediate sensitivities to drugs, it would seem a little premature to conclude from this limited data that reagins were being detected by inactivation of the penicilloylated phage. It will be interesting to see, therefore, whether reaginic antibodies can be detected by this method in the sera of patients showing well defined inhalant sensitivities using, for example, pollen allergen coupled to bacteriophage T4. As, however, in the case of the early hemagglutination systems employed in attempts to detect reagins (mentioned in the previous section), it should be recognised that the phage-inactivation technique will probably detect blocking antibodies and other non-reaginic antibodies of immunoglobulin classes other than E. For this reason, its application in its present form might prove to be restricted to the measurement of anti-hapten antibodies.

2.4.3.2 Passive platelet sensitisation. The release of serotonin labelled with ^{14}C has been used by Caspary and Comaish (1967) to detect antibodies in the sera of patients showing hypersensitivity to equine anti-tetanus serum or to penicillin. A particular advantage of the method is the avoidance of washing the platelets after labelling, which is possible because of the very great avidity of platelets for 5-hydroxytryptamine. The same criticism can be made of this work, however, as was levelled at the previously described phage-inactivation studies; namely, that allergic sera have been used which probably contain appreciable amounts of antibodies other than γE reagins. This difficulty is also raised by the observation that antibody can be passively transferred from the human allergic sera examined to normal rabbit platelets and, conversely, from rabbit antisera to normal human platelets. This effect would appear to resemble the in vitro damage of rabbit platelets (as revealed by histamine release) by an unrelated antigen–antibody (γG) reaction, which according to observations by Gocke and Osler (1965) begins in the fluid phase and not on the platelet surface. Both systems appear to require the presence of fresh plasma, suggesting the involvement of some additional factor in the elicitation of the platelet lysis resulting from antigen–antibody combination.

In contrast, studies by Barbaro and Zvaifler (1966) have shown that antigen-induced histamine release from washed platelets of rabbits producing homologous PCA antibody (similar to that described in ch. 6) occurs in the absence of plasma. As histamine is released under similar conditions, from human leucocytes sensitised with reagin, it is suggested that the rabbit PCA antibody sensitised rabbit platelets in a similar manner to the mode of sensitisation of human leucocytes by human reagins. The participation of plasma components adsorbed on the rabbit platelets has yet to be ruled out, however. Furthermore, it will be necessary to demonstrate that rabbit PCA mediating antibody is capable of in vitro sensitisation of normal platelets. Preliminary studies (Siraganian and Oliveira 1968), comparing the mechanism of in vitro histamine release from platelets and leucocytes of immunised rabbits, suggest that it is not. Washed platelets suspension (isolated from blood drawn at intervals during a 7 week period following a single injection of either egg albumin or human serum albumin) consistently failed to release histamine on addition of specific antigen, irrespective of the presence or absence of fresh plasma. In contrast, more than half of the immunised rabbits' blood samples yielded leucocytes which released significant amounts of histamine on the addition of antigen. The latter observation is consistent with the observations of Greaves and Mongar (1968), who demonstrated that substantial amounts of histamine were released from basophil-rich, platelet-free, suspensions of leucocytes from rabbits actively sensitised to ovalbumin on in vitro challenge with the specific antigen.

Human platelets contain appreciably lower contents of histamine than do rabbit platelets, but this need not be a disadvantage in their use as a vehicle for reagin–allergen interaction; because, as the work of Caspary and Comaish (1967) and others has shown, measurement of serotonin offers an alternative sensitive indication of lysis. As in the rabbit, however, there is no convincing evidence that isologous reagin-type antibodies are capable of sensitising human platelets; nor can it be concluded from published data that reagin–allergen complexes will initiate platelet agglutination under the appropriate conditions. The claims of Storck, Hoigné and Koller (1955) that a suspension of human platelets in non-allergic serum, containing a dialysate of allergic serum, was agglutinated on addition of allergen could not be substantiated by other investigators (Kleine, Mathes and Muller 1957; Taylor, Hayward and Augustin 1958). An explanation of the effect can possibly be found in the observations of Miescher and Cooper (1960) and

Siqueria and Nelson (1961), which have indicated that the aggregation of platelets (rabbit and guinea pig) by antigen–antibody (γG) complexes is probably attributable to combination of such complexes with one of the components of complement, the resulting complex then binding to the platelet surface. As there is no evidence, however, that γE reaginic antibodies bind complement, following their combination with specific allergen, platelet agglutination would not seem to be the most promising method to employ in their detection; particularly as both human and monkey platelets have been shown to lack in vitro reactivity with a variety of conventional antigen–antibody systems in the presence of either guinea pig, human or monkey complement. There is no denying, however, the value of in vitro platelet systems in the study of sensitivities to certain drugs (e.g. sedormid, quinidine) resulting in thrombocytopenic purpura (Ackroyd 1954; Bolton 1956); where platelet–drug complex is agglutinated by antibody in the patient's serum in the absence of complement, but is lysed when complement is present.

2.5 Radio-immunoassay of IgE

2.5.1 Early studies

Radio-immunoassay techniques have, of course, been used for some considerable time now in the estimation of trace amounts of hormones and hormone-binding antibodies in human sera. It is perhaps a little surprising, therefore, that they did not find a more rapid application to the estimation of reaginic antibodies in the sera of hypersensitive individuals.

I tried unsuccessfully some ten years ago (referred to in Stanworth 1963) to demonstrate directly the selective binding of ^{131}I-labelled inhalant allergen by the reaginic antibodies in the serum of a horse dandruff-sensitive individual (P.R.), using both 'overtaking electrophoresis' on cellulose acetate paper and density gradient ultracentrifugation. In retrospect, however, it is probable that these negative findings can be attributed to the use of a relatively weak allergic serum (and also a crude allergen preparation), because later investigators have succeeded in demonstrating labelled allergen–reagin combinations by means of indirect precipitation techniques.

Lidd and Farr (1962) were the first to adopt this approach, using the ammonium sulphate technique of Farr (1958) to measure the ragweed-binding antibody in the sera of rabbits immunised with ragweed pollen extract and in the sera of ragweed sensitive humans. This depends upon the insolubility of labelled allergen–antibody γG-globulin complexes in 40 per cent saturated ammonium sulphate, in contrast to the solubility of free allergen in solutions of this salt concentration. As, however, in the application of the 'red cell linked antigen' agglutination tests (§ 2.4.2), it is essential to distinguish specific reagin–allergen combination from the binding of allergen by other types of antibody present in allergic sera. Hence, although Lidd and Farr (1962) demonstrated that labelled allergen was bound specifically by antibody, rather than as a result of non-specific co-precipitation, it was quite likely that non-reaginic antibodies were contributing to the binding shown by their ragweed-sensitive individuals' sera. Moreover, some binding was even shown by non-allergic individuals' sera. Nevertheless, using a similar ammonium sulphate precipitation technique, Pruzansky, Patterson and Feinberg (1962) demonstrated a significant binding of ^{131}I-labelled purified ragweed antigen (King fraction) by untreated sensitive individuals' sera but not by the sera of untreated non-allergic individuals. This was confirmed by a later study by Lidd and Connell (1964), who found that the majority of sera from a group of untreated symptomatic ragweed-sensitive patients specifically bound ^{131}I-labelled purified ragweed pollen fraction, in contrast to the behaviour of the sera of non-allergic individuals. There was, however, a poor correlation between the specific binding capacities of these sera and their P–K dilution titres; contrary to expectation, if the radio-immunoassay procedure employed was measuring only reaginic antibodies.

A troublesome disadvantage of the Farr technique is the risk of bringing down labelled antigen non-specifically, on precipitation with ammonium sulphate. Pruzansky and Patterson (1964) have overcome this drawback by the use of a specific anti-human γ-globulin antiserum to precipitate labelled allergen–antibody complex. In this method, based on techniques first used by Feinberg (1954) and Skom and Talmage (1958) to detect non-precipitating antibodies, varying amounts of ^{131}I-labelled allergen of high specific activity is added to aliquots (0.5 ml) of diluted (1/10) human allergic serum. Addition in the reverse order, i.e. antigen to serum, is to be avoided as this results in adsorption of antigen to the test tubes. After incubation of the mixture at 37° for 2 hr, sufficient rabbit anti-human γ-globulin is added to precipitate all the human γ-globulin present. After further incubation at 37° for 1 hr the precipitate is separated by centrifugation, and the supernatant is counted in a NaI crystal well-type scintillation counter. The percentage of total counts, after correction for entrained supernatant, is also determined. It was found that the amount of radioactivity removed by washing the precipitate was almost constant, averaging 10 per cent of the counts in the original supernatant.

Sera from untreated ragweed-sensitive individuals assayed by this technique were shown to bind labelled purified allergen. Moreover, it was shown that the amount of labelled ragweed allergen bound by such sera increased following injection of the donors with ragweed extract in emulsion or saline; and that non-sensitive individuals injected with ragweed extract in emulsion produced similar quantities of antibodies against ragweed antigen irrespective of whether they subsequently developed immediate or delayed cutaneous sensitivity. These observations suggested that the radio-immunoassay procedure adopted did not provide a specific measure of reaginic antibodies, as was also indicated by the lack of correlation between labelled allergen binding and P–K activity of the allergic sera tested. Indeed, this could hardly be expected, in the light of more recent observations on the γE nature of reagins, as the precipitating antiserum employed was raised (in rabbits) against a commercial (Pentex) Cohn fraction II of human serum (which would mainly comprise γG-globulins).

In the circumstances, an obvious development of the specific precipitation technique was the use of antisera directed specifically against one or other of the various human immunoglobulin classes. Yagi et al. (1963) used radio-immunoelectrophoresis to demonstrate that ragweed antigen-binding antibodies were associated with all the (then known) major immunoglobulin classes (i.e. IgG, IgM and IgA). Similar observations were made by Reisman, Arbesman and Yagi (1965), who attempted a semi-quantitative assessment of the extent of labelled allergen binding based on the intensity of the precipitin arcs revealed by auto-radiography of the stained and dried agar immunoelectrophoresis slides (having previously added antibody against specific immunoglobulin, and ^{131}I-labelled short ragweed pollen allergen, to the longitudinal trough following electrophoresis of the allergic serum). Ishizaka, Ishizaka and Hornbrook (1967) employed an essentially similar radio-immunodiffusion procedure, where it was possible to titrate the amount of allergen-binding antibody by reacting serial dilutions of the allergic serum (in the peripheral wells of an Ouchterlony plate) with a mixture of antiserum specific for one of the human immunoglobulin classes and labelled allergen (1 mg/ml of ^{131}I-labelled ragweed allergen E) in the centre well. Rabbit antiserum raised against the same antigen preparation was used as standard, being titrated in the same way. Thus, it was shown that the γE antibody titre of a group of sera from ragweed-sensitive individuals, but not their γG, γA nor γM titres, correlated with their P–K titres.

The authors state, however, that the general diffuse appearance of the γE precipitin lines revealed in this manner, and their close proximity to the peripheral wells of the Ouchterlony plates, makes reading of the titration end-point difficult. Hence, it was necessary to compare the darkness of the γE lines on radio-autographs with that formed with a certain amount (0.0062 μgN/ml) of rabbit anti-ragweed antigen E antibody. This problem can be avoided by adoption of the other, quantitative, radio-immunoassay procedure employed by Ishizaka and associates (1967). This is based on a technique used by Newcomb and Ishizaka (1967) in the measurement of human γG and γA antibodies to diphtheria toxoid, and is an extension of the specific precipitation technique used by earlier workers. An essential precaution to be observed in using the technique is that the concentration of radioactive antigen for incubation should be in great excess (e.g. 5–10 times) compared with the antigen-binding activity of the total antibodies in the sera. Otherwise, antibodies which are associated with two or more immunoglobulin classes may form a single antigen–antibody complex, which may be precipitated with rabbit antibodies specific for either of these immunoglobulins. Another difficulty was the very low concentrations of γE antibodies in the sera tested with the result that only very small amounts of precipitate were formed. Consequently, in order to minimise loss from these precipitates on washing, they were formed in 0.5 per cent agarose. Aliquots (0.1 ml) of undiluted serum were incubated with an equal volume of appropriate dilutions of radio-active allergens at 3° for 24 hr. Equal volumes of anti-γE serum and 2 per cent agarose were mixed at 45°, and 0.2 ml of the mixture was added to each tube. A control series of mixtures contained normal rabbit serum in place of the anti-γE serum. After incubation at 37° for 1 hr and 3° for 48 hr, the agarose gel was removed from the bottom of the tubes and washed in 10 ml saline for 7 days at 3° with two changes per day. The gel was transferred to new tubes for radioactivity measurement, the amount of allergen specifically combined being calculated by subtracting the count of the control gel formed in the presence of the same concentration of radioactive allergen. (The presence of the gel was found to reduce the count by 5 per cent.)

Using this technique to test human allergic sera, it was found that the allergen-binding capacity of one immunoglobulin class was not significantly affected by the presence of antibodies of another class, and that the sum of allergen-binding activity of γG, γA and γE antibodies was in agreement with the total antibody level as determined by precipitation with specific anti-light chain antibodies. Furthermore, the skin sensitising activities of the ragweed-sensitive individuals' sera examined were again shown to correlate with the antigen-binding activities of their γE antibodies, but not with those of γG or γA antibodies.

The data of Ishizaka and his associates (1967) also provided some idea of the range of γE antibody concentration in allergic individuals' sera and of the minimum skin sensitising dose, by comparing allergen-binding activity with that of a specific rabbit antiserum containing a known amount of anti-ragweed antigen (E) antibody (i.e. 0.03–0.06 μg Ab N/ml). Thus, assuming that the avidity of human γE antibody is comparable to that of the rabbit antibody (which is not necessarily so), the minimum dose of skin sensitising antibody needed for a positive P–K reaction was calculated to be of the order of 10^{-6}–10^{-5} μg N. This is about 1/1000 of the minimum dose of guinea pig γ_1 antibodies and rabbit γG antibodies needed for the induction of PCA reactions in guinea pigs (Ovary 1958). Similarly, it was calculated that the range of γE antibody in the allergic sera investigated was equivalent to rabbit anti-ragweed allergen concentrations of 0.019–0.065 μg Ab N/ml, which corresponds to a range of antibody protein of 0.119–0.406 μg/ml (assuming the antibody contains 16 per cent N). This falls within the range of total γE-globulin levels (namely 122–4033 mμg/ml) of a group of allergic sera determined by Johansson (1967), by means of a radio-immunosorbent assay procedure to be described shortly.

The studies of Ishizaka and associates (1967) demonstrated that the sensitivity of their radio-immunoassay compares favourably with that of some of the other types of technique developed for the measurement of reaginic antibodies. But, the technique is still appreciably less sensitive than passive skin testing in humans or, indeed, in monkeys; and from this evidence, it would not appear to be as sensitive as the passive leucocyte and tissue sensitisation procedures already described (§ 2.3). Obviously, however, radio-immunoassay techniques possess advantages as routine assays, foremost amongst which is the lack of dependence on fresh viable tissue or leucocytes.

2.5.2 Radio-immunosorbent procedures

One of the big disadvantages of the radio-immunoassay technique described above, is the difficulty of retrieving minute amounts of γE-anti γE precipitates, even when these are formed in 0.5 per cent agarose. Moreover, the use of a great excess of radio-labelled allergen could presumably lead to dissociation of such complexes. This type of problem has been avoided by other investigators by the use of radio-immunosorbent techniques, where the antibody is coupled chemically to a solid phase. Its subsequent reaction with labelled antigen is an irreversible process, and consequently the time required to achieve such combination is diminished. The separation of free from bound antigen is accomplished merely by washing the solid phase, which also enhances the speed of the antibody–antigen reaction. Moreover, as in the radioimmunoassay procedure employed by Berson and Yalow (1962) in the measurement of hormones such as insulin, the sensitivity of the technique is sharpened considerably by using it as an inhibition system based on the competition of unlabelled antigen in the test sample and of radio-labelled antigen for the solid phase-linked antibody. Hence, in such systems, the amount of labelled antigen bound to the antibody varies inversely with the concentration of antigen in the test sample; the latter antigen being measured by its effect on the binding of a small quantity of the labelled antigen to a fixed quantity of specific antibody.

Catt, Nial and Tregear (1966) have developed this type of procedure for the measurement of human growth hormone in plasma, using as solid phase a synthetic copolymer of styrene and polytetra-fluoroethylene (Fluon G4), to which specific rabbit antihormone antibody was coupled by shaking with the isothiocyanate graft polymer in the presence of normal rabbit serum and bicarbonate buffer. Residual serum remaining after incubation of the test sample with the solid phase–antibody conjugate can be removed by washing prior to incubation with labelled antigen. This avoids dilution of the tracer antigen with excess of unlabelled antigen, resulting in a considerable increase in the number of radioactive antigen molecules which combine with unoccupied binding sites on the solid phase-antibody. It was demonstrated that this led to greater accuracy in the estimation of very small quantities of unlabelled antigen, because the effective specific activity of the tracer is much higher than when added to the system in the presence of unlabelled antigen to be measured.

Other advantages attributed by Catt and his associates (1966) to this system were its simplicity of operation and its superior sensitivity. The method merely involves the incubation (48 hr) of standard and unknown solutions with small quantities of the solid phase–antibody conjugate, followed by a series of washing steps before and after subsequent incubation (24 hr) with the labelled antigen. This entire procedure can be performed in a vial suitable for counting in a well-type γ-radiation counter; whilst a further simplification involves the use of antibody-coated solid phase in the form of thin wafers (discs) of uniform size and surface area, one of which can be dropped into the assay vial. The sensitivity of the method in the estimation of plasma growth hormone was found to be always 0.4 mμg/ml or less, frequently under 0.1 mμg/ml and even as low as 0.02 mμg/ml in the most sensitive assay recorded. But in trial experiments in my laboratory (McLaughlan 1971), using commercially available 'Protapol' discs (Catt, Niall and Tregear 1967), substantial amounts of radiolabelled antibody (sheep anti-human IgG) were found to be removed by subsequent washing; indicating that the discs did not bind antibody firmly enough to meet the requirements for a suitable solid phase support. *

Alternative, more successful, solid phase radio-immunoassay techniques are based on the use of the antibody carrier in particulate form. Of these, a method (Wide and Porath 1966) based on a technique devised originally for the assay of various protein hormones (and later γG-globulin) has proved particularly useful in the immediate hypersensitivity field. This involved first coupling the appropriate antibody covalently to ultrafine sephadex particles, in the form of the isothiocyanate-phenoxy hydroxy phenyl derivative. The antigen-binding capacity of the resultant antibody-polymer particles was found to be unaltered after 8 months storage at 40° in the dried state, or in a suspension ready for use. Thus, 10 g of the conjugate was sufficient for 10 000 tests, of which (it is claimed) 50–100 could be undertaken by a trained technician in one day. Moreover, the incubation and final separa-

* The successful use of filter paper discs, to which the antibody is coupled following activation by cyanogen bromide, has been recently reported (Wide 1971).

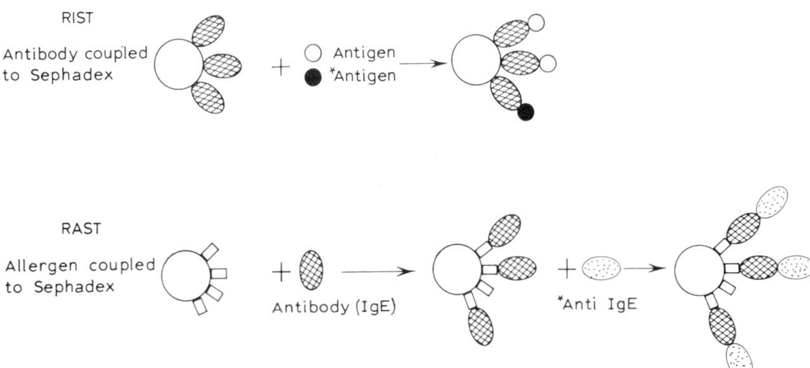

Fig. 2.29. Schematic illustration of the basic principles of the R.I.S.T. and R.A.S.T. methods of assaying total and antibody γE-globulin. * radio-labelled.

tion of free from antibody-bound antigen can be made in the same tube, thereby simplifying the manipulative procedures.

The discovery (Johansson and Bennich 1967) of a myeloma counterpart of the immunoglobulin class (i.e. γE) to which reaginic antibodies are now known to belong (ch. 4), has permitted the application of a modified form (fig. 2.29) of the radioimmunosorbent test of Wide and Porath to the direct estimation of the level of γE-globulin in allergic sera. This technique (now referred to as R.I.S.T.) involves the use of: (1) antibodies directed specifically against the Fc region of γE myeloma protein, covalently coupled to an insoluble dextran derivative activated by thiophosgene (and, more recently, cyanogen bromide), and (2) purified γE myeloma protein labelled with ^{125}I (to a specific activity of 100 μc/μg) by the chloramine T method (Hunter and Greenwood 1962). Furthermore, in order to make the assay specific, immunosorbent (0.05–0.10 mg) is suspended in buffer solution (1 ml) containing: normal pooled serum (diluted 1/250), IgG (11 μg/ml), Bence Jones protein (8 μg/ml) from the IgE myeloma patient himself and Fab fragment (0.1 μg/ml) derived from the whole myeloma IgE. The concentration of γ-globulin in the test sample is determined by comparing its capacity to inhibit the binding of ^{125}I-myeloma IgE with the inhibition produced by

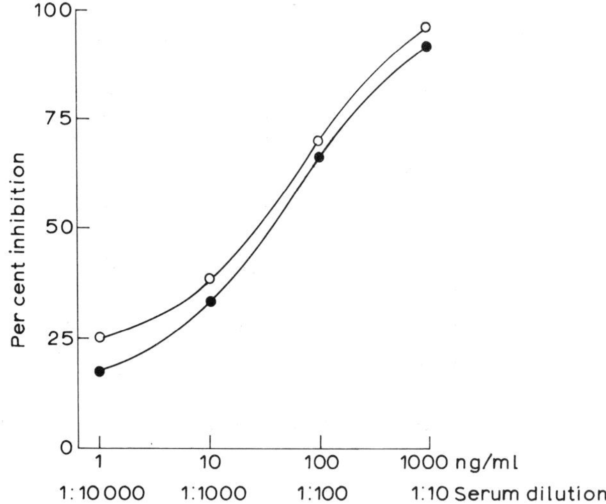

Fig. 2.30. Dose–response curves showing the inhibition of the binding of myeloma ^{125}I-IgE to immunosorbent by unlabelled myeloma IgE (•) and by normal serum (○). (Reproduced from Johansson et al. 1968, by permission of the authors.)

standard myeloma IgE solutions of known concentration. A typical inhibition dose–response curve, obtained in this manner, is reproduced in fig. 2.30; from which it will be seen that it is possible to measure γE-globulin levels as low as 0.005–0.10 μg/ml.

Here, at last, then is a method of measuring reaginic (γE) antibodies which does not require the use of suitable normal primate tissue or cells. It is important to recognise, however, that in this procedure the γE-globulin is being detected *as antigen* by the polymer-coupled anti-γE antibody (see master fig. 2.1). Nevertheless, by means of R.I.S.T. a significantly raised γE-globulin level has been observed in the serum of adult allergic asthmatics. For instance, as will be seen from table 2.6, 63 per cent of a group of 16 patients with allergic asthma (as diagnosed on the basis of skin and provocation tests, as well as on case history and physical examination), showed a significantly raised serum IgE level (Johansson 1967). The highest serum level observed was 4033 ng/ml, being about 2.5 times higher than the mean serum IgE level of 1589 ng/ml; and 8 out of the 16 patients in this group had abnormally high serum

TABLE 2.6
Serum IgE levels determined by R.I.S.T. (Johansson 1967).

No.	Mean	S.D.	< 700 ng per ml	> 700 ng per ml
Asthma, total (38)	828 (49–4033)	1146	27 (71%)	11 (29%)
A, Allergic (16)	1589 (122–4033)	1433	6 (37%)	10 (63%)
B, Non-allergic (22)	275 (49–1510)	293	21 (95%)	1 (5%)
Normal * (61)	330 (105–1394)	236	58 (95%)	3 (5%)

* Sera from healthy blood donors. Range in parentheses.

N.B. It has now become the custom to express total IgE levels in international units (IU). Originally one IU was approx. equivalent to 1 ng IgE, but one IU of the WHO ref. standard in current use is approx. equivalent to 2 ng IgE (see also page 124).

IgE levels, above 1000 ng/ml (Bennich and Johansson 1971). In contrast, only 5 per cent of 22 patients with 'non-allergic asthma' showed a similarly raised serum IgE level, as did 5 per cent of a group of healthy Swedish blood donors (table 2.6). The 61 normal individuals examined showed a mean serum IgE level of 330 ng/ml (range: 105–1394), which is somewhat higher than the mean serum IgE level (198 ng/ml; range: 100–420) of our 10 normal British leucocyte donors (referred to earlier in fig. 2.23). Moreover, a group of non-atopic patients (on ACTH therapy) were shown (McLaughlan 1970), by R.I.S.T., employing CNBr activated micro-crystalline cellulose (rather than sephadex) as anti-IgE antibody carrier, to possess a similar mean IgE level (i.e. 212 ng/ml), as will be discussed further later.

2.5.3 Serum IgE levels in various forms of immediate sensitivity

A comparison of the mean serum IgE levels of groups of adult atopic individuals showing clinical evidence of hypersensitivity to different-allergens is revealing[12] as will be seen from the data in table 2.7, obtained in a preliminary survey using R.I.S.T. The mean serum IgE level of 26 patients showing relatively clear-cut

TABLE 2.7

Serum IgE levels (R.I.S.T.) of groups of adults showing symptoms of hypersensitivity to various allergens (Stanworth and Johansson, unpublished data).

Predominant sensitising allergen	Number of adults in group	Mean serum IgE level (ng/ml)	Range (ng/ml)
Grass pollen	27	1503	118 – 4300
Aspergillus	5	2423	1150 – 4025
Animal danders	10	513	170 – 1300
Dust	5	577	170 – 1325
Mites	4	192	120 – 258
Food	4	155	60*– 270
Drugs	3	147	30 – 230
(Grass pollen †)	6	233	67 – 380

* 4 month baby † Sub-clinical symptoms

sensitivities to grass pollens, referred to us by 3 clinical allergist, was found to be 1503 ng/ml (range 118–4300). This is about 7 times higher than the normal adult levels mentioned above. Significantly high serum IgE levels were also observed, somewhat surprisingly, in a group of 5 allergic asthmatics with prominent symptoms of aspergillus sensitivity; a condition in which γG-type precipitating antibodies have been implicated.

In contrast, the mean serum IgE level of a group of 10 adults sensitive to various animal danders was only 513 ng/ml (range: 170–1300); and that of a small group (of 5) showing predominant sensitivity to house dust was of a similar order of magnitude, namely 577 ng/ml (range: 170–1325). Furthermore, it is interesting to note that the mean serum IgE level of 4 other patients in whom mite sensitivity had been diagnosed was only 192 ng/ml (i.e. not significantly different to the normal adult level). Similarly, no evidence of raised IgE levels has been found from R.I.S.T. measurement on the limited number of sera examined from individuals showing symptoms of immediate hypersensitivity to foods (e.g. flour, milk etc.) and drugs (antibiotics etc.). In the latter connection, however, it is worth mentioning that a significantly raised IgE level (i.e. 1080 ng/ml) was found in an autopsy specimen of serum from an individual who suffered a fatal anaphylactic reaction to benzyl penicillin; and this serum also proved capable of mediating PCA reactions in baboons, which were specifically inhibited by excess myeloma IgE (in a similar manner to the inhibition of sensitisation by sera from hayfever patients (ch. 5).

The smallness of the numbers in most of the groups examined so far in this preliminary study precludes, of course, serious statistical analysis of the findings. Nevertheless, they tend to support limited reports from other laboratories on, for instance, the low IgE levels in the sera of children showing symptoms of dust/mould sensitivity (Berg and Johansson 1969). Our findings (in table 2.7) could possibly be construed as substantiation of the suggestion (Bennich and Johansson 1971) that different types of allergen differ in their ability to stimulate IgE production, pollens being more effective than dusts.

Another significant point emerging from an examination of the data given in table 2.7, is that the mean serum IgE level of a group of University Staff (or their relations) claiming to be sensitive to grass pollens, but showing only weakly positive prick test reactions to extracts of allergens, was barely above the normal adult mean level.

TABLE 2.8

Serum IgE levels in children with atopic diseases [a] (Bennich and Johansson 1971).

Diagnosis	No. of children	No. of children with high levels [b]	Mean IgE concentration [c]
Bronchial asthma	13	10	563
Hay fever	22	8	297
Bronchial asthma and hay fever	28	15	350
Bronchial asthma and atopic eczema	8	7	744
Hay fever and atopic eczema	4	2	599
Negative allergologic investigation	7	1	111

a) Data from Berg and Johansson (1969).

b) IgE concentration higher than mean plus 2 S.D. for the age.

c) In per cent of the predicted arithmetic mean value for healthy children of the same age.

TABLE 2.9
Duplicate serum IgE levels (R.I.S.T.) in children with asthma or asthma + eczema (McLaughlan, Stanworth and Price, unpublished).

	IgE (ng/ml)			
	Asthma		Asthma + eczema	
	7400	7400	14300	13000
	680	700	1500	1480
	2040	2150	1280	1200
	1380	1220	350	350
	1040	1200	12500	11000
Mean	2522		5744	

The results of R.I.S.T. measurements (Bennich and Johansson 1971) on the sera of children with various forms of atopic disease are summarised in table 2.8. A radio-immunodiffusion technique has also been used to measure the IgE level in asthmatic childrens' sera, as a possible means of assessing the severity of their condition (§ 2.4.6). As will be seen, the children with perennial symptoms of asthma had a higher mean serum IgE level than the group of children whose symptoms occurred mainly during the pollination season. In children showing symptoms of atopic eczema (Prurigo Besnier) as well, the mean serum IgE levels was even higher. We have confirmed this in my own laboratory, by R.I.S.T. measurement on groups of 6 asthmatic children with and without eczema (table 2.9). The mean serum IgE level was 2522 ng/ml in the former group and 5746 ng/ml in the latter (McLaughlan, Stanworth and Price, unpublished). High serum IgE levels have also been reported in adult patients with pronounced atopic eczema (Juhlin et al. 1969), the mean IgE level of 2733 mg/ml (of a group of 28) being about 11 times the normal mean; whilst one patient who also suffered from severe asthma due to animal and pollen sensitivity was found to possess a serum IgE level as high as 31 000 ng/ml.

At the other end of the scale, IgE has been detected by R.I.S.T.

TABLE 2.10
Serum IgE levels in healthy adults, and children of various age groups (Bennich and and Johansson 1971).

	Geometric mean	Confidence limits (96% interval)	Range
Cord serum	36.3	12.9 – 102	16.0 – 97.5
Children			
1½–4½ months	60.6	43.5 – 84.5	50.0 – 86.0
3½–9 months	75.7	24.7 – 233	24.0 – 223
9 months–3 years	114	29.0 – 450	49.5 – 540
3–5 years	158	45.3 – 528	62.0 – 308
6–10 years	190	55.6 – 648	63.0 – 535
11–15 years	246	71.9 – 838	54.0 – 840
Adults	248	61.4 – 1000	66.0 – 1830

at very low levels (mean: 35 ng/ml) in the serum of new born infants, where it supposedly results from production by the foetus; since no correlation is seen (Johansson 1968) between the maternal serum IgE concentration and that of the new born, in keeping with the known failure of reaginic antibodies to get across the placenta of the allergic mother (ch. 4). The development of IgE in childhood seems to resemble most closely that of IgA (Berg and Johansson 1969); with a slow and even increase that does not reach maximal level until early adulthood (see table 2.10), followed by a slow but insignificant decline.

Turning again to the allergic state, urticaria – which along with hayfever and allergic asthma has been considered as a manifestation of immediate-type hypersensitivity – is another condition in which the serum IgE level has been found (unexpectedly) to be usually normal (Juhlin et al., 1969).

Two other disorders in which very high serum IgE levels have been observed are parasitic infections, in the absence of clinical manifestations of atopy, and non-atopic eosinophilia (table 2.11). The possible significance of these observations will be discussed further in later chapters. At this stage it should be mentioned that, in my own experience, not all cases of non-atopic eosinophilia show elevated serum IgE levels.

2.5.4 Serum IgE levels in other disorders

With the availability of a method of measuring the IgE concentration (as opposed to the reaginic antibody content) in serum and other body fluids, it has been interesting to ascertain whether there are any other conditions in which the levels are abnormally high. The findings from such studies are summarised in table 2.11. It was particularly interesting, for instance, to see whether the serum IgE level was raised in such conditions as ulcerative colitis; where a hypersensitivity factor has sometimes been invoked without any firm information about the nature of the offending 'allergen'. The grossly elevated serum IgE level (i.e. 13 800 ng/ml) of the first case examined in my own laboratory seemed highly suggestive, but this was subsequently attributed to a concommitant skin disorder as only 3 out of 49 patients with ulcerative colitis examined in

TABLE 2.11
Other conditions in which serum IgE levels have been measured (based mainly on Bennich and Johansson 1971).

Raised levels	Normal levels	Low levels
Parasitic infections e.g. with *Ascaris lumbricoides* *Toxacara canis* *Capillaria philippiensis* hook worm bilharziasis Wiskott-Aldrich syndrome Mononucleosis * Non-atopic eosinophilia	Autoimmune disease e.g. rheumatoid arthritis, S.L.E., ulcerative colitis Gastro-intestinal disturbances e.g. coeliac disease Myelomatosis (other than IgE) † Macroglobulinaemia † Acute pneumonia Malaria Syphilis 'Normal' IgA deficiency	Hypogammaglobulinaemia Ataxia telangiectasia

* In first serum sample taken (at 10d), but significant decrease in IgE level of later serum samples (taken over 50d period).

† IgE levels vary with levels of other immunoglobulins.

Sweden have proved to have raised serum IgE levels (Bennich and Johansson 1971). Similarly there is little convincing evidence of raised serum IgE levels in patients with other kinds of gastrointestinal disorder, including gluten- and milk-sensitive patients with acute coeliac disease (Stanworth and Asquith, unpublished).

As might have been expected, low IgE levels have been observed in the sera of patients with hypogammaglobulinaemia; but the extent of reduction of serum IgE is nowhere near as marked as that shown by immunoglobulins of the other classes. We have recently undertaken a survey of the serum IgE levels (determined by a modified R.I.S.T. procedure) of a relatively large group (i.e. 46) of hypogammaglobulinaemic patients, in an attempt to obtain evidence that the reaction to administered human γG-globulin shown by the occasional patient was of the immediate type; possibly directed against the substantial amount of aggregated material usually found in therapeutic γG-globulin preparations. But the serum IgE levels of 2 such patients (of 69 and 10 ng/ml) were well within the range of the group investigated (i.e. 4–38 ng/ml; mean: 61 ng/ml [13]). Moreover, it did not prove possible to evoke a PCA reaction in a baboon which had been injected with serum from a γ-globulin reactor, on challenge with a specimen of the therapeutic γ-globulin in unheated or heated (63°, 20 min) form.

Other deficiency states in which the measurement of serum IgE level is of some interest include ataxia telangiectasia (Ammann et al. 1969), where there is sometimes a lack of detectable amounts of serum IgA, and the IgA-deficient states seen occasionally in normal individuals. The finding of normal IgE levels in the latter individuals is of interest in relation to the paradoxical situation that arose at the time when reaginic antibodies were thought by some investigators to be associated with γA-globulins (ch. 4), despite the observation that some γA-deficient individuals were atopic.

2.5.5 Measurement of antibody IgE

Returning to the question of the estimation of reaginic antibodies by radio-immunosorbent techniques, it is of course essen-

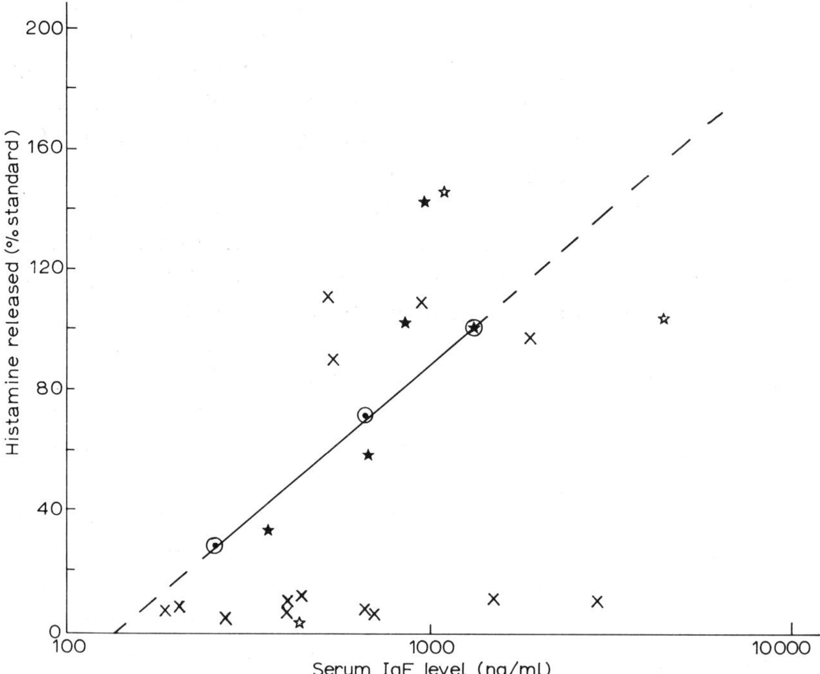

Fig. 2.31. Comparison of the capacity of various allergic sera to sensitise passively chopped human lung for allergen-induced histamine release (expressed as a percentage of the release mediated by a standard allergic serum) with their total IgE levels determined by R.I.S.T. (Stanworth, Johansson and Sheard, unpublished data). Key to symbols: the stars and crosses refer to chopped lung assays performed in 2 different laboratories; whilst the circles refer to different dilutions of the standard allergic serum.

tial to recognise that in this type of assay total IgE is being measured as antigen (fig. 2.1); and not as specific antibody IgE, as in the other in vitro assays discussed earlier. This is apparent from fig. 2.31, where the capacity of various groups of allergic sera to sensitise chopped human lung for allergen-induced histamine release (by the technique described in § 2.3.2.1) is compared with their total IgE levels determined by R.I.S.T. Although there is evidence of a relationship between the two parameters, the correlation is far from complete; presumably because the divergent cases possess a broad-range hypersensitivity to allergens other than the cocksfoot pollen protein used to initiate histamine release in the chopped lung assay. It might be anticipated, therefore, that the R.I.S.T. procedure would provide a summation of the serum concentrations of the whole spectrum of γE antibodies, directed against the entire range of allergens to which the patient in question is hypersensitive. But it should be added that the results of the preliminary absorption experiments mentioned earlier (§ 3.2.2) raise the possibility of the existence in allergic individuals' serum of 'non-antibody' γE-globulin, which is antigenically intact but incapable of sensitising isologous human tissue. Furthermore, studies of the response of other classes of antibody, namely rabbit IgG-directed against allotypic immunoglobulin, (Catty, personal communication), suggest that there are other situations where 'non-antibody' immunoglobulin might result from antigenic stimulation.

There is obviously a need, therefore, for radio-immunoassay procedures capable of estimating γE antibody specifically. The radio-allergosorbent test (R.A.S.T.), outlined in fig. 2.29, has been developed (by Wide et al. 1967), with this objective in mind. This involves reacting the allergic serum with Sephadex particles to which a particular allergen has been coupled following cyanogen bromide activation (as was used for coupling the anti-IgE in the R.I.S.T.). After incubation for 2–24 hr at room temperature, with slow vertical rotation of the test tube, the particles are repeatedly washed (by centrifuging) with saline containing 1 per cent Tween before the addition of specific radio-labelled (^{125}I) anti-IgE antibody (isolated by the use of bromoacetyl cellulose immunosorbent). The activity remaining bound after incubation, centrifugation and washing of the particles is found to be approximately proportional to the amount of reaginic (γE) antibody in the allergic serum; and the sensitivity of the technique is apparently of the same order as that of the P–K test. Furthermore, the dose response curves constructed from the results of tests on various dilutions of serum from different allergic individuals have been found to be roughly parallel (fig. 2.32).

In a preliminary application of R.A.S.T. to the estimation of reaginic (γE) antibodies in a group of adults with asthma and

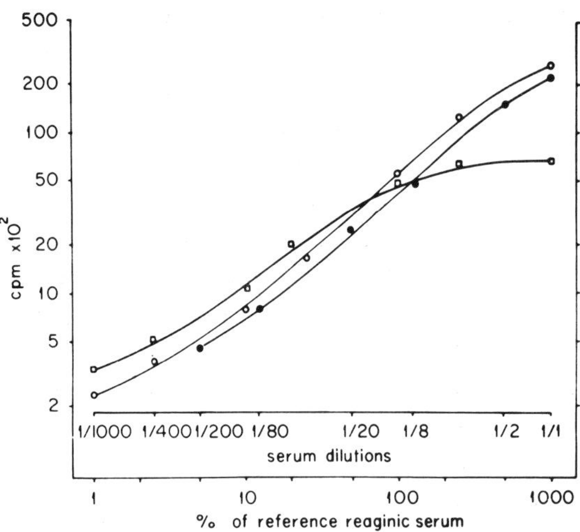

Fig. 2.32. Quantitation by R.A.S.T. of IgE antibodies in serum of a horse dandruff-sensitive patient (●) and of a dog dandruff-sensitive patient (□), who had been regularly hyposensitised, using serum from an untreated birch pollen-sensitive patient (○) as reference. (Reproduced from Bennich and Johansson 1971; by permission of the authors).

hayfever relatively poor agreement was observed with the results of direct skin tests (Wide et al. 1967), but a comparison with reactivity on provocation testing revealed a better correlation. Better correlations have been observed, too, on measurement of reaginic antibodies to pollens, house dust and danders, in more recent studies on larger groups of individuals (Berg et al. 1971); and the R.A.S.T. procedure has also been applied to the detection of γE antibodies directed against penicillin (Wide and Juhlin 1971), mite allergens in dust (Stenius and Wide 1969) and several parasite allergens (Bennich and Johansson 1971).

But it will be essential to resolve several difficult technical problems before the R.A.S.T. becomes established as an accurate and reliable method of measuring specific γE antibody. One area where complications arise concerns interference by antibodies of other immunoglobulin classes within the test serum, and the non-specific adsorption of γG-globulin molecules on to the allergen-coated particles can also lead to difficulties. There is also the demanding task of producing highly purified allergen preparations for coupling to the carrier particles, if the cross-reactivities encountered in the use of commercial allergen preparations (which are notoriously crude) are to be avoided. An example of this type of complication was the observation (Bennich and Johansson 1971) that Sephadex particles coupled with a commercial cow dander allergen preparation were detecting, in the serum of healthy children and adults, γG antibodies directed against bovine serum γ-globulin (occurring as a contaminant in the dander) as well as antibodies cross-reacting with the labelled sheep (anti-γE) γG-globulin antibodies used in the R.A.S.T. system. A similar situation might be anticipated with the use of crude horse dander allergen; which has been shown (Stanworth 1957) to be contaminated with trace amounts of serum albumin and γ-globulin extracted from the dried epidermal scales comprising the dandruff.

In preliminary studies in my laboratory which have yielded promising results (McLaughlan 1970) it was found that the R.I.S.T. method, which (as described earlier) provides a measure of total IgE level, can be adapted to the assay of specific antibody IgE by performing a preliminary absorption step with allergen (cocksfoot or Timothy pollen) coupled to immunosorbent. This avoids, therefore, the need for measuring the uptake of γE antibody on the particles by direct interaction with radio-labelled anti-IgE (fig. 2.29); and, presumably averts some of the complications of the conventional R.A.S.T. system outlined previously. It remains to be seen, however, whether there will be other disadvantages to this simpler approach, which is now being investigated more extensively.

2.5.6 Assay of IgE by immunodiffusion

Another type of radio-immunoassay of IgE which is beginning to find application in clinical laboratories, is based on the single radial diffusion method of Mancini et al. (1965) used widely for the quantitative estimation of the major immunoglobulin classes. This method (Rowe 1969), known as the 'radioactive single radial diffusion (R.S.R.D.)' procedure, involves the visualisation of the normally invisible precipitin zones formed by diffusing allergic sera through agar gel into which is incorporated anti-IgE; by application of a second antiserum containing a radio-labelled antibody directed against the antibody immunoglobulin in the γE-anti γE precipitate. The technique is about 40 times less sensitive than the R.I.S.T. procedure, and its reproducibility is not as good. Its greatest disadvantage, however, is the relatively long time (e.g. 5–10 days) taken to obtain a result (compared with 24 hr for the other methods), because of the daily manipulations (e.g. washing steps etc.) involved and the need for autoradiography to obtain visualisation of the precipitin rings. The process can be shortened by the incorporation of radio-labelled anti-IgE directly into the agar (Arbesman et al. 1972); but at the expense of having to handle larger amounts of radioactive material.[14]

Despite its disadvantages, the single radial diffusion method is beginning to find application in routine screening for raised IgE in clinical laboratories because, unlike the radio-immunosorbent techniques discussed previously, it does not depend upon a supply of pure monomeric IgE for isotope-labelling. For instance, it has been used recently in an attempt to assess the severity of asthma in children by comparison of their serum IgE level with their clinical grading in terms of frequency of episodes, persistence of history and clinical and physiological manifestations of the condition (Hogarth-Scott et al. 1971). The mean serum IgE level of each of the 4 grades examined was found to correspond with the severity of asthma in that grade, there being a significantly increased mean serum IgE level in children in the most severely affected grades. As in the case of measurement of total serum IgE level by the other methods already discussed, however, a few individuals with pronounced asthma were found to possess anomalously low serum IgE levels and conversely the occasional individual with no (or minimal) clinical evidence of asthma proved to have disproportionately high levels of IgE. But, as Hogarth-Scott and his associates point out, the apparently normal individuals (selected solely on the criterion of the presence or absence of asthma) might have had other allergic conditions such as nematodiosis;

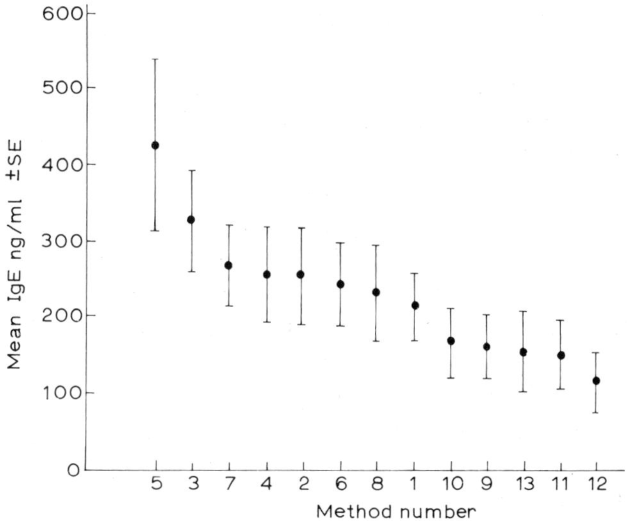

Fig. 2.33. Mean IgE level (± standard error) of the same 19 human sera determined by 13 radio-immunoassay procedures, employing as immunosorbents: (1) Sigmacell (25 μg); (2) cellulose carbonate (20 μg); (3) Sephadex (Seph.) G25 ultrafine (10 μg); (4) Seph. G25 ultrafine (5 μg); (5) Seph. G25 superfine (100 μg); (6) Seph. G25 ultrafine (10 μg); (7) bentonite (1 : 600 buffer-diluted anti-IgE); (8) bentonite (1 : 1600 calf serum-diluted anti-IgE); (9) RSRD method; (10–13) antibody (1 : 1600 diluted anti-IgE)-coated tubes, using as diluent buffered saline containing: (10) BSA (1%) (11) Tween (0.05%); (12) BSA (1%) and calf serum; (13) Tween (0.05%) and calf serum. Anti-IgE employed: anti-American (PS) myeloma IgE in every procedure except Nos. 4 and 6, where anti-Swedish (ND) myeloma IgE Fc fragment was used. (Reproduced from McLaughlan 1970.)

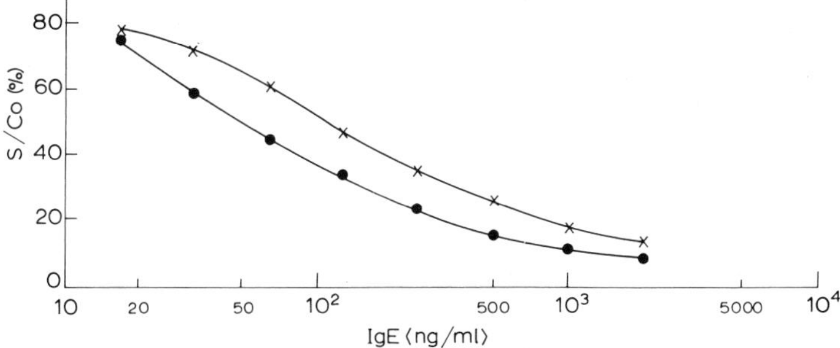

Fig. 2.34. R.I.S.T. assay of IgE in the allergic serum referred to in fig. 2.33: Standard curves obtained using cellulose carbonate (X) and CNBr-activated Sephadex (•) as immunosorbent (S/Co = ratio of activity of standard serum test over that of the control, lacking inhibitor.) (Reproduced from McLaughlan et al. 1971.)

and, besides, the cell-bound γE antibodies (rather than the circulating IgE) might well reflect a truer picture of the clinical condition of the patient.

2.5.7 Relative performance of various radio-immunoassay methods of estimating IgE

Finally, it might be worth making a few comments on the relative performances of the principal radio-immunoassay methods of measuring IgE, discussed in this section. A recent investigation conducted by my colleague P. McLaughlan (1970) is invaluable in this respect, because it has involved a most thorough direct comparison (with statistical analysis of the findings) of many different procedures using the same group of normal and allergic sera throughout. These have included radio-immunosorbent assays employing different types of antibody carrier, the antibody-coated tube and protapol disc techniques of Catt and Tregear (1967) referred to earlier; and the radio-single radial diffusion method (R.S.R.D.) mentioned in the previous section. Of these, the use of 'Enzite' (a carboxymethyl cellulose derivative marketed by Miles-Seravac) and protapol discs (obtainable from I.C.I. Australia) as antibody carriers proved unsatisfactory. Moreover, the R.S.R.D. and antibody-coated tube methods were found to give lower serum IgE levels than those obtained with particulate solid phases (as will be seen from fig. 2.33). On the other hand, bentonite, cyanogen-bromide-activated micro-crystalline cellulose ('Sigmacell') and cellulose carbonate all proved to be adequate alternatives to the ultrafine Sephadex G25 used in the conventional R.I.S.T. The cellulose carbonate derivative (McLaughlan et al. 1971) is particularly useful (see fig. 2.34), because it can be coupled with antibody directly (by virtue of nucleophilic attack of any free amino groups on the carbonate ring), thereby avoiding the use of the potentially hazardous cyanogen bromide as carrier-activating agent. Another point which emerged from McLaughlan's studies was that either anti-whole myeloma IgE or antiserum raised against the Fc fragment was suitable for the radio-immunoassay of IgE.

It was disappointing that the elegantly simple coated-tube technique did not prove as satisfactory as the immunosorbent methods (possibly, it's thought, because it is a 'static' system). A sandwich tube technique (Salmon et al. 1969), on the other hand, has been shown (Bennich and Johansson 1971) to be as accurate as R.I.S.T. in the estimation of serum IgE; but, as this requires a preliminary coating of each tube with a relatively large amount of pure antigen (in this case IgE), it is seriously handicapped at present by the limited availability of this essential reagent. This situation could alter, however, with the advent of the preparative immunosorption procedures now being developed in several laboratories for the isolation of workable amounts of IgE from the processing of large volumes of allergic sera. Such a practice would also overcome the limitation of the present procedure of relying upon only one or two γE myeloma proteins as antigenic standard.

2.6 Standard reagents for use in γE antibody estimation

If maximum accuracy and reliability is to be achieved from a biological assay it is essential to have available a stable reference standard, which can be used as a yard-stick in different laboratories. Fortunately, the World Health Organisation has taken on the task of establishing a standard for human γE-globulin estimation (Rowe et al. 1970) in the form of a pool of sera of high IgE content from 91 adult West African donors, which has already been distributed to many laboratories together with a sample of specific anti-IgE antiserum (raised in sheep by Bennich and Johansson, by immunisation with the Fc fragment of purified myeloma IgE).

The stability of the reference serum stored in lyophilised form under nitrogen in glass ampoules, has been investigated over a period of a year; during which time some of the ampoules were held at elevated temperatures (40° and 37°) to accelerate any tendency of the γE-globulin towards degradation. Radio-immunoassay (R.I.S.T. and R.S.R.D.) indicated that no significant change of potency had occurred in the IgE stored for a year under these conditions, compared with material kept in lyophilised form or in

TABLE 2.12
Influence of the time of storage (in lyophilised form) on the capacity of allergic sera to sensitise passively normal human leucocytes.

Donor leucocytes	Sensitising serum	Batch No.	Time stored in freeze dried form	Allergen	Specific histamine release % TAH
D.R.S.	P.R.	2	4 months	Horse dander	42
D.R.S.	P.R.	3	2 months	Horse dander	21
			4 months	Horse dander	20
			6 months	Horse dander	6
			8 months	Horse dander	0
R.D.	P.R.	3	3 weeks	Horse dander	68
			4 months	Horse dander	24
			7 months	Horse dander	63
M.H.	P.R.	3	1 week	Horse dander	20
M.H.	M.D.	2A	1 week	Timothy pollen	17
			2 months	Timothy pollen	17

the frozen state at –20°. It is important to realise, however, that neither of these assays are capable of revealing any change in the tissue-sensitising activity of the standard serum (fig. 2.1). This is a serious omission from the stability studies, because of all the properties of γE-globulin now measurable (by the methods outlined in this chapter) tissue sensitising activity is probably of most clinical significance. Moreover, this parameter might be expected, on 'a priori' grounds, to be more vulnerable to alteration during storage than would antigenicity (as measured by R.I.S.T. or R.S.R.D.).

In this connection, we were encouraged to find in our quantitative P–K studies (Stanworth and Kuhns 1965), mentioned earlier, that the standard horse dander-sensitive individual's (PR) serum appeared to retain its P–K activity during several months storage (of 5 ml aliquots) at 4° in lyophilised form under nitrogen in glass ampoules prior to reconstitution in sterile distilled water. Furthermore, we have since shown that these conditions of storage appear to have little effect on the capacity of the serum to sensitise normal individuals' leucocytes in vitro for allergen-induced histamine release (table 2.12, which should be considered in the light of the day-to-day variability of the technique as indicated by the data in fig. 2.20). As was pointed out earlier, however (§2.3.2), it is now known that it is essential to re-adjust the *p*H of the lyophilised serum following reconstitution in distilled water, if it is to be used for in vitro passive sensitisation purposes.

It is worth mentioning that other investigators (Perlman and Layton 1967) have obtained evidence of the stability of reaginic antibodies towards the effects of freezing and thawing and lyophilisation of the parent sera, on the basis of unchanged P–K and monkey PCA titres.

In a recent quantitative study (Stanworth and Johansson 1973) of the stability of γE antibodies in a pollen sensitive individual's

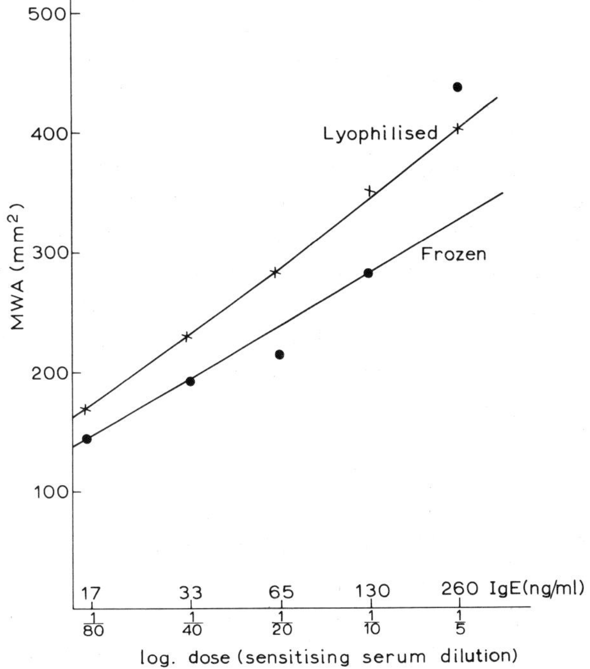

Fig. 2.35. Comparison of log(dose)-response curves obtained by baboon PCA testing of dilutions of the same standard allergic (pollen-sensitive) serum stored in lyophilised or frozen form.

serum stored in both lyophilised and frozen form for various time periods at 4°, the IgE concentration as measured by R.I.S.T. and R.A.S.T. has been compared with the tissue-sensitising activity of the serum as determined in vivo (by baboon PCA testing) and in vitro (by the chopped lung assay). It was concluded from these parallel studies, that lyophilisation (which is obviously more convenient) was not inferior to freezing (at −20°) as a method of preserving tissue-sensitising as well as the antigenic activity of γE-globulin. This is indicated, for example, by the baboon PCA log (dose)–response curves shown in fig. 2.35. On the other hand, it also became apparent that lyophilisation as well as storage for 4 weeks at temperatures of 4° or 25° rendered the γE antibodies more vulnerable to denaturation; as revealed by PCA testing of various dilutions of the allergic serum.

Nevertheless, the findings from this latest study are encouraging; suggesting that it should be possible to develop a lyophilised sensitising serum reference standard, for distribution to different laboratories. A more challenging problem, yet to be resolved, is the question of finding a source of sufficient quantities of such a serum. Ideally, it should originate from a single donor with a well-defined inhalant-hypersensitivity. But in practice it will probably prove necessary to pool allergic sera from individuals showing different specificities (e.g. to grass pollen, animal danders etc.); against which the investigator can compare his own working allergic serum standard, which is also stored under optimum stabilising conditions.

According to the recommendations of WHO, IgE concentration determined by comparison with their serum standard (which itself has been calibrated by reference to myeloma IgE) should be expressed as units of activity per ml of solution. For example, the arbitrary unitage assigned to their IgE serum standard 68/341 was such that 1 unit of activity is 'that present in 9.284×10^{-3} mg of freeze-dried powder'; or, in other words, each ampoule of 92.84 mg of lyophilised serum contains on average 10 000 units of IgE activity. It is to be hoped, however, that ultimately the availability of a highly purified non-myeloma IgE in sufficient quantities for general distribution will render this expediency no longer of any practical value.

2.7 Concluding comments

It will have become apparent from this appraisal of the various methods now available for the measurement of immediate hypersensitivity reactions that the situation is much more satisfactory than it was as recently as a decade ago, when P–K testing provided the only form of assay. Indeed, it might be argued that there is now a wider range of procedures available for the estimation of γE-globulins than for any other class of immunoglobulin.

Obviously there is a need for further assessment of the capabilities of many of the techniques discussed. It is hoped, however, that some benefit will have been gained by the emphasis which I have placed on the results of direct comparisons of the performances of different types of assay using the same standard allergic serum; a practice which has usually been neglected in the past. Furthermore, it is important to note that this approach has included a comparison of basic methods of measuring tissue-sensitising activity with the newly developed radio-immunoassay procedures, which provide a measurement of other parameters.

Despite the advantages of the latter techniques, it will have been recognised that there is still uncertainty about the clinical significance of the data which they provide. In this respect, even the measurement of tissue-sensitising activity of circulating γE antibody could prove to be less revealing than a method capable of determining the extent of tissue-binding. One possibility of accomplishing this was to exploit the ability of intradermally injected anti-human IgE antiserum to evoke immediate weal and flare reactions, presumably by cross-linking mast cell bound γE-globulin molecules (according to the mechanism discussed in ch. 5). But although the minimum effective dose of anti-IgE antiserum needed to evoke a standard skin reaction was found to be related inversely to the subjects' serum IgE level, measurement of this parameter failed to differentiate reliably between atopic and non-atopic persons (Newcomb and Ishizaka 1969); nor was any correlation observed between the results of similar tests and the severity of the disease in patients with atopic dermatitis, which did however correlate with the serum IgE (Ogawa et al. 1971).

Notes

[1] This can now be minimised by screening test sera for Australia antigen.

[2] But we have recently shown (Stanworth and Smith, Lancet, 1972, ii, 491) that local injection of human myeloma IgE 4, unlike myeloma proteins of the other three IgE sub-classes, is capable of inhibiting subsequent (+4 hr) skin sensitisation of baboons by human γE antibodies.

[3] This has recently been discontinued, unexpectedly, but another phencyclidine derivative Ketalar (Ketamine hydrochloride) is available as an alternative from the same manufacturers.

[4] Except that histamine was estimated by the spectrofluorometric procedure outlined in fig. 2.13 (p. 57).

[5] The time course of decline in responsiveness of monkey skin, stored at 4°, to antibody–allergen induced histamine release would seem to parallel that of the decrease of metabolic activity observed (Lawrence, J.C.; personal communication) in split-thickness quinea pig ear skin stored at this temperature.

[6] An in vitro method, based on the use of healthy-looking sliced human skin removed at mastectomy, has recently been described (Greaves, M.; Yamamoto, S.; Fairley, V.M.; B.M.J., 1972, *2*, 623).

[7] This number of assays can be performed in 1 hr by means of the fully automated procedures recently developed by Evans, D. and Thompson, D. (I.C.I.) and Martin, L.E. and Harrison, C. (Allen and Hanburys).

[8] It is interesting to note that recent electron microscopic studies (Sullivan, A.L.; Grimley, P.M.; Metzger, H.; J. Exp. Med., 1971, *134*, 1403) suggest that the amount of endogenous IgE on human basophils varies from individual to individual, and does not correlate with serum IgE level.

[9] Improvement of the reproducibility between assays performed on the same occasion can be achieved by always determining the total available histamine by addition of the specific release value (obtained by analysis of the supernatant) to that remaining in the sediment (retrieved in TCA).

[10] Ann Smith (working in my laboratory) has shown that by reverting to the buffy coat method of separating leucocytes, using a mechanical tube-slicer, it is possible to increase drastically the recovery of total wbc (from 6 to 11 × 10^6/ml) and the mean yield of basophils proportionately from 6.4 to 10.3 × 10^4/ml. Thus, a strong correlation can now be demonstrated between the basophil content of the working cell suspension and the total available histamine, which has been increased on average from 0.087 to 0.193 μg/ml reaction volume.

[11] A basophil separation technique has been recently described (Day, R.P.; Clinical Allergy, 1972, *2*, 205) which, reputedly, provides preparations of 93% purity at an average yield of 74%.

[12] But as with the measurement of other parameters, the IgE levels of *serial* serum samples from a patient are usually more illuminating.

[13] The mean IgE level of a later group of 19 hypogammaglobulinaemic sera investigated was only 14 ng/ml (range < 3–102) (McLaughlan, P.; Webster, A.C. and Stanworth, D.R.; to be published).

[14] This problem has recently been overcome (Brostoff, J. personal communication) by the use of enzyme-conjugated (as an alternative to radio-labelled) antibody in the R.S.R.D. technique; by analogy with the usage of similarly labelled protein antigen in the enzyme-linked immunosorbent assay (E.L.S.A.) (Engvall, E. and Perlmann, P.; Immunochem., 1971, *8*, 871) which is of comparable sensitivity to the R.I.S.T.

CHAPTER 3

Allergen structure and function

3.1 Introduction

It seems logical to consider the nature of the substances responsible for initiating hypersensitivity responses, before going on to discusss the characteristics of the antibodies which are produced and the manner in which these are thought to mediate the release of vasoactive agents.

The increase in tempo in the investigation of sensitising antibodies in recent years has tended to detract from the progress which is being made in the characterisation of the major antigens (allergens) responsible for their production. Yet, despite the complexity of most allergenic materials, substantial strides are being made in the isolation and characterisation of their active constituents; a process which is being facilitated by the emergence of physico-chemical techniques, such as iso-electric focusing and polyacrylamide disc electrophoresis with improved resolving power, and by the availability of highly sensitive serological methods for the detection of antigenic heterogeneity.

It is not the intention here, however, to provide an exhaustive account of the many and varied allergens which have been characterised in any detail, as a recent monography by Berrens (1971) has gone a long way to meeting this need. This chapter will be mainly concerned with comparing the characteristics of allergens from diverse sources, with the object of ascertaining whether there are underlying structural features in common which could be of significance in the initiation of a hypersensitive (rather than an immune) response. Discussion will also be concerned with possible roles of the allergen in the elicitation of anaphylactic reactions in pre-sensitised individuals; and in their isolated tissues and cells.

Firstly, however, it would perhaps be of some practical value to comment upon suitable methods of assaying allergenic activity; and to outline (for the benefit of future investigators in this field) a general approach to the isolation and characterisation of this type of antigen, based on my own experience in the study of horse dandruff allergen.

3.2 Assay of allergenic activity

The characterisation of allergens, like that of any other biologically active substance, rests heavily upon the reliability of the methods available for their assay.

Of these, direct skin testing in sensitive individuals is still the most convenient, despite its obvious limitations. Often, however, investigators refuse to push it to the limits of its accuracy; being content with a mere semi-quantitative assessment of the weal and flare responses produced, without recognising those factors which have been shown to influence accuracy and thereby ensuring that tests are performed under optimum conditions.

The series of careful quantitative skin test studies undertaken some time ago by Becker and his associates have provided valuable guide-lines in this respect (as mentioned in the previous chapter). For instance, these have shown that there is a decrease in responsiveness to the injected allergen as the forearm is descended, and that the radial side is less reactive than the ulnar side (Becker and Rappaport 1948). They have also indicated that increasing the volume of allergen injected intradermally from 0.01 to 0.02 ml (representing an actual volume increase of 0.005 to 0.010 ml) is equivalent to increasing the dose by 300 per cent; and that the accuracy is probably doubled by measurement of weal area rather than diameter (Rappaport and Becker 1949). Furthermore, they observed a linear dose–response relationship over only a very small dose range; and the slope of the log(dose)–log(response) plot was disappointingly small (Becker and Rappaport 1948).

I have preferred to use the direct prick test, in preference to intradermal allergen challenge, because this introduces considerably less potentially hazardous material and gives more clear-cut responses in the low concentration range. For instance, Squire (1950) estimated that as little as 3×10^{-6} ml of liquid is introduced into the skin by this procedure; with a fair degree of precision (± 16 per cent). My approach has been to perform duplicate prick tests, suitably spaced on the forearms of sensitive individuals to take into account the influence of site on the resultant weal and erythema response (an effect which can be avoided by use of the back of the recipient). First, a drop of the test allergen solution is placed on the centre of each site (previously outlined with a marking pen), then a sterile sewing needle is used to pierce the dermis through the drop (thus permitting the influx of the allergen). After 10 sec have elapsed, the excess fluid is carefully mopped up with cotton-wool. The outlines of the resultant weals are traced on transparent sheeting at precise intervals (e.g. 10, 20 min) after challenge, their areas being determined by super-imposition on to graph paper followed by the 'counting of squares'.

Ideally, tests should be performed on multiple dilutions (10-fold) of allergen solution, care always being taken to assess the response to a sufficiently high dilution before proceeding to test lower dilutions. It is also important to compare the activities of solutions of different allergen preparations or fractions, at comparable protein concentrations, directly by testing in the same recipient on the same occasion.

There have been numerous moves by clinical allergists towards the adoption of a standard unit of allergen activity, such as the 'Noon unit' (defined as the amount of allergen contained in 10^{-6} g of dry pollen) and the 'protein nitrogen unit' (being the activity associated with 10^{-8} g of pollen antigen). But obviously these are of no value to the experimentalist; because they fail to take into account non-allergenic (nitrogen-containing) contaminants, which are usually numerous and which often vary in proportion between different extracts of the same allergenic material.

On the other hand, it is useful to be able to relate the activity of highly purified allergen preparations to protein (or nitrogen) concentration. This is done, for instance, in the in vitro measurement of allergenic activity by means of the direct leucocyte test. For, as already mentioned in the previous chapter, it has been found (Lichenstein and Osler 1964) that an approximately linear relationship obtains between the amount of histamine released (measured spectrofluorometrically) and the log of the allergen concentration; which varies from donor to donor, thereby providing a means of assessing the degree of severity of his sensitivity to that particular allergen (expressed as the amount of allergen required to effect a 50 per cent response). Moreover, it has been shown (Lichenstein et al. 1966) that the same technique can be used to assay the activity of the allergen (e.g. ragweed) as well, with a sensitivity which exceeds that of the direct skin test by about 20 times (i.e. as little as 10^{-6} μg of allergen/ml was detectable in this manner). Despite recent refinements (mentioned in ch. 2), however, in vitro leucocyte assay is a lengthy and laborious procedure; which is not readily applicable to the simultaneous measurement of multiple allergen preparations.

Once an allergen has been identified and isolated in highly pure form it should be possible, of course, to estimate it as antigen; by quantitative immuno-diffusion or by a suitable radio-immunosorbent assay (by a similar principle to that employed in the R.I.S.T. method of assaying sensitising antibody, illustrated schematically in fig. 2.29). This supposes that antigenic determinants characteristic of the particular allergen survive the isolation process, and that an antiserum directed specifically against such determinants is available.

Because of the exquisite sensitivity of the direct skin test, and likewise that of the in vitro alternative mentioned above, it is always difficult to be certain that the activity shown by a particular allergen preparation is not due to the presence of a trace contaminant; which is not even detectable by the most sensitive method of antigenic analysis. There are, however, ways of tackling this problem as will be illustrated by the example considered in the next section.

Finally, it should be pointed out that my comments on assay have so far been largely restricted to the measurement of activity of inhalant-type allergens; although, as the classical work of Prausnitz and Küstner (1921) indicated, food sensitivities can also sometimes be demonstrated by direct prick testing. Any serious claim as to the allergenic nature of a particular ingestant should obviously be backed up, however, by the results of confirmatory feeding tests using both the whole substance and a range of proteolytic digestion products; as was done, for example, in recent studies on the nature of the major allergen in cod (Aas and Elsayed 1969), where passively sensitised normal recipients were fed isolated fish allergen fractions concealed in beef.

The possibility of metabolic, or other chemical changes, leading to the in vivo formation of an allergenically active derivative is more difficult to confirm. This problem is frequently encountered, of course, in drug sensitivity; and is often not resolved by attempts to demonstrate that the drug in question is converted to an allergenically-active form on reaction with a plasma protein constituent or some other arbitrarily selected protein 'carrier' (a topic which will be returned to, later).

3.3 Characteristics of major types of allergen

3.3.1 Horse dandruff

I first encountered the problem of allergen characterisation in 1949, when faced with the task of isolating the constituent of horse epidermal scales (dandruff) responsible for the relatively severe hypersensitivity reactions to horses shown by certain individuals. At its most dramatic, this was manifested as a fatal anaphylactic shock following the injection of diphtheria or tetanus antitoxin. Squire (1950) was of the opinion that the effect was caused by small amounts of horse serum albumin, present as contaminant in the antitoxin preparation injected, to which horse dandruff allergen was closely related structurally. But, after numerous abortive attempts to apply the known methods of isolation and crystallisation of horse serum albumin to the isolation of the active dandruff constituent, I decided it would be necessary to start by treating the horse dandruff extract as an unknown mixture of proteins of which one or more possessed allergenic activity.

I am outlining the outcome of my efforts here because they represented the first systematic study of an allergen system; which, despite subsequent development of protein fractionation techniques, might still serve as a guide in the investigation of other systems.

There had been many previous unsuccessful attempts to isolate pure allergen from extracts of other inhalant-type allergens (e.g. pollens, house dust etc.), besides animal danders. These usually proved to contain multiple protein components, pigment and innumerable low molecular weight substances; and, although the active fractions seemed to be of protein nature, they often showed an unusual stability to heat treatment (possibly attributable to a high content of conjugated carbohydrates) and some even appeared to resist proteolysis. But none of the active fractions obtained were properly characterised, the sole aim appearing to be the isolation of skin-reactive fractions regardless of the deleterious action of the reagents (e.g. strong acid, strong alkali, organic solvents) employed; a factor which no doubt contributed to the problem of retrieving pure active constituents in their native state. Another difficulty in allergen isolation has proved to be the nature of the constituents themselves; many of which are not as easily separable as the serum proteins, for example, because of their similarity in electric charge and size.

When I first started working on the horse dandruff system, immunodiffusion precipitin analysis had not been devised. Hence, far greater reliance had to be placed upon the limited physicochemical procedures available at that time. Nevertheless, as will be indicated, it was still possible by a process of *reductio ad absurdum* to make a preliminary identification of the active constituent. The purpose throughout was to apply conventional methods of globular protein fractionation, taking every care to avoid denaturing conditions and thereby preserving the native structure of the sensitising substances. This applied right from the extraction

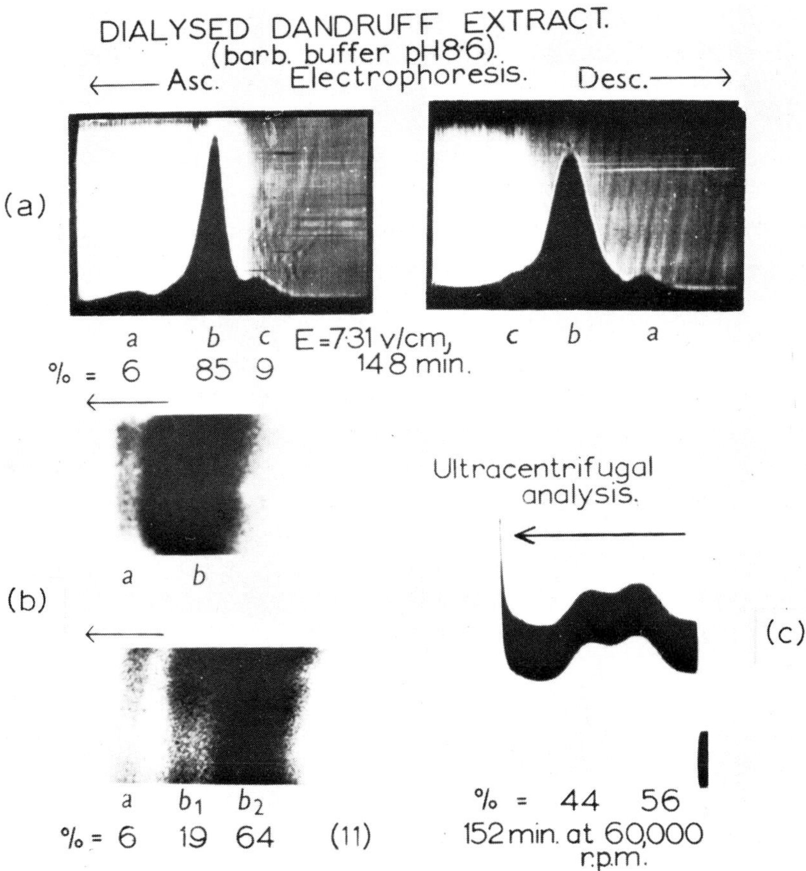

Fig. 3.1. Analysis of horse dandruff extract by: (a) free-solution electrophoresis; (b) paper electrophoresis; (c) free-solution ultracentrifugation (from Stanworth 1957A, B).

stage, where the acetone used in the initial defatting process was kept at reduced temperature (1°), and in subsequent extraction of the defatted epidermal material (where the use of saline was eventually abandoned in favour of buffered saline).

A preliminary purification step, involving exhaustive dialysis of the crude extract, removed about 40 per cent of the total solute to leave a light brown opalescent solution containing about 1 g per cent (w/v) protein i.e. a yield of 1 per cent of the starting epidermal material. Free solution electrophoresis revealed this to contain one major and two minor components (tentatively labelled a, b and c), as is indicated in fig. 3.1a. Unfortunately, only one of the minor components was separable by paper electrophoresis (fig. 3.1b), presumably because of the high rate of diffusion of the electrophoretically similar proteins through this medium. Analytical ultracentrifugation performed at a later stage (Stanworth 1957) proved even less resolving, showing 2 peaks of approximately equal size with sedimentation coefficients (S_{20}) of 3.7*S* and 1.9*S* (fig. 3.1c).

The leading question then was: with which of these components is allergenic activity associated? In attempting to answer this it should be pointed out that it is not necessary initially to isolate the components in pure form. Assuming that activity was only associated with one of them, all that was required was to obtain a sufficient number of different fractions in which the proportion of the various components differed; and then to compare their direct skin activities in horse dander-sensitive individuals on a constant weight basis.

Quantitative salt-precipitation (using sat.ammonium sulphate as

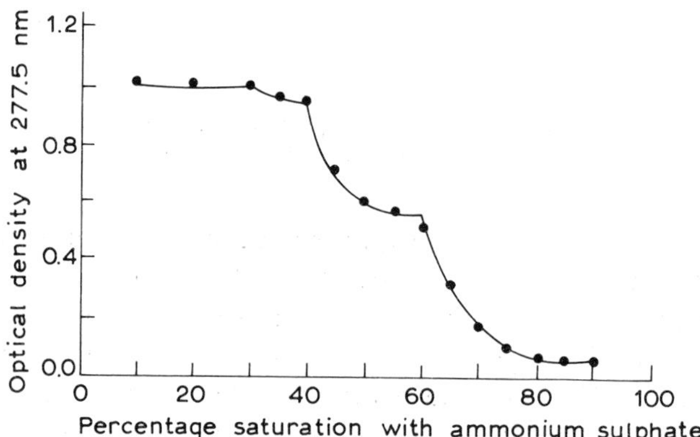

Fig. 3.2. Quantitative salt-precipitation analysis of horse dandruff extract, indicating the concentration limits between which the major components separated out (from Stanworth 1957A).

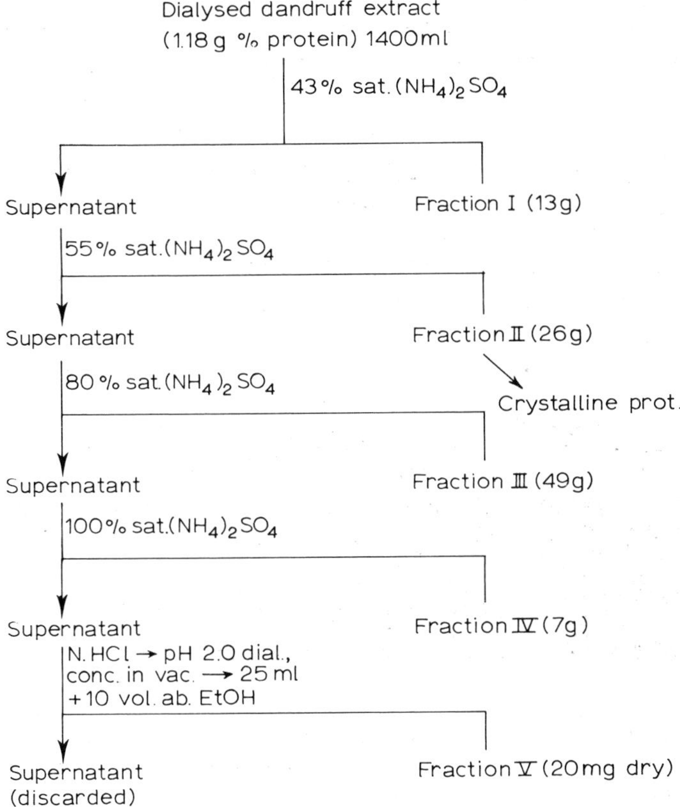

Fig. 3.3. Large scale ammonium sulphate precipitation scheme adopted in the fractionation of horse dandruff extract (from Stanworth 1957A).

precipitant) revealed the appropriate concentration limits between which to separate the fractions (fig. 3.2). Four major fractions were obtained from a subsequent large scale precipitation, as revealed by fig. 3.3. Moreover, paper electrophoretic analysis of these revealed that a substantial degree of separation of their various protein constituents had been achieved; an impression which was strengthened by the staining of halves of some strips for carbohydrate and by the determination of hexose/N ratios. Thus, the analysis of a prosthetic group had discerned differences between

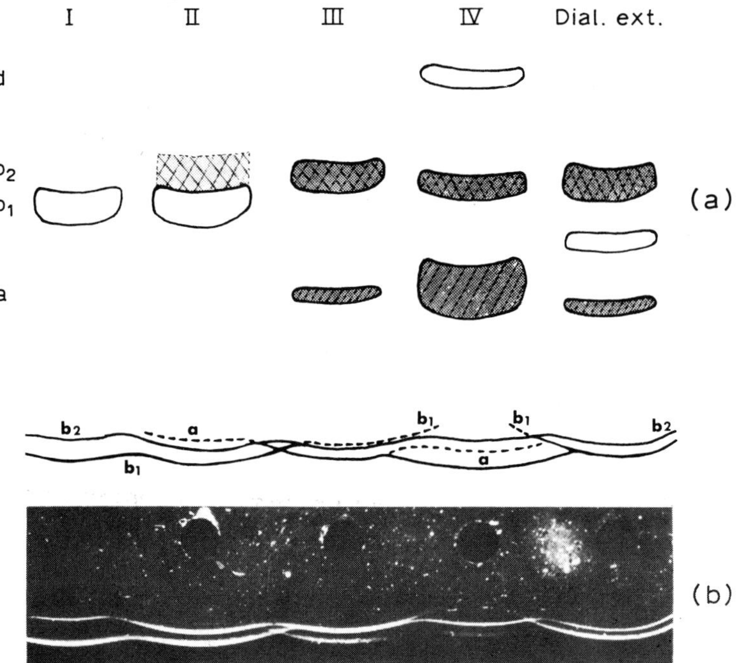

Fig. 3.4. Comparative analysis of major salt precipitation fractions of horse dandruff extract by: (a) paper electrophoresis, with staining for carbohydrate (indicated by the shading) as well as protein; (b) immunodiffusion in agar, against a rabbit anti-whole dander extract antiserum (from Stanworth 1957B).

certain components (e.g. those obtained in fractions I and II) which were not evident from protein staining alone; as will be seen from fig. 3.4a, in which the results of comparative paper electrophoretic analysis of the various salt precipitation fractions are represented schematically.

It was apparent, then, that if activity was confined to the b component, say, fraction I would be expected to prove the predominantly active one; whereas, if it were associated with component a, to take another example, the highest activity should have been seen in fraction IV. The results of the comparison of the direct skin activities of the fractions, in 4 different horse dandruff-sensitive individuals, with their electrophoretic composition

TABLE 3.1

Electrophoretic compositions and allergenic activities of salt-precipitated horse dandruff protein fractions (from Stanworth 1957A).

Protein fraction	Relative concentrations of electrophoretic constituents (%)				Site	Weal diameters elicited on duplicated sites					Mean	Standard error of mean
	a	b_1	b_2	Remainder (c, d, etc.)		Patient D.P. (mm)	Patient M.H. (2nd test) (mm)	Patient A.P. (mm)	Patient M.H. (1st test) (mm)	Patient R.V. (mm)		
Crude extract	6.0	18.8	64.4	10.8	1	18.2	15.4	10.4	10.5	7.4	–	–
						16.8	14.5	11.9	8.7	6.5		
					2	15.3	13.5	13.4	6.9	5.6		
						% mean diameters elicited by crude extract						
Dialysed extract	4.9	25.3	56.7	13.1	1	121.4	89.7	108.4	103.4	84.6	90.8	14.0
					2	67.9	61.4	145.4	62.1	63.1		
Fraction I	0.0	74.6	0.0	25.4	1	27.4	37.2	26.9	0.0	47.7	36.6	8.5
					2	48.2	42.1	42.0	34.5	60.0		
Fraction II	0.0	71.8	13.4	14.8	1	32.7	34.5	47.9	0.0	81.5	45.3	16.5
					2	50.0	40.7	62.2	17.2	86.2		
Fraction III	6.8	8.7	78.3	6.2	1	52.4	89.7	84.0	118.4	95.6	87.6	14.5
					2	128.0	104.1	75.6	67.8	60.0		
Fraction IV	52.3	0.0	40.0	7.7	1	74.4	86.8	84.0	69.0	55.4	76.5	5.3
				(4.2 = d)	2	69.6	86.9	83.2	71.3	84.6		
Fraction V	–	–	–	–	1	0.0	–	0.0	–	–	–	–
					2	0.0	–	0.0	–	–	–	–

determined by quantitative paper electrophoresis is shown in table 3.1. A careful scrutiny of the data there will reveal that allergenic activity is associated with the b_2 component, which comprised about 64 per cent of the total protein in horse dandruff extract; a conclusion which was later substantiated by further comparative skin tests on fractions comprised predominantly of a, b_2 and d components, separated by preparative paper or starch column electrophoresis.

The only discordant note seemed to be the detection of some skin activity in the salt precipitation fraction I, which according to paper electrophoresis appeared to be composed entirely of the b_1 component. But comparative gel-diffusion precipitin analysis (using antiserum against crude dander extract), performed later when the Ouchterlony technique became available, showed a readily detectable b_2 component line relatively near to the sample well (fig. 3.4b).

Further comparative immunodiffusion under optimum conditions revealed that the b_2 component line in the most active fraction (III) was in fact composite; corresponding to electrophoretically slow (b_2S) and fast (b_2F) components, which were only partially resolvable by acetylated cellulose column electrophoresis

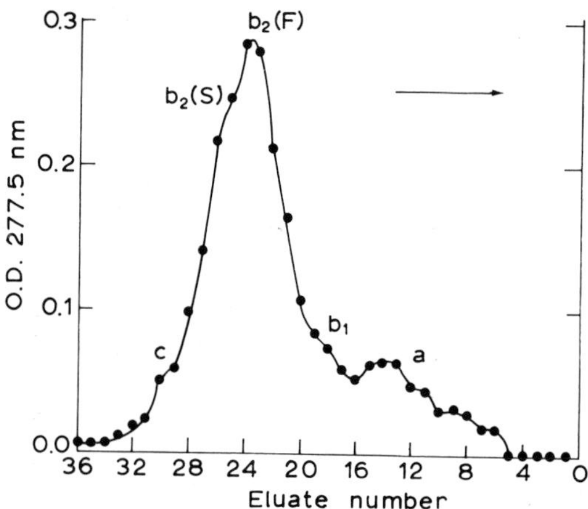

Fig. 3.5. Preparative column electrophoresis (on acetylated cellulose) profile of horse dandruff extract salt-precipitated fraction III (from Stanworth 1957B).

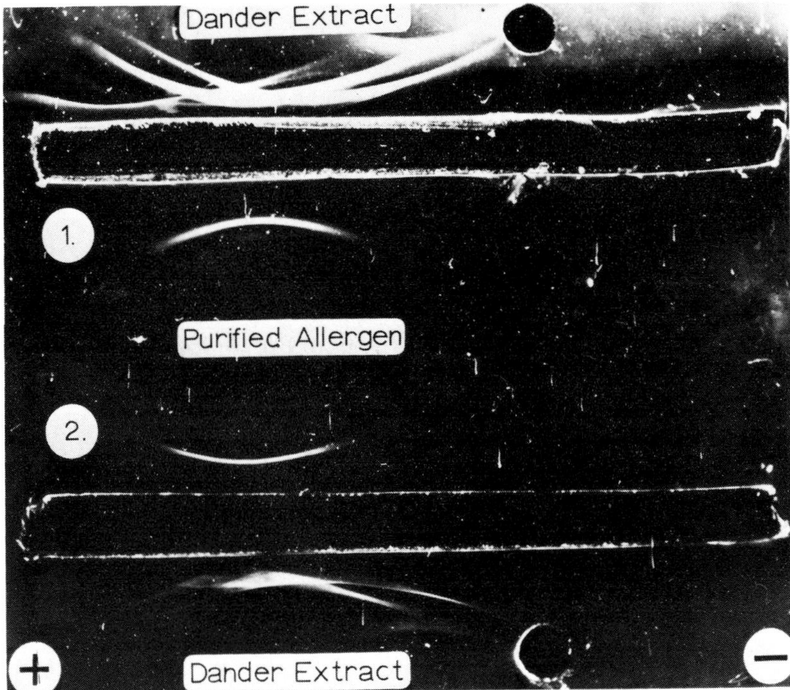

Fig. 3.6. Immunoelectrophoretic pattern of a purified horse dandruff allergen component compared with that of the parent dandruff extract (antiserum:rabbit anti-whole dander extract).

(fig. 3.5). Furthermore, repeated zone electrophoresis failed to resolve these two components. * One of the sub-components b_2S was ultimately purified (fig. 3.6), somewhat surprisingly, by a 2-stage gel filtration of the salt precipitation fraction III on Sephadex G75; an approach which also resulted in the separation of a non-reactive, electrophoretically fast, 'a' component in antigenically pure form (thus providing a valuable 'negative control' substance).

The finding of skin reactivity associated with the purified b_2S

* Recent studies suggest that preparative polyacrylamide electrophoresis might be more successful in this respect.

TABLE 3.2

Carbohydrate compositions of total horse dandruff protein and various sub-fractions, including a purified allergen preparation: b_2S (Stanworth and Willard, unpublished data).

Horse dander fraction	(Galactose + mannose)/2 (%)	Hexo-samine (%)	N.glycolyl neur-aminic acid (%)	Skin reactivity (of 20 mg% solns.) 20′ weal area (mm^2) 1	2	mean
Total protein (a, b_1, b_2F, b_2S, etc.)	4.08	2.66	2.42	29	31	30
Fraction III (a, b_2F, b_2S)	5.77	3.45	3.16	4	37	21
Purified allergen (b_2S)	13.90	1.50	3.52	12	21	17
Purified component (a)	(2.00)		0.00	0	0	0
Controls						
Buffered saline				0	0	0
Histamine (0.1 mg/ml)				6	7	7

component is contrary to my previous tentative suggestion (Stanworth 1957), based on studies of composite b_2 fractions, that only the faster (b_2F) component carried allergenic activity. It now seems probable, however, that both the b_2S and b_2F sub-components possess allergenic activity and that these are antigenically related. The carbohydrate compositions of a purified horse dander allergen component (b_2S) and the non-active component 'a' are compared in table 3.2, with those of the parent salt-precipitation fraction III and total horse dandruff extract. The presence of galactose and mannose (in a 1/1 ratio) was confirmed, but at a higher total level (i.e. of 13.9 per cent hexose) than that (i.e. 9 per cent hexose) reported earlier (Stanworth 1957A) for the composite b_2 component. This increase presumably reflected removal of a cabohydrate-poor b_2F component; thus providing – as does, for example, repeated hexose/N determination on progressively purer fractions – an independent indication of the final isolation of a pure component (i.e. when the hexose/N ratio no longer changes with further manipulation). The previous observation of the presence of traces of fucose was not confirmed, possibly because this was restricted to the b_2F component. A substantial amount of N-glycolyl neuramic acid was now detected, however. This was of interest, because the N-glycolyl derivative of neuraminic acid is also found in horse serum glycoproteins, in contrast to the N-acetyl derivative present in human serum and epithelial glycoproteins.

Another interesting observation was the absence of neuraminic acid from the non-allergenic 'a' component of horse dandruff extract which raised the exciting possibility that the neuraminic acid was directly associated with allergenic activity. But this was discounted in a subsequent experiment, in which removal of this derivative from purified allergen (b_2S component) by neuraminidase treatment, was found to have no obvious effect on its direct skin activity (table 3.3). This does not necessarily mean, however, that the N-glycolyl neuraminic acid constituent of the allergen does not play some essential role in the initial sensitisation of pre-disposed individuals to horse dandruff. It is possibly of some significance, in this connection, that similar studies on one of the few other allergens in which neuraminic acid has been found, namely in a glycoprotein constituent of human seminal fluid

TABLE 3.3

Effect of neuraminidase treatment on the skin reactivity of purified horse dandruff allergen (Stanworth and Willard, unpublished data).

Fraction		Protein concn. (mg %)	Skin reactivity (10 min weal areas)		
			1	2	mean
Total dander extract	untreated	1282	171	192	182
Purified allergen prep. 1	untreated	138	44	63	54
	treated		47	69	58
Purified allergen prep. 2	untreated	90	22	22	22
	treated		48	76	62

(Halpern et al. 1967), suggested that this derivative was involved in allergenic activity (Halpern 1967).

Ultracentrifugal analysis of solutions of the purified allergen at different solute concentrations revealed an S° value of 3.43S; in contrast with the lower $S_{20,w}$ value of 2.5S reported earlier (Stanworth, 1957B) for the total b_2 component preparation, which was shown to possess a molecular weight of 34 000 by osmotic pressure measurements. Electrophoretically it moved ahead of horse serum albumin, when a mixture of the two was analysed on paper.

It could be confidently concluded, therefore, that at least one major allergenic fraction retrievable from horse dandruff extract differed markedly in its properties from horse serum albumin, contrary to Squire's (1950) original expectations. Nevertheless, it was possible to show by immunodiffusion analysis of highly concentrated solutions (i.e. 20 g/100 ml) of horse dandruff protein that traces of albumin and other horse serum proteins (including α_2-macroglobulin) were present as contaminants; presumably originating from the skin cells, which had acquired them from the circulation. Hence, it seemed likely that those asthmatics who showed sensitivity to horse serum albumin as well as to horse dandruff had become hypersensitised to traces of serum proteins present in inhaled horse epidermal material; rather than that their anaphylactic reaction to injected antitoxin was due to a cross-reactivity between contaminating serum albumin and the horse dandruff allergen (as Squire had supposed). This offers an explanation of the observation (discussed by Beede et al. 1958) that animals sensitised to horse dander could be shocked by horse serum, but that the reverse situation did not obtain i.e. animals sensitised to horse serum could not be shocked by horse dander. On a clinical level, this means that patients developing serum sickness do not become 'horse asthmatics'; whereas horse asthmatics can react violently to horse serum (as already mentioned).

The various stages of my investigation of the horse dandruff system have been described chronologically, in some detail, because it is felt the findings are relevant to other allergen systems showing similar orders of complexity and contamination with allergenic substances from other sources. Of these, house dust is of course a classic example (which will be discussed further later). It is imperative that sufficiently sensitive immunological techniques should always be employed in a systematic manner in the characterisation of allergenic preparations, if one is to ensure that the observed activity is due to the protein in question and not to an unrelated contaminant.

Hypersensitivity to the dander of mammalian species other than the horse is not uncommon. These include laboratory animals, such as rabbits and guinea pigs, as some experimental biologists are well aware to their discomfort. The danders of common household pets can also prove troublesome to people. Yet little information is available about the chemical nature of the allergenic constituents responsible; presumably because of the problem of obtaining sufficient 'raw material' for any detailed investigation. It might be anticipated, however, that the danders of these other species will be found to contain an allergenic component bearing some structural similarity to the major allergen (b_2 component) of horse dandruff. Furthermore, fine structural differences of this component might prove to be responsible for cases of sensitivity to one species of cat (e.g. common cats) but not another (e.g. Siamese cats), to take one example.

The type of relationship envisaged between the dander allergen of different species would resemble the structural homology observed between certain serum proteins of various species. Of these, the α_2-macroglobulin constituent provides a particularly good example (James 1965). It is perhaps of some significance in this connection, too, that hyperimmunisation of rabbits with horse dandruff extract (Stanworth 1964) as well as with solutions of total egg white or cow's milk proteins (Stanworth, unpublished data) produced antibodies which cross-reacted with human serum α_2-macroglobulin. It is also interesting to note that some preliminary evidence has been obtained (Berrens 1971) to suggest that 2.5S α_2-glycoproteins found in human and horse dandruff may share antigenic determinants which are absent from the 'native' preparations, but which arise during the course of the exfoliation process.

The shedding of epidermal scales is a process which would be expected to lead to the antigenic alteration of constituent proteins; an effect which might also lead to the induction of allergenic properties. There is, however, no convincing evidence of the presence of specific reaginic antibodies in the sera of individuals showing skin reactivity to human dandruff. Fractionation of extracts of defatted human dandruff by precipitation with saturated ammonium sulphate, followed by acetone in HCl, has yielded a series of fractions, most of which show substantial skin activity in atopic patients in general (Berrens 1971). All of these have, however. proved to be highly heterogenous and contaminated by various serum proteins; so that attempts to demonstrate antigenic relationships with horse dandruff allergen have not been very fruitful. The possibility that some of the observed reactions to human dandruff are of an auto-immune type cannot be excluded at this stage.

3.3.2 Pollen allergens

It is perhaps not too surprising that techniques devised initially for the separation of globular serum proteins have not always proved particularly useful in the fractionation of plant protein constituents. The complexity of pollen extracts is most probably enhanced by the action of enzymes leached out of the granules, which are active at room temperature. Another problem is the variation in yield and composition of the protein constituents recovered from pollen of the same species harvested in different years (Goldfarb and Kaplan 1967). Factors such as these have no doubt been responsible for the considerable confusion which arose from early attempts to characterise pollen allergens; at a time when the isolation of dialysable (low molecular weight) active fractions were frequently reported, and when it was often difficult to form any firm conclusions about the relationship between the non-dialysable constituents studied in different laboratories. To add to the difficulties, investigators in this field have a habit of using their own personal systems of nomenclature [1] and, sometimes, even changing these in 'mid-stream'.

Fortunately, as in the isolation of reaginic antibodies discussed in the next chapter, the development of highly resolving protein fractionation techniques in the last few years has helped to overcome many of these problems; and a few pollen allergens have now been obtained in a relatively high state of purity. Even so, it is still not always easy to establish how the active allergenic components studied by one group are related to those described by another; and powerful techniques such as immunodiffusion are not always being applied as effectively as they might be.

Of the pollen allergens, ragweed has been studied most intensively, in the United States; whilst European investigators have confined their attentions mainly to those of common grasses (rye, cocksfoot and Timothy) and, to lesser extent, to that of the alder tree. The multi-step fractionation procedure adopted by King and his associates (e.g. King et al. 1964; King et al. 1967A), which incorporates diethyl amino ethyl (DEAE) and triethyl amino ethyl (TEAE) cellulose chromatography, salt precipitation and gel-filtration steps, has yielded 2 major allergens (designated E and K); and 2 minor components, which are chemically related to these and considered to be artifacts formed during isolation. The most active, E, allergen has been used widely in the studies of reaginic antibodies to be referred to in later chapters. It has been estimated to constitute 90 per cent of the total allergenic activity of ragweed pollen, although it only accounts for about 6 per cent of the pollen proteins. The second most active allergen (K) has been found to be, on average, about half as active as the allergen E; and its content in pollen extract is estimated to be half of that of allergen E. Although of similar molecular weight (around 38 000) and electric charge, the E and K allergens differ in amino acid composition and have been shown by immunodiffusion analysis to possess some distinctive antigenic determinants whilst sharing others.

It seems more than fortuitous that major (IB and IC) and minor (IIB and IIA) allergen fractions, showing similarities in molecular size and electrophoretic mobility to the major and minor ragweed allergen fractions, have been isolated from rye grass pollen extracts (Johnson and Marsh 1966A). The ragweed and rye pollen extracts show similar starch gel electrophoretic patterns, in which allergenic activity appears to be distributed amongst several rather than a single component. This has prompted Johnson and Marsh (1965) to refer to the members of the group as 'isoallergens', a possibly premature choice of terminology. As the IB and IC constituents of rye grass pollen appeared to differ only in their amide content, it has been suggested that the former is gradually converted to the latter by hydrolysis of amide groupings. The, electrophoretically faster, minor components (IIB, IIA) were assumed to be distinctive allergens on the dubious grounds that they are active in only a small proportion of individuals who are sensitive to the major allergen (IB/IC); and because they failed to inhibit precipitin formation between the major allergen and rabbit antiserum directed against rye pollen extract.

Further investigations would seem to be warranted before it can be concluded unequivocally that the minor rye pollen allergenic fractions bear no relation to the major (IIB/IIC) fraction. In this connection, it is interesting to note (somewhat surprisingly) that a purified low molecular (15 000) allergenic fraction (Ra3) has been recently isolated from aqueous extracts of short ragweed pollen (Underdown and Goodfriend 1969); and found to be antigenically unrelated to the major ragweed E allergen, with which it is claimed to share common allergenic determinants but differ in allergenic specificity. Moreover, as will be discussed further later, this preparation has been shown to possess a distinctive amino acid composition; and to be unusually basic compared to the well characterised allergens already referred to in this and the previous section. Despite these antigenic, physical and chemical dissimilarities, however, Underdown and Goodfriend (1969) have suggested the possibility that an Ra3 'region' is included within the allergen E molecule.

The allergenic constituents of Timothy and cocksfoot pollen extracts have not been characterised to anywhere near the same extent as have the ragweed and rye grass pollen allergens just discussed. Nevertheless, preliminary studies (e.g. Malley and Dobson 1966) would seem to suggest similarities in biological and physico-chemical properties, a conclusion which is supported by a recent interesting study (Marsh et al. 1970A) in which a direct comparison has been made of the allergenic fractions of 7 different grass pollens (representing 6 botanical tribes). This has involved comparative analysis of allergenicity by direct skin testing of fractions separated by starch gel electrophoresis (at *p*H 8.5), by leaving excised slices of gel containing the fractions for 20 min on circular scratches made on the backs of grass pollen-sensitive individuals; whilst the antigenicity of the electrophoretically separated fractions has been compared by immunodiffusion, using rabbit

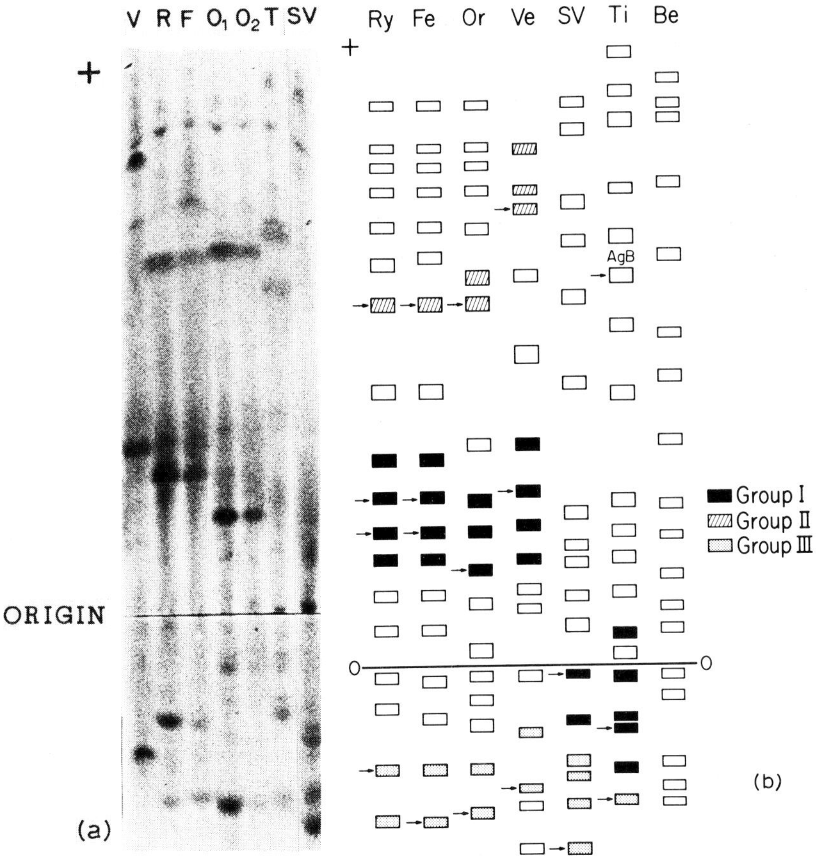

Fig. 3.7. Comparative starch gel electrophoresis patterns of solutions (20% w/v) of dialysed whole extracts of various types of grass pollen. (Reproduced from Marsh et al. 1970A, by permission of the authors.) Abbreviations: Ry, rye; Fe, fescue; Or, orchard; Ve, velvet; SV, sweet vernal; Ti, Timothy; Be, Bermuda.

antisera raised against rye grass fractions and crude pollen extracts. This approach has revealed 3 distinct groups of antigens, classified as Groups I, II and III (fig. 3.7) in most pollen extracts with the exception of Bermuda grass. Moreover, antigens from a particular group, but from different pollens, possessed similar allergenic properties in the individuals tested. In other words, components which were cross-antigenic in rabbits were cross-allergenic in man.

As the Group I components have been found previously to comprise the major rye grass allergens (IB/IC) it has been concluded that closely related antigens of fescue, orchard and velvet pollens are probably also the major allergens in these pollens. The Group II (IIB, IIA) fractions are also considered to be important allergens, despite the reservations discussed earlier; as are the Group III fractions which, it is interesting to note, are (like the ragweed Ra3 component mentioned earlier) relatively basic in nature, moving towards the cathode on electrophoresis at *p*H 8.5. Marsh and his associates (1970A) have gone as far as to suggest that grass-sensitive individuals can be broadly classified on the basis of skin reactivity to the different groups of antigen.

3.3.3 House dust

Of all allergenic materials studied in any detail this is by far the most heterogeneous, comprising a hotch-potch of substances of both animal and plant origin. Moreover, the dust from one household will contain agents not present in that from another and vice versa. It is not surprising, then, that there has been so much confusion and so many conflicting claims about the nature of allergens isolated from house dust.

Some idea of the extent of complexity of the system is indicated by studies (Berrens and Versie 1967) which have employed rabbit antisera raised against various fractions of house dust to demonstrate the presence of: glycoprotein constituents from human dandruff, kapok, cotton linters, feathers, hay and wool; whilst other studies have revealed the presence of several human serum proteins including immunoglobulins G and A (Versie and Brocteur 1967) and various blood group substances (Brocteur and

Versie 1967). There would seem to be some doubt, therefore, about the value of applying a rigorous general fractionation procedure to the attempted isolation of pure house dust allergen (such as that illustrated in Berrens 1971, page 146), under conditions which seem likely to contribute to the complexity of the system by promoting unwanted protein interactions and cleavage processes. Indeed, one wonders whether the 'intimate mixture of closely related glycoproteins', which according to Berrens and his associates (1965) constitute house dust allergen, did not originate as a result of such deleterious manipulative treatment during fractionation; and, in fact, these investigators have gone as far as to suggest that house dust 'allergens' represent cell wall glycopeptides solubilised during decomposition reactions of the Maillard type between free amino groups on glycoproteins and reducing sugars. Firm direct evidence in support of this idea, that house dust 'allergen' is a product of chemical processes occurring within decomposing dust, has yet to be provided however; and, as will be discussed further in §3.4, there seems to be no convincing reason for equating activity of allergenic substances in general with the presence of N-glycosidic protein-sugar linkages as Berrens (1971) has done.

If, on the other hand, a satisfactory systematic fractionation of house dust extract is to be achieved it would seem necessary first to try to remove – by the mildest possible treatment – all known allergenic substances, using adequate serological methods of control. In this connection, it is interesting to note that the claim that the allergenic component of house dust is a substance excreted (or secreted) by the mite *Dermatophagoides pteronyssinus* (Voorhorst et al. 1967) is gaining increased support from clinical allergists. It should be recognised, however, that such claims are based on the observation that skin reactions to extracts of house dust and *D. pteronyssinus* culture are seen in the same frequency in the same allergic patients; and that they show (semi-qualitatively) a high degree of correlation (Spieksma and Voorhorst 1969). In weighing the significance of this type of indirect evidence, however, it is important to bear in mind that the mites used in such studies are grown in media comprising human skin scales and powdered yeast or Gaines dog meal prepared from wheat, maize, soya bean, bone and fish meal, wheat by-products, animal fats and vitamins (many of which are, themselves, allergenic). Moreover, in this connection, it is interesting to note that it has been estimated that a man produces around 5 g of dandruff per week (Spieksma 1970); which is apparently enough food for the highest number of *Dermatophagoides* ever found (? in a single house-hold). Hence, it would seem to be important to consider whether the mite is perhaps merely a 'vehicle' capable of 'processing' allergenic material which is originally of human epidermal origin.

Only some very careful serological detective work, employing techniques of comparable specificity and sensitivity to those practiced in forensic science laboratories, would seem capable of establishing whether mite allergen is a constituent of the arthropod's excretum; or whether it is an intrinsic body constituent, which is shed into the atmosphere. It is hoped that work now being directed towards the large-scale culture of these organisms will lead to the production of specific antisera against characteristic intrinsic antigens.

It would seem to be significant that the mite genus *Dermatophagoides* has been found to be present in much higher numbers than any other genera in house dust (Spieksma 1970); and also that a seasonal periodicity is apparent in the numbers of mites in dust, and that this number differs considerably from one household to another depending upon the relative humidity, temperature etc. But, it would seem to be stretching this type of inductive reasoning a little far to imply, as Spieksma has done, that the lower prevalence of house dust allergy in higher mountain areas in Switzerland can be equated with the lower numbers of mites found there.

In summary, the question as to whether the principal allergenic components of house dusts are of chemical or biological origin is far from being answered yet. Indeed, it has yet to be established that allergens peculiar to house dust are responsible for the substantial evidence of human hypersensitivity to this material. Under the circumstances, therefore, it would seem to be a little premature to attempt to couple house dust extract (and dried extracts of mites and mite culture medium) to activated Sephadex for use in a highly sophisticated procedure like R.A.S.T. (Stenius and Wide 1969); in an effort to measure reaginic antibodies directed against allergenic constituents of these materials.

3.3.4 Food allergens

Common foods comprise protein systems just as complex as those found in many inhalant allergenic materials. For instance, at least 20 protein constituents have been identified in cow's milk (Hanson and Johansson 1961). The identification of active allergens amongst these presents additional problems, however; for, as mentioned earlier, skin testing does not always reveal a reactivity which is directed against a digestion product of the ingested material. Such a possibility is supported by a recent study (Spies et al. 1970) in which it was demonstrated that new antigenic determinants are generated in milk proteins as a result of pepsin hydrolysis at *p*H 2.0 for 8 min.

There have been innumerable attempts to incriminate precipitating antibodies directed against milk proteins, in conditions of adult intolerance to milk; as well as in cases of cot death and other infantile conditions, where ingested foreign milk antigens have been under suspicion. Moreover, it has been shown that a larger proportion of sera from such patients sensitise guinea pigs for PCA reactions, than do sera from normal adults or infants (Parish 1969). But this heterologous tissue-sensitising activity has been attributed to the presence of γG-type antibodies measurable by the R.C.L.A.A.R technique, in which milk (and egg) proteins were linked to the carrier erythrocytes by photo-oxidation. In fact, there have been several reports of the occurrence of antibodies to various milk proteins in the sera of healthy adults and children; and in various gastro-intestinal disorders (such as adult coeliac disease and ulcerative colitis) and chronic respiratory conditions, where there is no obvious evidence of γE-mediated hypersensitivity.

On the other hand, there have been few attempts yet to demonstrate that suspected cases of milk sensitivity contain anti-milk γE antibodies in their circulation. In one such recent study (Kletter et al. 1971), γE antibodies to cow's milk proteins were detected in the sera of infants by means of a radio-immunodiffusion technique, (which measures antigen binding, rather than tissue sensitising activity); but similar antibodies were also detected in some patients who failed to show clear-cut symptoms of milk allergy, notably amongst infants who suffered from milk aspiration or recurrent respiratory disease. Perhaps, therefore, the suggestion of Bleumink and Young (1968) is justifiable; that a distinction can be made as far as milk allergy is concerned between hypersensitivity in which precipitating antibodies (presumably of the non-γE-type) directed against milk protein antigens are involved, and atopic conditions mediated by γE antibodies. In support of this idea, they quote the findings of Goldman et al. (1963); which indicate that atopic children showing clinical symptoms of rhinitis, asthma and atopic dermatitis – in whom there was a close correlation between skin reactivity to milk protein fractions and reactions to oral challenge with the same proteins – did not possess a higher incidence of milk precipitating antibodies than normal (non-allergic) individuals and non-milk sensitive atopic individuals.

It could yet turn out, however, that non-γE-type sensitising antibodies were involved, similar to those suspected of being implicated in some cases of drug allergy; and, in this case, it is possibly of some significance that total serum IgE levels (estimated by R.I.S.T) have not been found raised in the small number of milk-sensitive individuals' sera so far examined in my laboratory (referred to in the previous chapter). Furthermore, PCA testing in monkeys detected reaginic (γE) antibodies in only about a third of a group of sera from milk-sensitive individuals (Parish 1969); although this might merely reflect the relative insensitivity of this type of assay compared with P–K testing, for example.

It is against this back-ground of uncertainty about the nature and role of the mediating antibody, that attempts have been made to identify and characterise the allergenic constituents of milk and other prominent food stuffs such as eggs and fish. The findings from such studies have often been confused, however, as a result of the use of ill-defined commercial protein fractions in dubious states of purity; Vaughan and Kabat's (1953) serological demonstration of at least 2 minor contaminating antigens in repeatedly crystallised ovalbumin obviously not having been heeded as a warning.

Hence, it was encouraging to see recent reports of comprehensive fractionations of cow milk (Bleumink and Young 1968) and egg white (Bleumink and Young 1969); where processed (i.e. pasteurised) milk and boiled eggs have been used as starting materials as well as the raw protein mixtures. Because, in this type of study, it has not always been recognised seriously that the protein is usually ingested in a denatured (or, at least, partly denatured) form; and that degradation products resulting from such denaturation might be involved in allergenicity.

The 'balance sheet' from a fractionation of pasteurised cow milk is reproduced in table 3.4; which clearly points to the major allergenic activity being associated with the β-lactoglobulin fraction (of 36 000 molecular weight, containing 0.1–1.0 per cent hexose), and substantiates earlier observations of the involvement

TABLE 3.4
Yields, protein compositions and skin reactivities of fractions obtained from pasteurised cow's milk [1] (from Beumink and Young 1968).

Fraction	Yield [2]	Protein composition [3]	Skin reactivity [4] (units/mg)
VM 1	32.5 g	casein and traces of whey proteins	<100
VM 2	2.5 g	whey proteins	500
VM 3	750 mg	(eu)globulins, serum albumin, [5] α-lactalbumin [5], β-lactoglobulin [5]	<100
VM 4	850 mg	serum albumin, α-lactalbumin, two not further identified components and small amounts of β-lactoglobulin	500
VM 5	500 mg	β-lactoglobulin	2500
VM 8	800 mg	proteose fraction [5]	<100

[1] Commercially pasteurized milk.
[2] Yields per litre of milk.
[3] As identified with the aid of agar and starch gel electrophoresis and immuno-electrophoresis.
[4] Average skin reactivities of 5 atopic patients with a positive skin test to milk.
[5] (Partly) denaturated components.

TABLE 3.5
Yields and skin reactivities of protein fractions from fresh egg white (from Bleumink and Young 1969).

Fraction	Eluted at *p*H	Identified protein components [1]	Yield	Skin reactivity (units/mg) [2]	Total activity
VE 8	starting material	egg white	200	50000	100 $\times 10^5$
VE 9	*p*H 4.4	ovomucoid	15	360000	54 $\times 10^5$
VE 10	4.6–5.0	ovalbumin A 1, 2 and 3	115	15000	17 $\times 10^5$
VE 11	7.0	conalbumin, 1 and 2 traces of ovalbumin	20	<1000	<0.2 $\times 10^5$
VE 12	8.0	ovoglobulins	5	5000	0.25 $\times 10^5$
VE 13	10.0	ovoglobulins, lysozyme, traces of ovalbumin and conalbumin	10	60000	6 $\times 10^5$
ovalbumin A 1, 2 and 3 3 times recrystallized				5000	

[1] Identified with the aid of starch- and agar gel electrophoresis.
[2] Average activity in 6 patients.

of this constituent based on oral provocation and skin testing (Goldman et al. 1963A and B) and on PCA testing in baboons (Parish 1967). Crystalline β-lactoglobulin, on the other hand, showed a much lower activity in atopic individuals giving positive skin reactions to cow milk. This observation is explicable in terms of the hypothesis (Bleumink and Young 1968) that browning reactions, occurring between lactose and proteins during pasteurisation, storage and household handling, can lead to the formation of N-glycosidic linkages which greatly enchance the allergenic activity of the β-lactoglobulin constituent (an idea which will be returned to later, in § 3.4).

A similar approach to the isolation of allergenic components of boiled eggs (Bleumink and Young 1969) has shown (tables 3.5 and 3.6) that activity is associated mainly with an ovomucoid fraction, on the basis of skin tests performed in 33 egg-sensitive individuals.

TABLE 3.6
Carbohydrate compositions of skin reactive fractions from fresh egg white (from Bleumink and Young 1969).

Preparation	Isolated from	Skin reactivity (units/mg)	Inhibitor activity [1]	Hexose content [2]	Hexosamine content [3]	Sialic-acid content [4]
VE 1	white from boiled eggs	200000	5.7	5.1	n.d.	n.d.
VE 6	ibidem purified	300000	6.6	7.1	14.9	0.63
VE 8	white from fresh eggs	50000	1.0	2.7	n.d.	n.d.
VE 9	ibidem purified	360000	8.0	6.3	14.7	0.60
ovomucoid	prepared after Lineweaver and Murray		8–9	6.0	14.5	0.60
Literature values			9–10	6–8	15.4	0.50

[1] Trypsin inhibitor activity, expressed in units/mg dry weight; one unit is defined as the activity of one mg of freeze-dried egg white. BAAE was used as substrate.
[2] Assayed after Bruckner, expressed as percentage galactose.
[3] Assayed after Antonopoulos, expressed as percentage N-acetylglucosamine.
[4] Assayed after Warren, expressed as percentage N-acetylneuraminic acid.

This substance, interestingly, possesses a molecular weight (31 500) of a similar order to that of β-lactoglobulin and it contains small amounts (0.6 per cent) of N-acetyl neuraminic acid as well as about 6 per cent hexose and 14.5 hexosamine. In addition to the ovomucoid fraction, the lysozyme component of fresh egg white also appeared to show allergenic activity. This was attributable, however, to a non-specific irritant effect; a conclusion which is supported by observations made in my own laboratory (Keogh and Stanworth 1972) during attempts to induce isologous PCA reactions in rabbits using lysozyme as antigen.

Of the other principal food allergens, by far the most information is available about the chemical characteristics of the active constituents of fish, as a result of the thorough and painstaking investigations of Aas (1968) and his associate in Norway. A highly active allergenic fraction (DS 22) has been isolated from cod

(*Gadus callarias* L) white muscle tissue, being a protein of the myogen (sarcoplasmic) group; and identified by oral ingestion tests as well as by direct skin testing and cross-neutralisation P–K tests. N-terminal (Arg) and C-terminal (Arg, Asp and Glu) amino acid analyses have been performed (Elsayed and Aas 1970); and it has been shown by gas liquid chromatography to contain small amounts of pentose and hexoses but not neuraminic (sialic) acid. Like most well characterised allergens, from other sources, it has been found to be relatively acidic; but its molecular weight was calculated (from S and D values) to be only about 14 500. More recently (Elsayed and Aas, 1971A) an even purer allergenic component (designated M), with an I.E.P. of 4.75, has been separated from 5 minor sub-constituents by iso-electric focusing and found to be representative of the parent DS 22 fraction. But it still appeared to be antigenically inhomogeneous, as indicated by the formation of multiple precipitin lines on immuno-diffusion testing against certain antisera raised against it; which, the authors feel, may represent molecular variants of a single protein. This highly purified protein was found to have retained the small amounts of pentose and hexoses present in the parent DS 22 fraction; but one of the minor highly allergenic components (with an I.E.P: of 4.85), separated from it by iso-electric focusing, was found to be completely devoid of any carbohydrate detectable by gas liquid chromatography (Elsayed et al. 1971).

This is an important observation because it suggests that a 'bound sugar' moiety is not directly involved in allergenic activity; contrary to my speculation of some years ago (Stanworth 1963), when considerably less data was available on the chemical composition of allergenic substances. It also casts considerable doubt on Berrens and Bleumink's (1965) proposal that allergens are characterised by the incorporation of 2-ketose sugars, and derivatives, linked to the amino groups of protein lysine residues through the carbon atom one position.

3.3.5 Allergenic drugs

Drug allergy presents problems to the investigator, at both the clinical and laboratory level, not encountered in other types of immediate hypersensitivity.

Throughout their life-spans most individuals are exposed to a wide array of prophylactic and therapeutic agents, varying from simple chemical compounds with haptenic potential to antigenic macromolecules such as natural and synthetic polypeptide hormones and polysaccharides like dextran. These are acquired not only directly, by injection or oral administration, but also accidentally by inhalation and ingestion (in milk and meat and other dairy products). Such exposure, over a latent period which can vary from a few weeks to a period of years, results in hypersensitisation in a small percentage of cases; and very occasionally the response takes the form of a fatal anaphylactic shock.

Consequently clinicians are wary of performing direct skin or provocation tests within the patient himself, a situation which gives rise to a sense of urgency to the current search for suitable in vitro alternative methods of diagnosing drug sensitivity. As already mentioned (in the previous chapter), however, simple techniques such as basophil degranulation have not proved as satisfactory for this purpose as was hoped, despite their early promise.

One can never be certain that negative findings from diagnostic tests are not due to a failure to challenge with allergen in a form in which it is active in the sensitised individual. To add to the difficulties, there is growing evidence that some drug reactions are not mediated in a classical manner by γE antibodies. Another complicating factor is the histamine liberating activity shown by certain drugs themselves. A particularly interesting example of this problem has been encountered in investigations in my own laboratory into the nature of the reactions seen in some patients who have been receiving a synthetic ACTH preparation (Synacthen) for rheumatoid and asthmatic conditions. Synthesis of this β^{1-24} polypeptide (see fig. 8.6a) provided a compound which, whilst retaining hormonal activity, was lacking those amino acid residues (25–39) with which the major antigenic activity of porcine ACTH was associated. But, unfortunately, this new compound was found to possess substantially greater histamine liberating activity than the whole β^{1-39} polypeptide (fig. 8.6a); because, whereas the de-

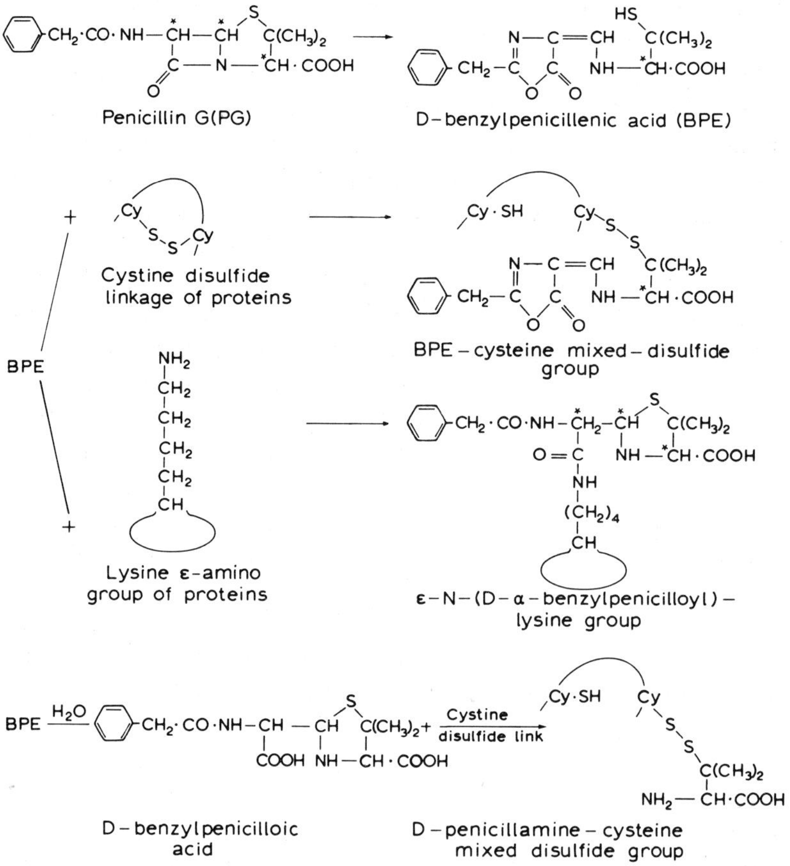

Fig. 3.8. Postulated routes of formation of several possible penicillin antigenic determinant groups. (Reproduced from Levine and Ovary 1961, by permission of the authors.)

leted amino acid residues were predominantly acidic, the residual 1–24 sequence contained a gross excess of basic residues.

Hence, the problem of identifying the true allergen is forever looming large over studies of drug allergy. This has been particularly so, of course, in the case of penicillin sensitivity; where it is supposed that various antigenic or haptenic forms arise in vivo (in a manner similar to that outlined in fig. 3.8). Studies on the mechanism of formation of antigenic penicillin in rabbits (Levine and Ovary 1961) have indicated that the N-(D-α-benzyl penicilloyl) group (BPO) is a major immunogenic determinant, being supposedly formed as a result of dissociation of penicillin G to D-benzyl penicillanic acid, which has the capacity to react directly with ϵ-amino groups of protein lysine residues to form a ϵ-N-(D-α-benzyl penicilloyl) lysine substituent (fig. 3.8). Further degradation of benzyl penicillanic acid leads to the formation of D-benzyl penicilloic acid which can react with free SH groups of proteins to form mixed disulphides of D-penicillamine (fig. 3.8). Moreover, it should be noted that penicilloic acid is but one of several derivatives (which include penicillanic disulphide, penicilloaldehyde and penicillamine) which are known to accumulate in penicillin preparations in vitro besides possibly forming from penicillin in vivo.

There is other chemical evidence to suggest, however, that penicillin itself may react directly with amino or hydroxyl groups, at neutral *p*H under physiological conditions, to form BPO determinants (Schneider and De Weck 1965, 1966; Batchelor et al. 1965); a consideration which is obviously pertinent to the problem of allergy to those penicillins (e.g. Penicillin V) which do not readily form penicillanic acid (Batchelor and Dewdney 1968). Moreover, the rate of direct reaction between penicillin and amino groups carriers measured in vitro is apparently sufficient to account for the formation of significant amounts of immunogenic conjugates over a period of several hours (De Weck 1968). But, as De Weck has also pointed out, rates of penicillin–carrier conjugation measured in vitro may have little relevance to the effective rates of conjugation in vivo; about which there is little information yet available.

To complicate the picture even further, there is evidence that a heterogeneous mixture of protein impurities, derived from the enzyme used in the manufacture of the highly purified 6-aminopenicillanic acid (6-APA) and from the fermentation of penicillin, could be important in the induction of allergenic reactions to the antibiotic (De Weck 1968; Batchelor and Dewdney 1968); as it has been shown to be strongly antigenic in animals and to be capable of evoking skin reactions in baboons and humans passively sensitised with penicillin sensitive individuals' sera (Stewart 1967). But, like the penicillin derivatives already mentioned, the haptenic specificity of this material is predominantly benzyl penicillolyl.

Yet another potential source of allergenicity are the 'polymer' forms, which have been observed in preparations of 6-APA and benzyl penicillin after removal of the penicilloylated protein impurity, and which rapidly appear in pure 6-APA preparations on solubilisation. It seems that such forms could also be involved in the elicitation of allergic responses, without being conjugated to a protein carrier (Batchelor and Dewdney 1968).

In any consideration of allergenic forms of penicillin it is also important to note that cross-reactivity with another group of antibiotics, the cephalosporins (Batchelor et al. 1965), might also be of some consequence.

In view of this wide variety of potential allergenic forms of penicillin, is not too surprising that the antibody response is also far from homogeneous. Although the benzyl penicilloyl grouping has been observed to be the major immunogenic determinant, at least 2 minor determinants are also effective. This underlines the importance, therefore, of allergen testing with both the major metabolite (BPO) and the minor ones (e.g. a mixture comprising benzyl penicillin G, benzyl penicilloate and benzyl penilloate); particularly as there is evidence that immediate allergic reactions are mediated by skin sensitising antibodies directed against minor determinants, whereas late urticarial reactions are mediated by BPO-specific sensitising antibodies (Levine 1966). In other words, patients showing positive responses to specific skin testing against minor determinants appear to be those with the highest risk of an immediate allergic reaction (including anaphylaxis) to penicillin (Levine and Zolov 1969).

The nature of the antibody involvement in allergic reactions to penicillin is still far from clear. There has been a tendency to attach too much weight to the findings from direct skin testing; and to rely on in vitro systems, such as lymphocyte transformation testing, which are unlikely to provide a measure of the atopic state of the patient. Moreover, even established passive sensitisation systems for the measurement of γE-type antibodies such as monkey ileum preparations in organ baths (Kunz et al. 1967), have not always been used to greatest effect.

It is interesting to note that in an investigation of 53 patients with proven penicillin allergy, only 16 (i.e. 30 per cent) were found to possess γE antibodies in their sera as indicated by PCA testing in baboons (Pedersen–Bjergaard 1969); whilst 29 of the patients' sera produced P–K reactions in normal human recipients. It seemed that reaginic antibodies are often present in such low titres in the sera of penicillin-sensitive individuals that they are only demonstrable by P–K testing; but even then in only 55 per cent of the cases investigated in this study. Similar findings resulted from attempts to sensitise human and monkey lung preparations with penicillin-sensitive individuals' sera, a poor correlation being found between direct skin reactivity to benzyl penicillin or penicilloyl-polylysine (Assem and Schild 1968). As these authors have suggested, therefore, it would seem to be important in the investigation of penicillin sensitivity to obtain a measure of tissue-bound reaginic antibody (by direct skin testing and leucocyte testing) as well as of circulating reagin. The practice which they have adopted of performing a passive lung sensitisation test (with the patient's blood) and direct leucocyte challenge in sequence, only proceeding to direct skin testing if the latter assay is negative, has been devised to ensure maximum safety and convenience to the patient.

As already mentioned in ch. 2, radio-immunosorbent assay of total serum IgE levels in the sera of drug-sensitive individuals has not proved very revealing. We have, however, observed an elevated IgE level of 1080 ng/ml (determined by R.I.S.T.) in a post-mortem serum specimen from a patient who suffered a fatal anaphylactic reaction to benzyl penicillin (Crystapen). Moreover, although PCA reactions were induced in baboons after short term sensitisation (3 hr) with the patient's serum on subsequent challenge with benzyl penicillin (Solupen), much more intense blueing reactions were observed by challenge after the longer sensitisation period (e.g. 27 hr) used for detection of γE antibodies. Taking the elevated serum IgE levels and the results of the PCA testing together, therefore, it seemed reasonable to conclude that this particular case of penicillin sensitivity was mediated by γE-type antibodies; a conclusion which was later substantiated by the demonstration that PCA activity could be blocked by co-administration of excess human myeloma γE-globulin with the sensitising serum. It seems likely, however, that non-γE-type sensitising antibodies might prove to be implicated in other cases; and that these would be detectable perhaps by their capacity for the short-term (2–4 hr) sensitisation of primate tissue; and in their stability towards heat treatment (Kunz et al. 1967). It is certainly not sufficient to conclude, as some investigators of potential cases of drug allergy tend to do, that the mere presence in the serum of drug-binding antibodies is indicative of hypersensitivity.

Another factor which could well be contributing to the difficulty of demonstrating sensitising antibody responses in some penicillin-sensitive individuals might well be the presence of inhibitory monovalent (haptenic) molecules in the challenge preparations; which have a capacity to combine with antibodies directed against the allergenic compound but lack the ability to elicit an immediate hypersensitivity response (De Weck 1968). As the sensitising antibodies in the sera of different penicillin-sensitive individuals have been shown to vary in their specificity for various penicillin derivatives, it is conceivable that such an inhibitory effect might be effective in some cases but not others. Moreover, it has been suggested that it is also operative in vivo, thus explaining the observation that penicillin may be tolerated even in patients who have clear-cut immediate type hypersensitivity to the BPO group (as revealed by skin testing with BPO polylysine).

Whilst on the subject of drug sensitivity, it is worth considering another aspect, which so far has received little attention. This concerns the suspicion that certain adjuvants used in drug preparations, although supposedly inert, might play some role in the induction of allergic reactions. For instance, it has been noticeable that reactions to the ACTH preparation 'Synacthen' have been recorded in patients who have received long-acting preparations incorporating a zinc phosphate complex (depot). Owing to its insolubility it is difficult to analyse, but it is conceivable that such a compound would under certain circumstances be capable of forming soluble 'multi-valent' aggregates of the hormonal polypeptide. Moreover, the slow release necessary for efficient hormone action will also tend to encourage the production of anaphylactic antibodies (as will become apparent from recent studies of the experimental induction of immediate hypersensitivity discussed in ch. 6).

In this connection, it is also interesting to note that hypersensitivity to carboxy methyl cellulose (CMC), a weak cation-exchanger used in the laboratory for protein fractionation purposes, has been incriminated in fatal anaphylactic reactions occurring in cattle which had received commercial penicillin preparations in which the CMC had been incorporated to stabilise suspensions or to facilitate dissolution of crystalline penicillin (Leemann et al. 1969). As the incidence of such reactions in cattle increased markedly in the months following a foot-and-mouth vaccination campaign, it was considered possible that penicilloyl-protein conjugate formed during the preparation of the vaccine could be responsible for sensitisation of the cows to penicillin. Skin testing in allergic and non-allergic cows indicated, however, that hypersensitivity was directed primarily against CMC alone; and not even against the penicilloyl groups with which it conjugates.

This apparently strong allergenicity of CMC in cows, despite its lack of immunogenicity in man and weak immunogenicity in rodents, is attributed to a difference in capacity to metabolize the substituted cellulose derivative. In support of this interpretation, the authors quote findings from studies with synthetic polypeptides (Gill et al. 1967), which point to a striking relationship between the ability of a compound to be metabolized and its capacity to induce an immune response. The requirements for 'sensitogenicty' are not necessarily the same as those for immunogenicity, however; although an ability to be metabolized might be important for this activity, too.

The sensitising properties of pure polysaccharides, such as the dextrans (fig. 3.9) used as plasma volume extenders (and for other clinical purposes) are interesting in this respect; because of their absence of immunogenic impurities on the basis of testing in rabbits (Richter 1970) and because of their relative inertness. It was

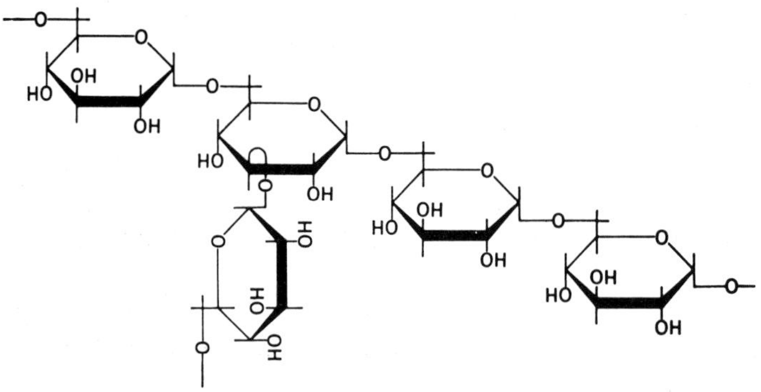

Fig. 3.9. Part of the structure of a typical dextran (a polymer of D-glucopyranose with predominantly α-(1–6) glucosidic linkages and α(1–3) cross-linkages).

found that the incidence of direct skin reactivity to straight chain dextrans is less than the incidence of reactivity to dextrans with more complex branched structures, from tests performed in individuals taken from among the high proportion of the population who have developed a reactivity to the polysaccharide naturally in the absence of deliberate contact (Kabat et al. 1957). Moreover, the ability of dextrans to induce sensitisation in humans has been found to be dependent upon molecular weight (Kabat and Bezer 1958). This has led to the development of a relatively low molecular weight dextran, with the result that anaphylactic reactions following clinical infusion have become very rare.

It is interesting that the mechanism governing such reactions in humans has been likened to hypersensitivity reactions induced in rats (Ingelman et al. 1969), presumably involving anaphylatoxin formation (table 8.2). This could explain the failure to demonstrate isologous tissue sensitising antibodies in the sera of dextran-sensitive humans. But in this connection the observations of Yount et al. (1968), to be referred to again in ch. 5, would seem to be of some significance. These have indicated that the inability of dextran-sensitive individuals' sera to induce PCA reactions in heterologous guinea pig tissue is due to the whole of the anti-dextran response being confined to the only one of the 4 human γG subclasses (i.e. γG2) which lacks the ability to fix to guinea pig tissue.

It is tempting to speculate that antibodies of a similar sub-class are in some way implicated in the allergic reactions observed within dextran-sensitive individuals. It is also of possible significance in this connection that it appears to be impossible to induce an antibody response to pure (peptide free) dextran in rabbits; a species which seems to lack the capacity to produce immunoglobulin of a sub-class analogous to the γG2 sub-class of humans (Keogh and Stanworth 1972).

Nevertheless, high titred anti-dextran antisera have been produced in this species by prolonged immunisation with dextran covalently conjugated to protein, and used in some interesting studies (Richter 1971) on the structural basis of anaphylactogenic and antigenic activity of dextran fractions. In guinea pigs maximally sensitised passively with such antisera, fractions of molecular weight ($\overline{MW}$) 3 600 or larger proved anaphylactogenic; whereas non-anaphylactogenic fractions of lower molecular weight (e.g. 1 430) conferred protection from anaphylactic shock due to injection of higher molecular weight fractions. It remains to be established, however, whether this system is an acceptable model for the study of mechanisms of immediate hypersensitivity reactions to polysaccharides in humans.

3.3.6 Other allergenic substances

Allergenic substances originate, of course, from many other sources; such as vegetable dusts and fibres, seeds, moulds, insects and helminths to mention just a few.

The problems of chemical characterisation of the active constituents of these materials are similar to those encountered in the study of the allergens already discussed. Here, too, cross-contamination with allergenic substances of different origin can complicate investigations. To take an example, individuals showing clinical indications of sensitivity to cotton products have been found to give skin reactions to medium used in the culture of micro-organisms (such as the fungus *Stachybotrius*) which are known to frequent cotton fibres (Taylor, G. personal communication). Furthermore, bacteria and moulds such as *Aspergillus niger* and *Peni-*

cillium, have been detected in samples of fine dust obtained from waste material removed from cleaning machines used in the processing of different grades of cotton (Furness and Maitland 1952); observations which have attracted the interest of investigators of aetiological factors involved in byssinosis.

As none of the allergenic constituents of the materials mentioned above have been adequately identified or characterised yet they will not be considered further in the context of the present discussion; which is concerned particularly with comparisons of the structures and properties of allergens derived from different sources. In this connection it is worth mentioning briefly, however, an allergenic constituent of the mould *Trichophyton* which has been investigated chemically in some detail (Barker et al. 1963); as this seems to differ strikingly in composition from all the other well characterised inhalant and food allergens (listed in table 3.7). Surprisingly, the main allergenic component of *Trichophyton mentagrophytes*, which apparently possessed the ability to induce both immediate and delayed types of hypersensitivity reactions in individuals infected by the dermatophyte, is a galactomannan-peptide comprising D-galactose (9 per cent), D-mannose (73 per cent) and peptide (9 per cent). Moreover, chemical and enzymic degradation studies suggested that the carbohydrate rather than the peptide was involved in immediate allergenic activity; whereas, in contrast, the protein portion of other well characterised glycoprotein allergens seems to be implicated in allergenic activity. It will obviously be important, therefore, to investigate this system further, in the light of more recently acquired knowledge about the mechanism of immediate hypersensitivity reactions, to establish that a true γE-mediated response is involved.

Finally, it would seem to be appropriate to mention here the question of new types of allergenic material to which individuals are becoming exposed for the first time. Ultimately, of course, it is to be hoped that the work discussed in this chapter will lead to the possibility of predicting the allergenic potential of new commercial products on the basis of their known structures. Until then, the approach adopted is inevitably an arbitrary one. Even so, it might have been anticipated that proteolytic enzyme preparations (whether originating from *B.subtilis* or other organisms) would contain or produce protein cleavage fractions with similar structural characteristics to those of typical allergenic substances; particularly if such preparations are contaminated with fragments of the parent bacteria themselves (as is claimed by Dubos 1971). Moreover, it could be expected that the inclusion of detergents in these mixtures would contribute to the formation and deleterious effects of such products, by promoting denaturation and cleavage besides facilitating their ready entry into the nasal passages of exposed individuals. It is not altogether surprising, therefore, that reports have appeared in the literature under such titles as 'Enzyme asthma, an occupational disease of laundry detergent workers' (Slavin and Lewis 1971).

Although such factory workers as well as the occasional housewife have been shown to give positive reactions to direct skin testing with alkaline proteinases of *B.subtilis* (Belin et al. 1970), it has yet to be established that their clinical manifestations are mediated by γE antibodies. An alternative suggestion that precipitating antibodies are in some way implicated (Pepys et al. 1969), in a similar manner to their supposed involvement in the allergic reactions shown by patients with bronchopulmonary aspergillosis and related conditions, also needs further investigation. It will be important, too, to consider the possibility that individuals with deficiencies in trypsin-inhibitors are more vulnerable to sensitisation by *B.subtilis* enzyme preparations; because there is some evidence that the sensitogenicity of these proteinases is enhanced by their proteolytic activity.

3.4 Structural basis of allergenic activity

In the light of my observations in the previous section (3.3) it is reasonable to ask whether there are structural characteristics common to all allergens, despite their diverse origins, which distinguish them from other types of antigenic substances.

It is possible to start to answer fundamental questions of this sort by two approaches. Firstly, by comparing the characteristics of

TABLE 3.7

Summary table, comparing properties of well-defined allergens from different sources (referred to in § 3.3).

Allergen	Symbol	Mol. wt.	S^0 ($S \times 10^{13}$)	% N	Acidic/ basic amino acid ratio	Carbohydrate composition			Enrich- ment factor	Reference
						%	hexose-pentose components	other sugar derivatives		
Horse dander	b_2S	34 000	3.43	10.2	2.6	13.9	Gal, Man	Nac. Glu (1.50%); NGNA (3.52%)	1.3	Stanworth (1957)
Ragweed pollen	E	37 800	3.05	17.1	1.9	0.5	Ara		40	King et al. (1964)
Ragweed pollen	K	38 200		16.6	1.7	0.6	Ara			King et al. (1967)
Ragweed pollen	Ra3	15 000	1.80	13.5	1.1	12.4	Ara			Underdown and Goodfriend (1966)
Rye grass pollen	IB	34 000	2.89	13.2	1.3	5.4	Gal, Man (Xyl)			Johnson and Marsh (1966A,B)
Rye grass pollen	IIB	11 000	1.36		1.3					
Cod myogen	DS 22	14 500	1.4		1.7	0.7–1.3	Gal, Glu, Man			Elsayed and Aas (1970)
	M Comp						Rib, Gal, Glu, Rib			Elsayed et al. (1971)
Cow milk	VM 5	38 000	2.7			3.0	Gal		5	Bleumink and Young (1968)
(β lacto-globulin)		36 000	2.7		1.9	0.1				
Egg white	VE 9	31 500	2.62			6.3	Gal, Man	Nac. Glu (14.7%); NANA (0.60%)	~ 7	Bleumink and Young (1969)
(Ovomucoid)						6.0	Gal, Man	Nac. Glu (14.5%); NANA (0.60%)		

those naturally occurring allergens which have been investigated in some detail, along the lines outlined already; and, secondly, by studying the reactivity of model allergenic compounds in humans and animals. In the latter approach it is, of course, essential to ensure that the anaphylactic-type reactions observed are mediated in the same fashion as true immediate hypersensitivity responses; a requirement which is not always fulfilled.

Turning first to an examination of the properties of the well-characterised allergens, referred to in table 3.7, it is apparent that these substances are by no means structurally identical as far as amino acid and carbohydrate composition is concerned. A variability in primary amino acid sequence is also indicated by differences in their susceptibility to proteolytic digestion; for example, unlike rye grass pollen allergenicity (Marsh et al. 1966), the activity of ragweed allergens is destroyed by pepsin (King and Norman 1962). A high degree of qualitative, as well as quantitative, variation is seen also in the carbohydrate moieties of the purified allergens; and, as mentioned earlier, a highly purified allergenic constituent has now been isolated from cod fish which appears to be completely devoid of any carbohydrate.

It seems reasonable to conclude, therefore, that there is no common primary structural denominator as far as allergenic activity is concerned; despite the claims of Berrens and his associates (Berrens 1971) that N-glycosidic protein-sugar linkages incorporated into the allergen structure during decomposition reactions of the Maillard type fulfil such a role. The evidence put forward in support of this hypothesis, based mainly on spectral analysis and enzyme-susceptibility testing of natural allergens and synthetic model compounds, needs substantiation by more direct investigations. Admittedly, it is interesting to note that the allergenic activity of the β-lactoglobulin constituent of cow milk, as measured by direct skin testing in milk-sensitive individuals, is increased as a result of synthetically incorporating N-glycosidically-bound lactose into the molecule (Bleumink and Berrens 1966). It is probably not without significance, however, that the blocking of free amino groups of the protein with reducing sugar profoundly influenced its net charge and charge distribution; and, moreover, heat changes occurring during the substitution process resulted in the unmasking of protein groupings and an increase in the sedimentation coefficient (S_{20}) from 2.8*S* to 3.7*S*. It seems perhaps a little premature, therefore, to attribute the observed change in skin reactivity of the β-lactoglobulin, following such treatment, to the presence of N-substituted 1 amino-l-deoxy-2 ketoses rather than to some secondary effect of the substitution process. If there is any real substance in such a claim it should be possible to show that any protein substituted in this manner becomes a potent allergen, as revealed by hypersensitisation testing in genetically suitable groups of experimental animals.

The well characterised allergens, nevertheless, show certain similarities in physico-chemical behaviour which probably reflect a similarity of tertiary and quaternary structure; and which, I am going to suggest, have an important bearing on their allergenic activity. As I pointed out in an earlier article (Stanworth 1963), it seemed more than coincidental that the sedimentation coefficients (and, therefore, the molecular size) of purified natural allergens invariably fell within a narrow range (of approximately 2–4*S*). Moreover, this conclusion has been strengthened by the sedimentation and molecular weight data reported for purified allergens which have been characterised since then (table 3.7); and even the molecular weights of the allergenic fractions of nematodes used in the experimental sensitisation of rabbits have been found to fall within a similar range (10–50 000).

Admittedly there appears to be one or two notable exceptions (i.e. ragweed allergen Ra3 and fish allergen M) to this rule, but it is possibly of some significance that both of these substances possess molecular weights which are approximately half of that of the allergens falling in the major molecular size group (of approximately 32–38 000). Could it be that they represent monomeric sub-units, which have become dissociated from a dimeric allergen during their isolation; but which have a capacity to re-associate under physiological conditions obtaining in the elicitation of immediate sensitivity reactions? It seems particularly interesting, in this connection, that β-lactoglobulin (the principal allergenic constituent of cow milk), although existing in a dimeric form (of

36 000 mol. wt) at moderate concentrations near its iso-electric point, has a tendency to dissociate into its monomeric sub-units (of 18 000 mol. wt) at certain *p*H values, temperatures and ionic strengths; whilst under other conditions (i.e. *p*H 4.6 and low temperatures) it octamerizes.

In view of these observations, it would be interesting to see whether other well-characterised allergens of similar molecular weight, such as horse dander allergen and ragweed allergen E, similarly dissociate into two sub-units under certain conditions; during, for instance, electrophoresis in SDS-polyacrylamide gels in the absence or presence of reducing agent. Pending the availability of such information, it is tempting to speculate that a 'dimeric' structure is an essential requirement for allergenicity; by analogy, for example, with the 2-unit structure which appears to be responsible for the hemagglutinating activity of the mitogenic constituents of certain lectins. Such an idea is entirely consistent with currently held views that the bridging by allergen molecules of adjacent cell-bound antibody molecules (fig. 3.10) is the crucial step in the initiation of anaphylactic reactions; a theme which will be returned to again in this section, and developed further in later chapters dealing with the role of the antibody in the mediation of immediate hypersensitivity reactions.

The suggestion that conformation factors play an important part in allergenic activity is supported by observations (King et al.

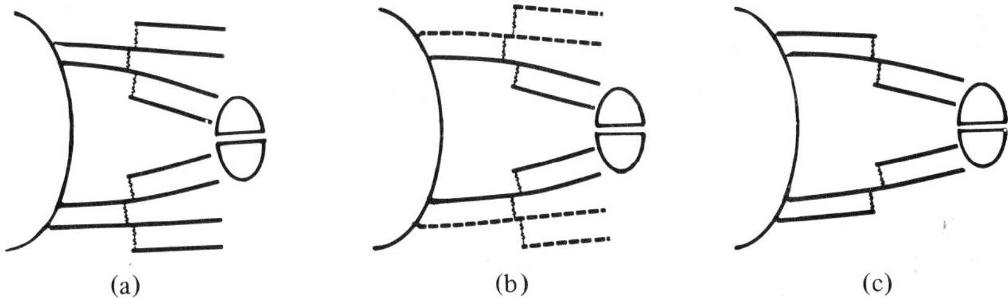

Fig. 3.10. Schematic illustration of the role of allergen in bridging adjacent cell-bound antibody in the initiation of anaphylactic reactions in the system comprising: (a) intact antibody; (b) hybrid antibody molecules, half of which comprise non-antibody sub-unit; (c) antibody molecules deficient in a Fab region (based on observations referred to in ch. 5).

1967) that the direct skin activity of ragweed allergen E is reduced by 10 000-fold, and its capacity to induce histamine release from sensitised human leucocytes is lost, as a result of reduction of its 3 disulphide bonds followed by alkylation. On the other hand, it should be mentioned that some evidence has been put forward (on the basis of inadequately controlled experiments) to suggest that the allergenic (and antigenic) activity of the cod fish allergen DS 22 is retained after reduction and alkylation (Elsayed and Aas 1971B). Obviously there is scope for more searching physico-chemical investigations of this and other highly purified allergens, to ascertain the precise role of quaternary structure in allergenicity. There seems to be no firm evidence in the literature of the occurrence of more than one type of polypeptide chain within an allergen structure; although, as mentioned earlier, end-terminal analysis revealed multiple C-terminal residues in cod allergen (DS22).

Apart from the suggestion of special quaternary structural characteristics, are there other requirements for allergenicity? Are there other structural features which distinguish allergens from the non-active antigenic proteins present in large amounts in most allergenic materials? Substitution of a high proportion of the ϵ-amino groups of the lysyl residues of ragweed allergen E by succinylation or acetylation, which greatly altered the charge as well as the conformation of the molecule, decreased both skin activity and the capacity for precipitin formation with specific rabbit anti-sera (King et al. 1967). This suggests that the allergenicity like the antigenicity depends upon the intactness of the ragweed E component structure. There are, on the other hand, reports of related types of investigation (notably by Marsh et al. 1970B), which, on cursory examination, seem to suggest that allergenicity can be divorced from antigenicity. It would seem to me, however, that the change effected in this work by treatment of rye grass allergen (Group I component) with formaldehyde and other amino-reactive agents, are of a quantitative rather than a qualitative nature; and that the production of 'allergoids' (with a view to the immunotherapy of atopic humans) is essentially a question of modifying a sufficient number of antigenic determinants on the allergen molecule, but without destroying all of the original determinants.

It is, therefore, still conceivable that one of the main requirements for allergenicity is that of a minimum number of antibody-binding (i.e. antigenic) determinants on the provoking molecule. In the light of my earlier suggestion, of a dual sub-unit allergen structure, the minimum number of antigenic determinants would be one on each of the 2 sub-units. This is entirely consistent with the 'bridging' idea (Ovary and Taranta 1963); which specifies that it is necessary to cross-link pairs of antibody molecules of similar antigen specificity, on adjacent sites on the target cell, by spanning them with a single antigen (allergen) molecule in order to initiate an anaphylactic response. Evidence in support of a mechanism of this type has come both from observations on the anaphylactic properties of artificial 'univalent' γG-type antibodies (an aspect which is summarised schematically in fig. 3.10, and which will be considered further in ch. 5); as well as from studies of the allergenicity in sensitised humans and animals of single and multivalent hapten-polypeptide conjugates. Penicilloyl-polylysine conjugates (Levine 1965A and B; De Weck and Schneider 1968) have featured prominently in the latter approach; which has indicated that neither the degree of substitution, nor the size of the carrier, markedly influence the efficiency of the allergen provided that it possesses at least 2 antigenic determinants.[2] Equimolecular concentrations of divalent and multivalent hapten-carriers (of the type illustrated in fig. 3.11) were found to be equally effective in inducing PCA reactions in guinea pigs passively sensitised with rabbit antibodies of comparatively high binding affinity; but for effective elicitation of PCA reactions in animals sensitised with antibodies of low affinity more than 2 (and preferably 3 to 6) haptenic groups per allergen molecule were required (Levine 1965B). Moreover, these should be sited relatively close together. In contrast, precipitin formation and the induction of passive Arthus reactions depended upon the formation of large cross-linked antibody–antigen complexes.

Similar observations have been made from studies of the weal and erythema responses of penicillin-sensitive humans to multi-

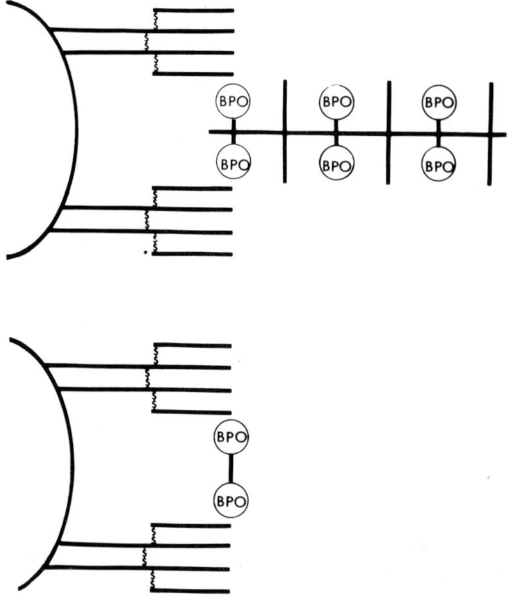

Fig. 3.11. Hapten-carrier conjugates used in the study of the structural requirements for allergenicity.

functional derivatives of penicillanic acid (Parker et al. 1962B). Multivalent penicilloyl-lysine conjugates were found to be about as effective as penicilloyl-protein conjugates (e.g. penicilloyl$_{60}$ bovine γG-globulin); but small divalent derivatives (e.g. bis-penicilloyl cystine) of molecular weights less than 1500 were relatively ineffective, as likewise were bis-DNP lysine derivatives, in evoking PCA reactions in sensitised guinea pigs because of the relatively low hapten-affinity of the antibodies involved (Parker et al. 1962A, C).

On the other hand, there have been reports that monovalent haptens are capable of eliciting anaphylactic reactions in sensitised guinea pigs; but all of these observations have been attributed to a capacity of the compounds tested to aggregate in vivo and to some extent in vitro (De Weck and Schneider 1969). In other words, they are thought not to be truly monovalent. Another possible complicating factor in the interpretation of results obtained from these sort of studies is the capacity of polylysines, and lowly substituted polylysines, to enter into electrostatic interactions with proteins as a consequence of their strongly cationic nature; which might perhaps lead to the formation of mixed 'specific antibody-polypeptide-non-specific protein' complexes in vivo (De Weck and Schneider 1968). The polycationic nature of polylysines is also responsible for their capacity to evoke non-specific release of histamine from mast cells (ch. 8); which probably explains why the non-specific skin reactivity shown by some hapten-polylysine conjugates could be abolished by succinylation of their free ϵ-amino groups.

Nevertheless, despite these reservations, and with the qualification that non-γE antibodies are quite probably operative in some of the skin reactions observed in drug-sensitive humans as well as in artificially sensitised animals, the studies with model allergenic compounds have contributed new knowledge about the structural basis of the activity of natural allergens; besides indicating possible areas of practical application in the field of drug allergy.

The elicitation of PCA reactions (in sensitised guinea pigs) by divalent hapten conjugates as small as di-benzyl-penicilloyl hexamethylene diamine (fig. 3.11), with a molecular weight as small as 788, as well as with much larger multivalent haptens (e.g. $BPO_{88}-PLL_{402}S$) might seem to be in conflict with my earlier observation that natural allergens possessed molecular sizes falling within a relatively narrow range. But this possibly reflects less stringent configurational requirements for γG-mediated anaphylactic reactions than those involving γE antibodies, a topic which will be considered in some depth in ch. 5. Even discounting this factor, however, the two observations are not necessarily incompatible. It could be that all natural allergens are of such a size and shape that they possess duplicate antigenic determinants, with strong affinities for γE antibodies, symmetrically sited at the critical distance for cross-linking of adjacent cell-bound antibody molecules; a requirement which would be most readily met by the possession of a 'dimeric' structure like that of β-lactoglobulin (as was discussed earlier). This is, of course, precisely the situation which obtains in the elicitation of reverse PCA reactions by rabbit γG antibodies against γG-globulin; because these antibody molecules possess one combining site for the cell-bound immunoglobulin in each half (i.e. in each Fab region) as is illustrated schematically in fig. 5.9. The obvious implication is that natural allergens are likewise symmetrical molecules, with the 2 halves each containing one or more γ-globulin-reactive (i.e. antigenic) determinant, and linked perhaps by an inter-chain disulphide bridge as are the half molecules of rabbit IgG.

Recent observations made in my own laboratory (Stanworth et al. 1971) are possibly of some relevance in this connection. We were able to show that anaphylactic reactions could be induced in ileum preparations of guinea pigs which had been sensitised specifically to aggregated (20–40*S*) human IgG only by challenge with the polymerised protein which contained aggregate-specific determinants. Monomeric (7*S*) IgG was, however, capable of inhibiting such reactions; presumably because it was acting like a monovalent 'hapten', such as monovalent penicilloyl conjugates which have been shown to inhibit anaphylactic reactions in guinea pigs elicited by multivalent derivatives (De Weck and Schneider 1969). Hence, despite their relatively huge size (of the order of $1-2 \times 10^6$ molecular weight), and lack of artificially substituted hapten groups, polymerised forms of IgG seem to be capable of initiating histamine release from sensitised cells by bridging adjacently sited antibody molecules in a similar manner to the supposed mode of action of small divalent hapten(BPO)-conjugates in BPO sensitised animals. This suggests that the polymerisation process brings together 'monovalent' monomer γG molecules into a polyvalent allergenic form; and that steric factors do not preclude cross-linking of cell-bound antibody molecules by this aggregate.

Low molecular weight, multivalent, benzyl penicilloyl-polylysine conjugates (e.g. containing 10–15 lysyl residues) have found practical application in the diagnosis of penicillin allergy because, whilst possessing the capacity to elicit skin reactions in the manner just discussed, they are nevertheless incapable of inducing anaphylactic antibody formation and thereby sensitising the patient (Levine 1966). They are, therefore, acting as true allergens but not as sensitogens.

There seems no reason to suppose, therefore, that the antibody-binding sites of allergens are in any way different chemically to those of antigens; but their manner of distribution on the protein back-bone could be of prime importance.

Another physico-chemical property common to most natural allergens is their acidic nature, indicated by their relatively high ratio of acidic (Glu, Asp) to basic (Lys, Arg, Hist) amino acid residues (table 3.7). An apparent exception to this generalisation is the low molecular weight ragweed pollen allergen fraction Ra3 (Underdown and Goodfriend 1969); which is a relatively basic glycoprotein, possessing some allergenic determinants in common with the major ragweed E allergen.

In view of the relationship which has been observed between the net electrical charge of antigens and specific (γG and γM) antibodies raised in rabbits (Sela and Mozes 1966), it is tempting to speculate that the relative similarity of electrical charge observed in natural allergens might reflect a role in determining the properties of the type of antibody which they elicit; particularly as Benaceraff and associates (1969) have proposed that a charged antigen exerts its effect by preferentially selecting and stimulating cells synthesising specific antibody of the opposite charge. Applying this idea indiscriminately to stimulation by allergens, however, it would be expected that the antibodies produced would be relatively basic, i.e. relatively slow moving on electrophoresis at *p*H 8.6 (and not fast γ-globulins as observed).

Nevertheless, in this connection, it is interesting to note the claims of Underdown and Goodfriend (1970), who have interpreted differences in the elution distribution patterns from DEAE Sephadex of human reaginic antibodies against ragweed allergens Ra3 and E as consistent with the assumption that their charges elicit preferentially the formation of γE antibodies of opposite charge (in agreement with the Sela and Mozes postulate, appertaining to γG antibodies of other species). Their claims would seem to be a little extravagant, however, because Sela and Mozes (1966) only observed clear-cut differences when using a common protein carrier substituted with positively or negatively charged haptens. In contrast, the amino acid composition of ragweed allergen Ra3 was found to be distinct from that of the ragweed allergen E (Underdown and Goodfriend 1969). Hence, the authors' alternative suggestion, that they were observing differences in antibody affinity rather than antibody concentration in the various chromatographic fractions, would seem to be a more plausible interpretation. It should also be mentioned that there has been a recent report of a lack of correlation between the net charge of antigen and antibody in guinea pigs immunised with charged DNB conjugates of polyamino acids (Nussenzweig and Green 1971).

This does not necessarily mean, however, that the charge on the allergen plays no role in its immunological activity in humans. On the contrary, it might facilitate its access to antibody bound on the negatively-charged target cell surface; which, incidentally, offers another explanation as to why substitution of the ϵ-NH_2 groups of the lysyl residues in β-lactoglobulin was found to potentiate its skin reactivity in milk sensitive individuals (Bleumink and Berrens 1966) as discussed earlier. Moreover, it seems particularly significant in this connection that studies of experimentally induced sensitivity to *Ascaris* in rats (Strejan and Campbell 1968) have indicated that homocytotropic antibodies are produced only against certain fractions, which display a negative charge at *p*H 8.6; and, furthermore, the intensity of the PCA response shown by such animals has been shown to increase with the electrophoretic mobility of the fraction (DEAE cellulose) used.

Attempts in my own laboratory to use the rabbit γG-globulin system for investigating the relationship between charge of antigens and specific isologous tissue sensitising antibodies were unsuccessful (Keogh and Stanworth 1972); although antibodies directed against positively and negatively charged hapten-protein conjugates were found to differ in composition as revealed by their susceptibility to digestion by papain under carefully controlled conditions. It was hoped, however, that it might have been possible to demonstrate the production of rabbit γ_1 isologous tissue sensitising antibody analogous to that found in the guinea pig. Moreover, if this had been found to be produced against antigens of one particular charge (a basic one, say) it would have been necessary to conclude that the nature of the antigen can influence an activity located in the Fc region of the antibody molecule; in contrast to its more usual effect on antigen-binding activity located in the Fab regions.

In summary, if one were asked to predict the structural characteristics of an ideal allergen on the basis of present evidence, one could justifiably suggest that it would be predominantly protein in nature, of relatively small molecular size (30–40 000 molecular weight) with a preponderance of acidic over basic amino acid residues; and probably with similar antigenic determinants, distributed in symmetrical fashion in 2 halves of the molecule, which were capable of inducing the formation of high affinity antibodies.

This does not preclude the possibility that 'common denominators', meeting these requirements, are widely distributed in a whole range of different allergenic materials. In this connection, it is perhaps worth referring back to my earlier comments (§ 3.3) about the detection of an α_2-macroglobulin in allergenic materials of widely different origin (horse dandruff, milk and egg white); all of which were shown to possess a constituent which cross-reacted serologically with human serum α_2-macroglobulin. For, it is probable that the same human serum macroglobulin component is also present in human dandruff, and might therefore be 'processed' in some way by mites growing on it; although, it should be added, that α_2-macroglobulin appeared to be absent from a human dandruff 'allergen' fraction isolated by Berrens (1971). In this connection, however, it is of considerable interest that a recent report (Slavin and Lewis 1971) suggests that potential allergenic determinants arise in bacillopeptidases (e.g. subtilopeptidase and subtilisin), used in enzyme-washing powder preparations, as a result of their interaction with the human α_2-macroglobulin component (as well as with α_1 trypsin inhibitor). All attempts in my laboratory to demonstrate α_2M-related antigens in pollen extracts have failed, however.

3.5 The nature of sensitogens

There is a tendency to equate 'allergenicity' with a capacity to sensitise, as well as with an ability to evoke immediate hypersensitivity reactions in pre-sensitised individuals. As I suggested in the Introduction, however, it seems to be more logical to refer to substances possessing the former property as 'sensitogens', by analogy with usage of the term immunogen.

The recent development of animal models of γE-mediated hypersensitivity (to be discussed in detail in ch. 6) is beginning to offer for the first time a direct means of defining those characteristics which are peculiar to sensitogens. In the meantime, one can only formulate a tentative picture of their structural and physical features, based on indirect observations.

It can be reasonably assumed that the physical size of inhalant sensitogens is of some importance; and, in particular, a capacity to become air-borne and to gain ready access to the nasal passages. Presumably inhalant sensitogens such as fragments of animal epidermal scales, cotton dust and other offending materials[3] behave in this respect like grass pollen grains (which have particles sizes ranging from about 16–58 μ diam.). Moreover, as mentioned earlier, such materials are most probably the 'vehicles' responsible for transport through the atmosphere of other sensitogenic substances (for example: micro-organisms, serum proteins etc.); which themselves might not possess the appropriate physical characteristics. From personal experience, it is remarkable how quickly an inhalant allergenic material such as horse dandruff can emanate through a laboratory and evoke an immediate reaction in the unsuspecting recipient; even when great care has been taken in opening its container. It is also of some relevance, in this connection, that at least one food allergen (the cod fish myogen component DS 22) has been found to be present in steam collected during its cooking (Aas and Jebsen 1967).

Present knowledge about the nature of the allergens referred to in the previous section has been obtained entirely from studies of soluble components isolated from aqueous extracts of the raw inhalant or ingestant material. It will be important to establish, however, the location of the active constituents within pollen grains (to take an example); and to determine whether they are directly involved in the initial sensitisation of suitably pre-disposed individuals, whilst still in their native form in the intact grain.

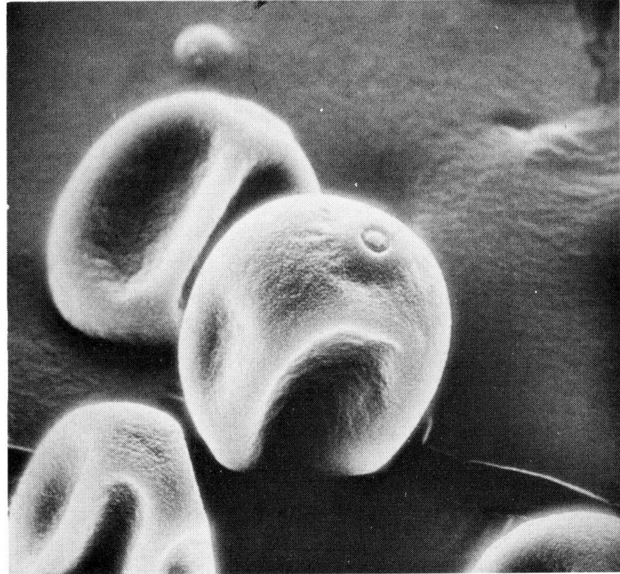

Fig. 3.12(a)

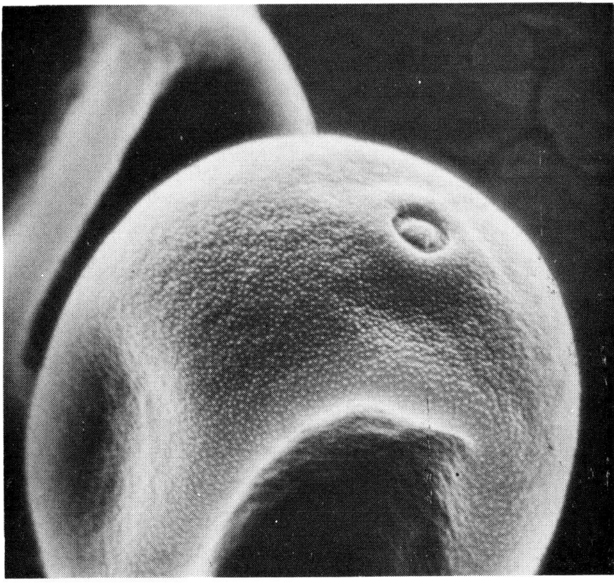

Fig. 3.12(b)

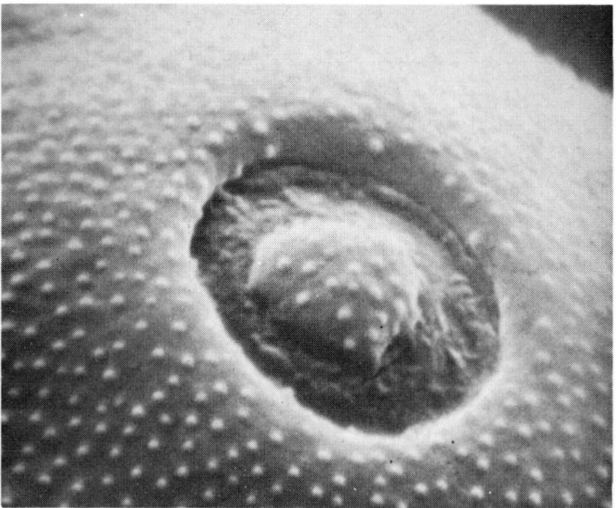

Fig. 3.12(c)

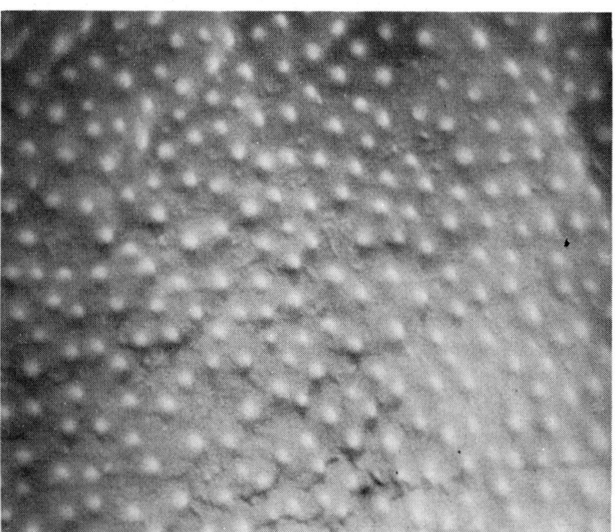

Fig. 3.12(d)

Fig. 3.12. Scanning electron microscope pictures of *P. pratensis* pollen grain: – (a) and (b) complete (× 1 200 and × 3 000); (c) showing germ pore (× 12 000); (d) surface detail (× 20 000) (kindly taken by Dr. A. Johnson).

The membranes of pollen and related spores are remarkably stable, both in a chemical and morphological sense (fig. 3.12); a property which is, of course, exploited in fossil pollen analysis. This can be attributed presumably to their predominant lipo-polysaccharide composition (Shaw and Yeadon 1966) which, in a wide variety of pollen and spore membranes, includes a relatively inert lignin-like fraction (in addition to 10–15 per cent cellulose and 55–65 per cent lipid). Consequently it seems unlikely that the allergenic constituents, which are globular proteins, are located on the outer membranes of the pollen grains (i.e. in the exine).

Despite, however, the chemical stability of the pollen membrane there is considerable evidence to suggest that these active constituents are readily accessible to extraction, in vivo as well as in vitro. This was apparent from the pioneering skin test studies performed a hundred years ago by Blackley (1873), who was himself a hayfever sufferer and who succeeded in evoking skin reactions on his forearms merely by rubbing grass pollen grains into abraded areas. It is also evident from much more recent studies (Johnson and Thorne 1958); which indicated that, even when extraction is performed on pollen grains without prior defatting, the allergenic constituents readily pass into aqueous solutions leaving the cell wall unimpaired (as revealed by microscopic examination).

In this connection, it is interesting to note that recent immunofluorescence studies (Knox et al. 1970) have confirmed earlier cytochemical observations (Knox and Heslop-Harrison 1969) that much of the protein detectable in short term (i.e. within minutes) leachates from intact pollen grains has probably been released from the inner layer of the wall (the cellulose intine); where proteins including enzymes such as acid phosphatase and RNA-ase can be detected by cytochemical procedures (Knox and Heslop-Harrison 1969). It seems possible therefore, that allergenic constituents of pollen grains are likewise located on the inner wall sites[4], rather than originating from within the cells; a point which would seem to be verifiable by immunofluorescence studies, using specific anti-allergen antisera. Perhaps they diffuse out through the germinal pores (fig. 3.12), through which a tube of protoplasm eventually passes at the time of fertilisation of the ovum; a possibility which would seem to be plausible in the light of recent observations (Knox and Heslop-Harrison 1971) that an important function of the pollen proteins appears to be concerned with sexual recognition.

Presumably a similar leaching out of allergenic constituents occurs from pollen grains which become lodged in the nasal mucosa, and in other potential sites of induction of a hypersensitivity response. It is conceivable that a relatively slow leaching out there, for example into the mucosal fluid, might represent a source of antigenic stimulation; which is potentiated perhaps by an adjuvant effect of the liposaccharide material in the walls of the pollen grains. Furthermore, protein antigen adsorbed on to aluminium hydroxide particles, an artificial sensitogen which has proved particularly effective in inducing anaphylactic antibody formation in experimental animals (ch. 6), could be mimicing this process.

But it should be noted that studies (Wilson et al. 1971) in which the fate of inhaled pollen (*Poa pratensis*), with its exine tagged with 99^{m}Tc (technetium), was followed for several hours in 5 asthmatics, indicated that the pollen was always deposited in the oropharynx and was rapidly swallowed; being detected almost immediately in the esophagus, stomach and later in the blood and urine. Radio-pollen was, however, never demonstrated in the lungs.

Notes

[1] Following a workshop held at the First International Immunology Congress (Washington, 1971) there has been a move amongst those actively involved in allergen characterisation to establish a universally acceptable nomenclature system for purified allergens.

[2] In this connection it is interesting to note that Richter, W. (Int. Arch. Allergy in Press) has recently shown that isomaltodecaose is the smallest oligosaccharide unit capable of eliciting PCA reactions in guinea pigs maximally sensitised with rabbit antibody against dextran-protein conjugate.

[3] Eg. mite faecal pellets (20 μ diam.) are very similar in size to pollen grains and become air-borne in the same way (McAllen. M; personal communication).

[4] Experimental evidence of this in the case of the localization of the allergenic constituents in the pollen-grain walls of *Ambrosia* spp. (ragweeds) has recently been obtained by adoption of the approach suggested (Knox R.B. and Heslop-Harrison J.; Cytobios. 1971, *4*, 49).

CHAPTER 4

Isolation and characterisation of reagins

In the study of any immunological process it is, of course, essential to establish whether the phenomenon observed is antibody (as opposed to cell) mediated and, if so, to go on and characterise the antibodies concerned.

4.1 Background studies

Since Prausnitz (1921) first demonstrated the transfer of immediate hypersensitivity by local injection of hypersensitive individuals' sera, innumerable attempts have been made to isolate and identify the humoral sensitising factor. Practically every technique developed by the protein chemist for the fractionation of plasma proteins has been applied to this task, at some time or other. Until recently, however, progress was frustratingly slow, in comparison with the great strides which have been made in the isolation and characterisation of other types of antibody. This was due to the extremely low level of reaginic antibodies in allergic sera, and to an inability to assay their activity by conventional methods of measuring antibody–antigen combination. The lability of isolated reagin preparations has also presented problems.

The early application of physico-chemical techniques, such as free-solution electrophoresis and electrophoresis–convection, to the analysis of allergic sera provided conflicting information about the nature of their constituent reagins. Activity was found, by different investigators, to be associated with α, β and γ constituents (see summary table, page 206, in my review on reaginic antibodies, Stanworth 1963). Similarly, equivocal results were obtained by free-solution ultracentrifugal analysis of allergic sera (Stanworth 1963), involving the use of partition cells to retrieve active fractions. The limitations of this method of ultracentrifugal separation have been discussed elsewhere (Stanworth 1967).

In retrospect, it is not very surprising that such experimental procedures failed to provide definitive information about the physico-chemical characteristics of the minute amounts of reagins present in the sera fractionated. The protein detection systems employed in these essentially analytical methods were relatively insensitive. For instance, it is now calculated (on the basis of IgE levels determined accurately by the radio-immunosorbent test) that the schlieren optical system employed in commercial electrophoresis and ultracentrifugation apparatuses is about 3000 times too insensitive to detect the reaginic antibodies in human allergic sera. Hence, in all the early physico-chemical studies of these antibodies it was necessary to adopt a correlative approach (despite its many pitfalls), in which the distribution of skin sensitising activity amongst fractions of allergic sera obtained by various procedures was compared with the composition of readily definable components.

The emergence of zone-separation techniques has helped to overcome this problem. Their advantages, as far as the fractionation of reagins is concerned, lies in their greater resolution and in the stabilisation afforded to the boundaries of minor protein constituents by the use of solid media or density gradients. On the debit side, reagins have a tendency to become irreversibly adsorbed to some solid media such as starch and substituted celluloses. Nevertheless, application of such techniques provided the first convincing evidence that reagins moved in the fast γ (i.e. γ_1) region on electrophoresis, and in the $7S$ region on ultracentrifugation.

The information about the electrophoretic mobility was obtained by examination of the distribution of P–K activity in starch block electrophoresis fractions of allergic sera (Brattsten et al. 1955; Sehon et al. 1956); and in fractions separated by chromatography on diethyl amino ethyl (DEAE) cellulose (Humphrey and Porter 1957; Stanworth 1959). The sedimentation characteristics were deduced, also, by examination of the distribution of P–K activity in chromatographic fractions and in fractions obtained by a relatively crude zone-centrifugation procedure employing buffered sucrose gradients (Stanworth 1967); which confirmed that reagins were not macroglobulins as had been suggested by some investigators (on the grounds of their failure to get across the placenta). Moreover, it soon became apparent that the buffered sucrose medium exerted a useful protective effect on the separated reagin molecules.

These investigations were the beginning of many attempts to show that reaginic antibodies are representative of a particular class of immunoglobulin. Initially, the choice appeared to be between the 7*S* and macroglobulin (i.e. 19*S*) classes; although it was quite conceivable, from a knowledge of the behaviour of other types of antibody, that activity would prove to be associated with more than one class. The classification of human immunoglobulins was simplified, at around this time, by studies (e.g. Franklin and Stanworth 1961) of their pathological counterparts (isolated from the sera of patients with monoclonal gammopathies). This led to the development of specific antisera capable of distinguishing between immunoglobulins on the basis of the distinctive antigenic determinants located within their heavy chains. By use of these highly specific reagents in quantitative immunodiffusion procedures, it was now possible to measure accurately the amounts of different immunoglobulins within fractions of allergic sera; and to compare the results with the P–K activities of the same fractions.

This was the approach which I adopted, for example, in the studies of the properties of reagin against horse dandruff allergen referred to earlier (Stanworth 1959). Thus, I was able to show that the activity in zone-centrifugation fractions correlated reasonably well with the distribution of the γG component and not with the γM component. Similarly, it could be shown that maximal P–K activity was eluted from DEAE cellulose with a γG fraction (albeit after the major, electrophoretically slow, fraction had already been eluted) and not with the γM fraction, which could only be retrieved at a much later stage of the elution procedure by a drastic lowering of the *p*H and increasing of the ionic strength (fig. 4.1).

The discovery by Heremans (1960) of yet a third major class of immunoglobulin, the IgA or γA (originally termed β_2A and later γ_1A) immediately raised the question of reagins being representative of this class (Heremans and Vaerman, 1962). This was an attractive idea, in many ways, for here was a type of immunoglobulin which was found to be prevalent in nasal fluid, saliva and other body secretions where it was thought to be involved in a 'front-line' defence mechanism; and, moreover, like reagins, it was difficult to detect in cord blood. Physico-chemically, too, γA-globulin appeared to possess the right 'credentials', i.e. it moved in the fast γ region on electrophoresis and in the 7*S* region on ultracentrifugation, showing a tendency to polymerise on isolation which seemed to offer an explanation of the apparently divergent sedimentation characteristics revealed by the early partition-sedimentation analysis of allergic sera in free solution (referred to earlier in this chapter).

Immunological studies appeared to provide even more convincing evidence that reagins were γA-globulins. For instance, reaginic antibody activity was demonstrated in purified γA-globulin fractions isolated from allergic sera (Vaerman et al. 1964); and the removal of this immunoglobulin from such sera by absorption with specific (sheep) anti-γA-globulin antiserum removed also their reagin activity (Fireman et al. 1963), in contrast to absorption with antisera directed against the other major immunoglobulin classes. By means of the radio-immunoelectrophoresis technique, Yagi and associates (1963) detected γA-globulin antibodies directed against ragweed E allergen, in the sera of hypersensitive individuals. Moreover, it was shown that P–K activity could be blocked by normal human γA-globulin (Ishizaka et al. 1963), and by purified α chain (Ishizaka et al. 1964), if this was injected into a normal recipient's skin before passive sensitisation or simultaneously with the transferred reagin.

Admittedly, it was disconcerting to come across pollen-sensitive

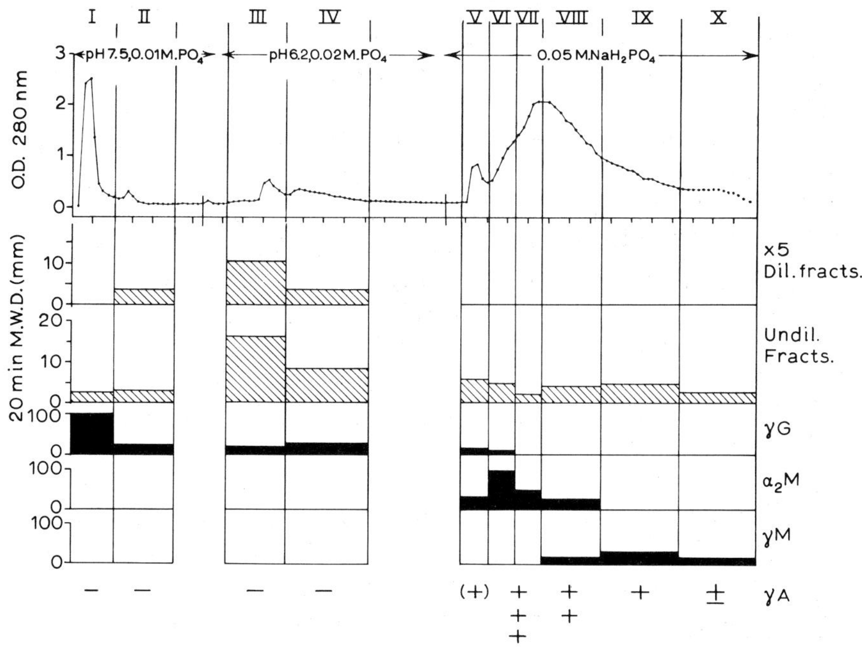

Fig. 4.1. Immunoglobulin composition and P–K activity of fractions of serum from a horse dandruff-sensitive individual, separated by DEAE cellulose chromatography using a step-wise elution procedure. (Reproduced from Stanworth 1965.)

individuals who contained no detectable γA-globulin in their serum (Loveless 1964), but this could always be attributed to the relative insensitivity of the immunodiffusion technique compared with the exquisitely sensitive P–K indicator system. There was, however, one other discordant note, as I pointed out at the time (Stanworth 1965A and B). As is seen in fig. 4.1, the maximum recovery of reagin (i.e. P–K) activity in fractions of allergic sera separated by DEAE cellulose chromatography occurred in a fraction in which γA-globulin could not be detected by means of rabbit antiserum directed specifically against this class of immunoglobulin. In my experience, the γA-globulin component could only be retrieved from the ion-exchange column (in a step-wise elution procedure) by lowering the *p*H (below 6.2) and by increasing the ionic strength (above a phosphate molarity of 0.02 M).

Could it be, then, that reagin was, after all, a unique class of immunoglobulin – a prospect which I suggested sometime ago in a review article (Stanworth 1963)? In attempting to reconcile the apparently conflicting chromatographic data with the evidence supporting the IgA nature of reagins, which I have already outlined, it is important to recognise that the findings on which the evidence was based were not unequivocal. For, owing to the far superior sensitivity of the P–K test, it was quite conceivable that reagin was present in active IgA fractions from allergic sera at a level far below the limit of detection of a conventional immunodiffusion technique. Conversely, antisera raised against such fractions might contain (unsuspectingly) antibodies directed against a reagin contaminant, which would not be demonstrable by the ordinary Ouchterlony or immunoelectrophoresis procedures.

Later studies by Ishizaka and his associates showed that this was, indeed, the probable explanation of their own and other investigators' observations on the supposed γA nature of reaginic antibodies. When rabbit anti-human IgA antiserum (rather than sheep anti-IgA) was used in absorption studies, reagin was not removed from allergic individuals' sera (Ishizaka et al. 1966C). Moreover, the anti-ragweed γA antibody demonstrable in allergic individuals' sera by radio-immunoelectrophoresis was shown not to correlate with their skin sensitivity activities (Ishizaka et al. 1966A; Reisman et al. 1965). Ishizaka and Ishizaka (1966), confirmed my own earlier observations on the lack of correlation between reagin activity and γA-globulin distribution in DEAE cellulose chromatographic fractions of allergic sera; and showed that essentially all P–K activity remained in the supernatant fluid after precipitation of the γA-globulin from reagin-rich fractions by means of specific antiserum. Their earlier findings on the P–K blocking activity of γA-globulin were also reversed, it now being shown (Ishizaka and Ishizaka 1966) that none of a group of γA myeloma proteins tested were inhibitory. Furthermore, the blocking activity shown by solutions of γA-globulin fractions isolated from allergic sera was found not to correlate with their protein concentrations.

Hence it was concluded that reaginic antibodies were associated with a minor component of allergic sera, which was included as a contaminant in supposedly pure γA-globulin preparations. Even before all this extra data was obtained, however, other pieces of evidence were emerging to indicate that reagins possessed unusual physico-chemical characteristics (for immunoglobulins), to match their distinctive biological properties. For instance, in gel filtration fractionation of allergic individuals' sera maximal P–K activity was eluted from Sephadex G200 columns slightly ahead of the 7*S* peak (Fireman et al. 1963; Terr and Bentz 1964; Stanworth 1965A). At the time, some investigators interpreted these observations as additional evidence in support of the γA nature of reagins. It was puzzling, however, that polymerised forms of γA-globulin were usually found in protein synthesised by neoplastic cells; whereas the high molecular weight material (i.e. $> 7S$) found in γA-globulin preparations isolated from normal human sera had been attributed to an artificial aggregation process occurring during isolation (Heremans 1960). Rockey and Kunkel (1962) had previously described density-gradient ultracentrifugation studies which showed that skin sensitising antibody against a purified glucagon preparation had a sedimentation coefficient in the 8–11*S* range. It was particularly significant, therefore, when the careful and accurate density-gradient studies undertaken by Andersen and Vannier (1964), on reagins in ragweed sensitive individuals' sera, revealed a sedimentation coefficient of 7.7*S* (7.4–7.9*S* range). Furthermore, in later sedimentation studies, on an artificial mixture of reagin and γA isoagglutinin, Ishizaka et al. (1966B) observed that the reagin sedimented between the 7*S* and 10*S* forms of the added γA antibody.

I had observed in 1960 (Stanworth 1963), by application of a sucrose density gradient procedure involving the recovery of fractions by tube-slicing (Stanworth et al. 1961), that the peak of P–K activity in ultracentrifugation fractions of serum from a horse dandruff-sensitive individual was slightly ahead of the γG-globulin peak as measured by quantitative immunodiffusion. I dismissed this observation, at the time, as due to experimental inaccuracy and failed to repeat it owing to a transfer of laboratory (to the U.S.A.). I mention it here as a warning against bias in interpreting experimental observations.

The discovery by Rowe and Fahey (1965) of a myeloma form of yet another class of human immunoglobulin (IgD or γD) inevitably raised the question as to whether reagin represented an antibody form of this protein. IgD was detected also in normal human sera (at a median level of 0.03 mg/ml) and observed to move in the fast γ region on zone-electrophoresis (fig. 4.2a). Furthermore, like reagin, it was eluted ahead of the γG peak on gel filtration through Sephadex G200 and ahead of the γA-globulin from DEAE Sephadex (fig. 4.2b, c). Several attempts to show P–K activity to be associated with this class of immunoglobulin have, however, proved unsuccessful (Ishizaka et al. 1966C; Coombs et al. 1968); nor was it possible to inhibit passive skin sensitisation by injection of IgD[1] (Rowe 1968).

The possibility had also been considered that reagin represents an antibody form of one of the 4 heavy chain sub-classes of human IgG, but Ishizaka et al. (1967) showed by chromatographic and immunosorption studies that reagin activity in the sera of ragweed-sensitive individuals is not associated with the γG-2, γG-3 or γG-4 sub-classes; and other absorption data would seem to suggest that it is unlikely to be associated with the major γG-1 sub-class. This does not exclude the possibility, however, that certain types of human skin sensitising antibody are representative of a particular γG sub-class (as will be discussed later).

4.2 Evidence of a new immunoglobulin class

In an attempt to provide more convincing evidence that reagins were a unique class of immunoglobulin Ishizaka and his associates set about the formidable task of isolating sufficient antibody from the sera of hypersensitive patients, for characterisation studies. They (Ishizaka et al. 1967A) accomplished this by application of a multi-step fractionation procedure – comprising salt precipitation, ion-exchange chromatography and gel filtration steps – to large pools of sera from individuals showing marked sensitivity to ragweed pollen; and by exploitation of sensitive radio-immunoassay procedures in the measurement of the reagin contents of the fractions isolated. These techniques (assessed in ch. 2), which provide a valuable in vitro alternative to P–K testing, rely upon rabbit antisera which have been raised against reagin-rich fractions and absorbed with normal IgG as well as with myeloma γA- and γD-globulins. Such antisera gave a precipitin line with reagin-rich fractions in the γ_1 region, on immunoelectrophoresis; and radio-labelled (^{131}I) ragweed E allergen was shown to combined specifically with this line. Moreover, the radio-labelled allergen binding capacity of allergic sera and reagin fractions, thus measured, was shown to correlate with their skin sensitising activity in normal humans and in monkeys (Ishizaka et al. 1967B); whereas absorption of allergic serum and reagin-rich fractions with the specific 'anti-reagin' antiserum removed these activities.

The purified reagin preparation obtained by the procedure evolved by the Ishizaka group was found to be 1000 times more active than the parent allergic serum (i.e. a positive P–K test was obtained with as little as 0.001 μg N, being equivalent to a P–K dilution of 180 000). It was shown by radio-immunoelectrophoretic analysis to contain light polypeptide chains of both K and L type (Ishizaka and Ishizaka 1966), and also IgD (Ishizaka et al. 1966B) on radio-immunodiffusion testing with specific antisera. Conversely, the anti-reagin serum (prepared as already indicated) failed to give precipitin lines with myeloma γG-, γA- and γD-globulins and with macroglobulinaemic γM-globulin.

On the basis of this type of finding, Ishizaka and his associates proposed that reagin activity in ragweed-sensitive individuals' sera was carried by a unique immunoglobulin, which they tentatively designated 'γE' (in view of its specific binding capacity for ragweed allergen E). Despite the mass of data presented in support of this idea, however, some of us felt that perhaps it was a little premature to make such claims until chemical evidence was available to confirm the existence of a unique type of heavy polypeptide chain. After all, absorption experiments with supposedly specific antisera directed against the well-defined immunoglobulin classes had already proved misleading, when claims were being made of an association between reagin and γA-globulin (Fireman et al. 1963).

Before the Ishizaka group had reported the results of their later studies on the isolation and characterisation of ragweed reagin, I had suggested (Stanworth 1965A) that the observed lack of correlation between distribution of P–K activity and γA-globulin in chromatographic fractions of allergic serum might be attributable to the mixed dimeric (i.e. γG–γA) nature of this antibody. This could possibly have accounted for the chromatographic elution position of reagin from DEAE cellulose and for its unusual sedimentation characteristics, besides providing a structural basis for its bi-specificity (i.e. its combining capacities for both antigen and tissues). The results of the later absorption studies with specific anti-γG and anti-γA antisera, already mentioned, suggested however that such a structure was unlikely to have been present in the reagin fractions studied by Ishizaka; unless, by chance, the mixed dimerisation process had resulted in the masking of the specific antigenic determinants on both the γ and α chains of the 2 monomer units.

4.3 Discovery of a myeloma form

The final evidence needed to confirm that reaginic antibodies are, indeed, unique immunoglobulins resulted from the perceptive observations of Johansson and Bennich (1967) working in Uppsala. They isolated an atypical myeloma protein (originally designated IgND), from the serum of a patient (N.D.) with myelomatosis and Bence Jones proteinuria, which lacked antigenic determinants characteristic of α, δ, γ and μ chains (i.e. the heavy polypeptide chains of the then known immunoglobulin classes) whilst possessing light chain determinants of type L. Substantial evidence has since been obtained from various types of investigation to indicate that this protein is a pathological counterpart of reaginic antibody; and of an antigenically similar protein detectable in extremely small amounts (e.g. 100–700 ng/ml) in normal individuals' sera by means of the sensitive radio-immunosorbent technique (R.I.S.T.) described in ch. 2, employing antisera raised against the myeloma protein.

Like myeloma γA- and γD-globulins, this atypical protein

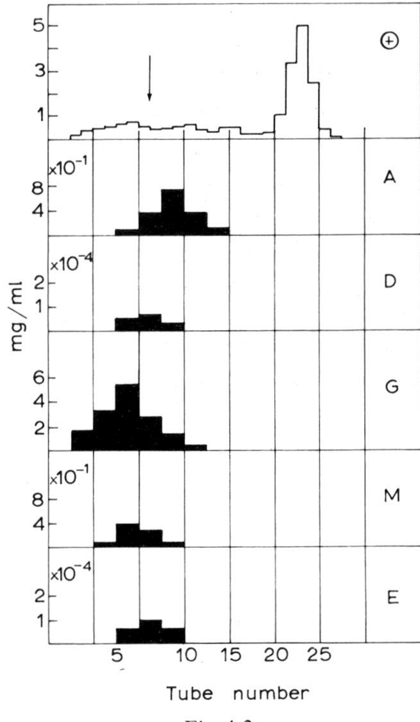

Fig. 4.2a.

Fig. 4.2. Comparison of the physico-chemical properties of the 5 major immunoglobulin classes. (a) zone-electrophoresis in starch (barbital buffer: *p*H 8.6, I = 0.05); (b) gel filtration on Sephadex G200 (0.1 M Tris-HCl-0.5 M NaCl, *p*H 8.0); (c) chromatography on DEAE Sephadex (0.1 M Tris-HCl, *p*H 8.0 with salt gradient). (Reproduced from Johansson et al. 1968, by permission of the authors.)

moved in the 'fast γ region' on zone-electrophoresis (fig. 4.2a). It was, however, eluted slightly ahead of these classes of immunoglobulin during chromatographic analysis of normal human sera on DEAE Sephadex (fig. 4.2c); and after them, although just ahead of the γ-globulin, during gel-filtration on Sephadex G200 (fig. 4.2b). Furthermore, free-solution ultracentrifugal analysis showed the atypical myeloma protein (IgND) to possess a sedimentation coefficient ($S^{\circ}_{20,\,w}$) of 7.92*S* (and M.W. = 190 000), i.e. very similar to the sedimentation coefficient assigned by Anderson and Vannier (1963) to the reaginic antibodies in ragweed-sensitive indi-

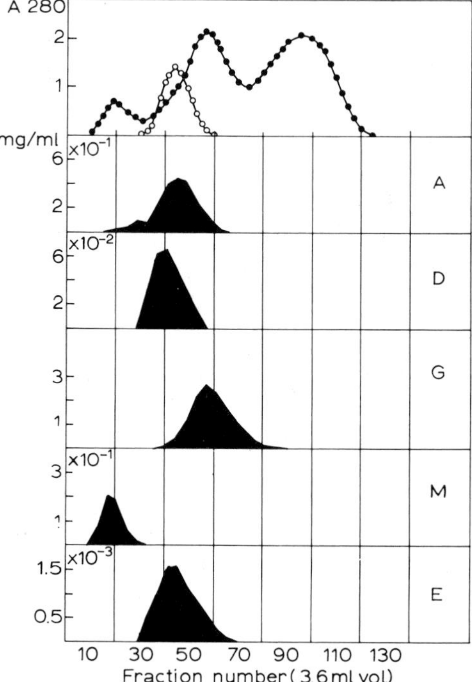

Fig. 4.2b.

viduals' sera on the basis of the observed rate of movement of the P–K activity in buffered sucrose gradients.

It was possible, of course, that this similarity of sedimentation behaviour was fortuitous, although it did seem significant that the myeloma protein isolated from the serum of patient N.D. was the first known type of immunoglobulin to show similar size characteristics to skin sensitising antibodies. Moreover, other observations were being made which suggested a relationship between the new class of immunoglobulin and reagin. For instance, a significantly elevated level (namely, 5 900 ng/ml) of an immunoglobulin antigenically related to IgND was detected in the serum of an individual with proven allergy to dog dander; although, admittedly, no allergic symptoms were apparent in 3 other individuals showing high serum IgND levels.

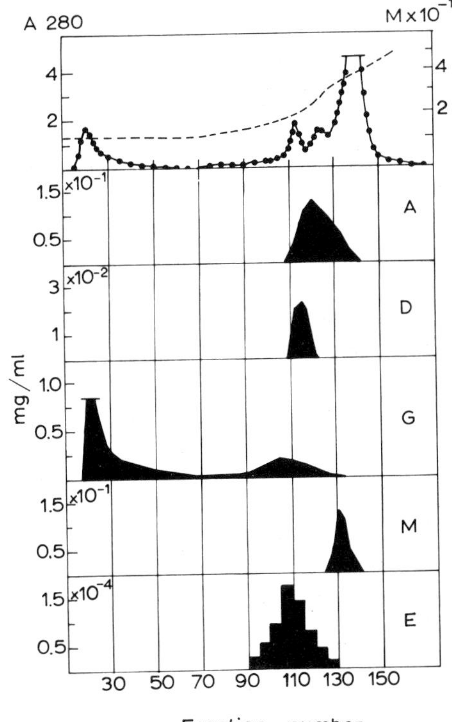

Fig. 4.2c.

Absorption of the serum of a horse dander-sensitive individual (P.R.) with a rabbit antiserum directed specifically against IgND appeared to remove its leucocyte sensitising capacity, but control tests with samples of the allergic serum which had been treated with normal rabbit serum showed only minimal histamine release (i.e. 6 per cent of the total available histamine).

More substantial evidence of a close structural relationship between the atypical myeloma protein and reagin was provided by comparative studies of the antigenic characteristics of a purified IgND preparation and the reagin-rich fraction (designated γE, referred to earlier), which Ishizaka and his associates had isolated from the sera of ragweed-sensitive individuals (Bennich et al.

1969). It was shown that antiserum directed specifically against the Fc portion of the myeloma protein and the antiserum raised against the γE reagin preparation gave a single precipitin line of identical specificity, and that this line bound radio-labelled ragweed allergen. Furthermore, anti-γE antisera precipitated the myeloma protein (IgND).

The most convincing evidence that the myeloma protein was a pathological counterpart of reaginic antibody was obtained, however, from inhibition P–K testing in a normal human recipient (Stanworth et al. 1967). As is seen from the data in table 4.1, intradermal injection of a dose of myeloma protein of between 300–3 000 ng mixed with the serum of a horse dander-sensitive individual (P.R.) was sufficient to effect complete competitive inhibition of P–K activity as revealed by subsequent challenge with allergen 24 hr later. In contrast, injection of a similar amount of a normal human IgG preparation had no such effect. Similarly, inhibition could be accomplished by prior intradermal injection of the myeloma protein into skin sites (on the forearms) in which P–K testing was subsequently performed 24–48 hr later (table 4.2).

Thus, not only is the myeloma protein antigenically related to reaginic antibody, but it also appears to possess the strong affinity of that antibody for primate tissues (fig. 4.3). This can be concluded, too, by the demonstration (ch. 9.3) that a general refractory state can be induced in baboons by the systemic administration of myeloma IgE. Moreover, it was significant that the myeloma patient (N.D.) showed none of the symptoms of immediate hypersensitivity, nor did he respond to skin tests with a whole range of commercial allergen extracts; presumably because, with such a massive level of tissue-binding immunoglobulin in his circulation, any reaginic antibodies which he might produce would be expected to be blocked in a similar manner to the inhibition of passive skin sensitisation in normal human recipients.

Hence, it was concluded that the myeloma protein was closely related structurally to reagin, without possessing the allergen-binding property demonstrable by this type of antibody (fig. 4.3). This would appear to be analogous to the situation obtaining with regard to the relationship between conventional IgG antibodies and their myeloma counterparts, where, except in certain rare

TABLE 4.1

Results of testing for competitive inhibition of the P–K reaction by the myeloma IgE (ND) protein (from Stanworth et al. 1967).

Test solution no.	Composition (one volume : one volume)		Amount of added Ig injected (ng)	Proportion of reagin-ND in total IgND injected* (%)	Results of duplicate P–K tests					
					10-min weal areas (mm^2)			26-min weal areas (mm^2)		
					1	2	mean	1	2	mean
1	Allergic serum (undiluted)	Saline solution	0	–	77	50	64	143	86	115
2	idem	IgND (600 μg ml)	30000	0.1	–	–	–	–	–	–
3	idem	IgND (60 μg ml)	3000	1.0	–	–	–	–	–	–
4	idem	IgND (6 μg ml)	300	9.0	10	13	12	28	44	36
5	idem	IgG (600 μg ml)	30000	0.1	43	44	44	119	106	113
6	idem	IgG (60 μg ml)	3000	1.0	43	61	52	89	130	110

Allergic serum, P.R.; Allergen, horse dander; normal recipient, J.H.; test site, back; interval between transfer and challenge, 18 hr.
* Based on a mean ($n = 6$) level of 615 ng ml of IgND in the P.R. allergic serum, as estimated by the radioimmunosorbent assay.

TABLE 4.2

Results of testing the ability of pre-injected myeloma IgE (ND) protein to inhibit the P–K reaction (from Stanworth et al. 1967).

Test solution no.	Composition of solution first injected (in duplicate as 0.1 ml aliquots)	Ig-concentration (μg protein/ml)	Results of subsequent PK testing with undiluted allergic serum (24-hr interval between transfer and challenge)					
			10-min weal areas (mm^2)			20-min weal areas (mm^2)		
			Left arm	Right arm	Mean	Left arm	Right arm	Mean
7	IgND	600	–	–	–	–	–	–
8	IgND	60	–	–	–	2	6	4
9	IgND	6	19	64	42	44	75	60
10	IgG	600	28	72	50	76	84	80
11	IgG	60	45	55	50	71	64	68
12	Saline	–	70	64	67	90	111	101

Test conditions as in table 1, except that sites on forearms used.

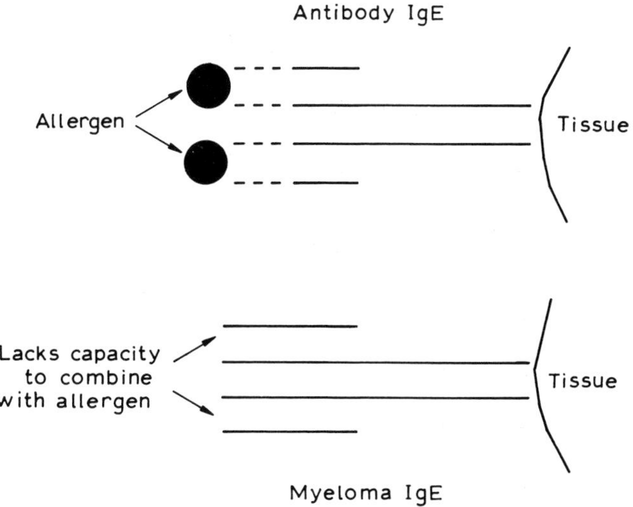

Fig. 4.3. Schematic representation of the structural basis of the difference in biological activity between antibody and myeloma IgE.

cases (e.g. Eisen et al. 1967), the myeloma proteins fail to show any capacity to bind antigen specifically (i.e. to sites located within their Fab regions).

Further immunological studies of the myeloma protein IgND (Bennich and Johansson 1968) provided evidence that its unique determinants were located in an Fc type of fragment produced by papain digestion. Its light chain determinants, on the other hand, were confined to Fab fragments. Chemical studies revealed that the IgND molecule is comprised of heavy and light polypeptide chains with respective molecular weights of 72 500 and 22 600. This means that it possesses an appreciably larger Fc region than the IgG molecule which, as will be discussed later (ch. 5), appears to contain the structure responsible for the distinctive biological properties of IgE antibodies.

On the basis of this substantial weight of evidence, resulting from extensive studies on both purified reagin and its myeloma counterpart (table 4.3), a memorandum was drafted in Lausanne in 1968 (Bennich et al. 1968) in which it was proposed that re-

TABLE 4.3
Comparison of physico-chemical and immunological properties of myeloma IgE and reaginic antibodies (from Bennich and Johansson 1970).

	IgE *	Reaginic antibodies
Molecular weight	190 000	–
Sedimentation rate (S)	8.2	8
Carbohydrate (%)	11.5	–
Light chain	λ(22,600)	κ, λ
Heavy chain	ϵ(72,500)	–
Antibody activity	+	+
Sensitisation homologous tissue	+	+
Heat (56°C, 30 min)	labile	labile
Reduction (0.1 M 2-ME)	labile	labile
Complement-binding	0	0
Electrophoretic mobility	γ_1	γ_1

* Physico-chemical data refer to E myeloma protein ND.

agins should be considered as representative of a new class of immunoglobulin to be designated IgE or γE (fig. 4.4); and that the heavy polypeptide chains of this protein be referred to as epsilon (ϵ) chains. Thus, the end has been reached of a crucial phase in the work on the isolation and characterisation of reagin, which started with the convincing demonstration by Prausnitz in 1921 of the involvement of this circulating antibody in the mediation of immediate-type hypersensitivity and culminated in 1968 with the conferring upon it of a unique immunoglobulin status.

A second case of γE myelomatosis has since been reported from America (Ogawa et al. 1969)[2] showing striking clinical similarities to the Swedish patient in that both had plasma cell leukemia and diffuse osteolytic lesions; besides showing a prominent M-component of antigenic Type L on electrophoresis of the serum, and Bence Jones protein in the urine. Already first reports of the primary amino acid sequence of the heavy (ϵ) polypeptide chains of these 2 myeloma proteins are appearing in the literature (e.g. Terry et al. 1970); and other studies are concerned with the nature and location of their carbohydrate prosthetic groups. Hence, with automated sequencing machines now available commercially, we

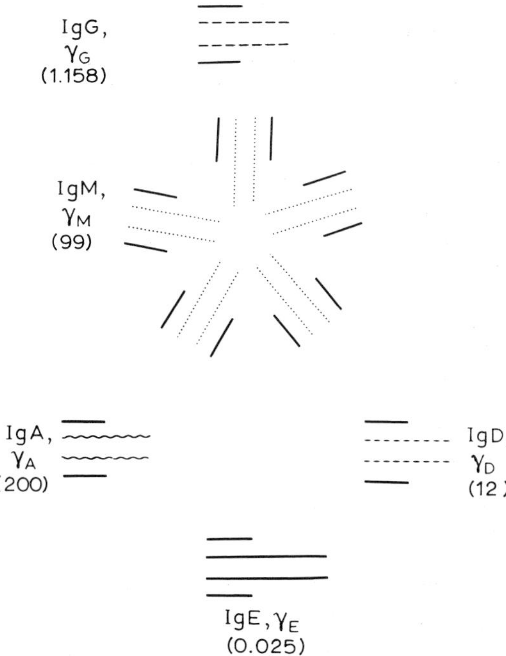

Fig. 4.4. Diagrammatic representation of structural relationship between the major immunoglobulin classes. The normal range of each (in mg/100 ml) in adult human serum is given in brackets.

should not have to wait too long for the elucidation of the complete primary structure of a γE-globulin molecule.

Yet despite the magnitude of such achievements, which will obviously lead to a much better understanding of the structural basis of reaginic antibody activity, it is important to recognise that in some cases of immediate hypersensitivity in humans, antibodies representative of classes other than IgE are probably involved. Furthermore, evidence is accumulating to suggest that there is heterogeneity within the immunoglobulin E class itself (as, indeed, there is in other immunoglobulin classes) which could prove to be of considerable clinical significance.

4.4 Heterogeneity of skin sensitising antibodies

It is important to get recent claims of reagin heterogeneity in proper perspective. These are based mainly on the demonstration of a polydisperse distribution of P–K activity within chromatographically separated fractions of allergic sera, and are thus corroborating the findings of earlier studies in which ion-exchange chromatography was first applied to the isolation of reagins. For example, the initial application of DEAE cellulose chromatography to the fractionation of the sera of grass pollen-sensitive (Humphrey and Porter 1957) and horse dander-sensitive individuals (Stanworth 1959) had shown that some P–K activity was recovered in fractions eluted before and after the one containing the maximum amount of reagins (eluted with 0.02 M phosphate buffer, *p*H 6.2, in a step-wise procedure, as is seen in fig. 4.1).

Several other groups (e.g. Goodfriend et al. 1966; Reid et al. 1966; Fireman et al. 1967; Goodfriend and Perelmutter 1968; Reid et al. 1968) have made essentially similar observations, in studies of the chromatographic behaviour of reagins directed against many different allergens; whilst other investigators (e.g. Malley and Perlman 1966; Radermecker 1969) have claimed to have isolated pure IgG chromatographic fractions with reagin activity. It is important to recognise, however, that many of these investigations were undertaken before convincing evidence (already considered) was obtained to indicate that reagin activity is associated with a new class of immunoglobulin; and, of course, before the sensitive radio-immunoassay techniques had been developed for the measurement of the distribution of this immunoglobulin in fractions of allergic sera separated by ion-exchange chromatography and by other procedures. Application of these types of assay by Ishizaka and Ishizaka (1967) to the analysis of DEAE Sephadex fractions of ragweed-sensitive individuals' sera, obtained by step-wise elution with Tris-HCl buffer (*p*H 8.0) of increasing molarity, detected IgE in 2 different fractions (eluted at 0.025 M and 0.035 M). Moreover, gradient elution of a reagin-rich, salt precipitated (50 per cent sat. $(NH_4)_2SO_4$) globulin fraction from a ragweed-sensitive individual's serum on DEAE Sephadex produced several P–K-reactive fractions containing IgE detectable by radio-immunodiffusion.

It is quite conceivable, therefore, that the other investigators listed above were observing a similar spread of reagin, undetected by the relatively insensitive conventional immunodiffusion techniques which they employed; particularly as they also adopted different chromatographic elution conditions to those used by Ishizaka and Ishizaka (1967). This is probably the explanation, for instance, of the observations of Perelmutter et al. (1966) and Goodfriend et al. (1966); who observed that part of the reaginic activity in their allergic sera was eluted with relatively strong (i.e. 0.1 M) Tris-HCl buffer (*p*H 8.0), in a 'pre-gradient fraction', whilst the rest was retrieved on application of a gradient using 0.5 M buffer (of the same *p*H). It is significant that studies by Ishizaka and his associates (1967) on the same allergic serum failed to demonstrate the resolution of reagin activity into separate peaks; and they found that those fractions of Perelmutter and his associates (1966) which appeared to lack reagin activity possessed the highest P–K activity on a weight basis. This apparent discrepancy is attributed to the practice of Perelmutter et al. (1966), and of others, of performing their P–K tests on fractions which have been concentrated to the same volume as the starting serum rather than to the same protein concentration. It is also significant that Ishizaka and Ishizaka (1966) found that the reaginic antibody activity in both pre- and post-gradient fractions was precipitated by specific anti-IgE antiserum.

It is perhaps not too surprising that a chromatographic procedure involving first step-wise and then gradient elution should yield more than one fraction of a particular immunoglobulin class. This is to be expected from the studies which James and I (James and Stanworth 1965) carried out some time ago on the chromatographic behaviour of isolated purified serum protein constituents. Evidence was obtained that the occurrence of reversible protein denaturation on the column could lead to spurious elution behaviour.

The question to be answered, therefore, as far as skin sensitising antibodies are concerned, is whether an apparent polydisperse distribution of P–K activity amongst chromatographic fractions of allergic sera represents an intra-immunoglobulin class heterogeneity, or whether it reflects the association of sensitising activity with more than one major immunoglobulin class. With regard to the former possibility, it is important to establish that the observed effect is not an artifact brought about by the chromatographic procedure adopted. If this can be satisfactorily excluded, it would be reasonable to conclude that activity is associated with immunoglobulin molecules of a particular class which differ in electrophoretic mobility. I demonstrated sometime ago (Stanworth 1959) that IgG fractions of differing electrophoretic mobility were retrievable by DEAE cellulose chromatographic fractionation of allergic sera, and there is now evidence (Ishizaka and Ishizaka 1968B) that IgE shows similar electrophoretic heterogeneity.

Recent iso-electric focusing studies of human and rabbit IgG (Howard and Virella 1970) suggest that such charge differences might be associated with sub-class heterogeneity; and it is not inconceivable that similarly distinguishable IgE sub-classes also exist. It is interesting, therefore, that Sela and Mozes (1966) have observed the chromatographic behaviour (i.e. the overall net charge) of rabbit antibody IgG appears to be related to the charge on the evoking antigen. For instance, acidic antigens (such as acidic multichain polyaminoacids) evoke the production of positively charged antibody (which is eluted relatively late from DEAE sephadex at *p*H 8.0, using a salt gradient of 0.02 M-0.3 M phosphate) and vice versa. This raises speculation (Reid et al. 1968; Ishizaka and Ishizaka 1968) as to whether what appear to be true heterogeneities in reagin activity in the sera of individuals showing sensitivities to a range of different allergens (e.g. Reid et al. 1968) might not represent an electrophoretically heterogeneous response to allergens of differing surface charge. In this connection, however, it is important to note that every inhalant allergen of those which have been characterised to any extent has proved to possess a relatively fast electrophoretic mobility at *p*H 8.6, i.e. a low iso-electric point, due to a relatively high proportion of dibasic amino acids. This is true of ragweed allergen E (King et al. 1967), for example, and of the purified horse dander allergen which I have been studying (which has been found to contain between 2–3 times as many acid as basic amino acid residues). It is also important to recognise that Sela and Mozes (1966) only observed a clear-cut relationship between antibody mobility and net charge of the antigen when the latter was presented as a single component. Complex antigens, such as diphtheria toxoid, evoked an antibody response which was much less readily resolvable by DEAE sephadex chromatography of the parent rabbit antiserum. It is not unreasonable to suppose, therefore, that a similarly heterogeneous antibody response would result from inhalation of antigenically complex pollen granules, to consider but one example of common type of inhalant. In this connection, it is interesting to note that Underdown and Goodfriend (1970) have recently published the results of a preliminary investigation which indicate that reaginic antibodies directed against a basic ragweed pollen component (Ra3) are eluted from a DEAE sephadex column later than the reaginic antibodies directed against the acidic ragweed allergen component (E); but it is necessary to interpret these observations with some caution, for the reasons mentioned in the previous chapter (§ 3.4).

Reid and associates (1968) demonstrated that the differing elution behaviour shown by the reaginic antibodies in the allergic sera which they examined by DEAE cellulose chromatography was not due to a procedural artifact, by carrying out re-fractionations of the relatively pure fractions in similar ion-exchange columns employing a slightly different buffer system. As, however, they employed only the relatively insensitive radial-diffusion technique to determine the immunoglobulin composition of their chromatographic fractions, the possibility cannot be ruled out that the heterogeneous distribution of reagin activity which they observed was due to a spread of IgE antibodies with differing iso-electric points.

Obviously in any future attempts to demonstrate a true heterogeneity in the reaginic antibody class this possibility must first be excluded, by carrying out a careful comparison of the distribution of the P–K activity in allergic serum fractions with their IgE content as determined by a sensitive and specific radio-immunoassay procedure. Although this type of investigation was not undertaken by Reid and associates (1968), it seems significant that these workers observed (in some cases) such widely different distributions of P–K activity within chromatographic fractions obtained under apparently standardised elution conditions from the sera of patients showing different specificities of hypersensitivity. For instance, it is interesting that a major portion of the reaginic activity in the sera of individuals showing sensitivities to ingestants was eluted in earlier fractions than the bulk of the activity in the sera of pollen and dust-sensitive individuals. Other preliminary evidence in favour of the existence of sensitising antibodies with different chemical properties was provided by studies (Reid et al. 1968) of the susceptibility of the P–K activity of allergic sera to treatment with 0.1 M mercaptoethanol (followed by alkylation with 0.01 M iodoacetate). This treatment was found to have little effect on the P–K activity of serum from a patient sensitive to bovine serum albumin, whereas it destroyed most sensitising antibody activity against Bermuda grass pollen. But it is possible that the treatment of the complex mixture of proteins in serum (rather than purified components) with reducing agents had initiated S–S interchange reactions, which could lead to spurious observations.

It is quite conceivable, of course, that the route of administration of allergen (as well as its chemical nature) is an important factor influencing the type of sensitising antibody produced. In this connnection, it seems significant that in those cases of immediate hypersensitivity in which an antibody mediator other than IgE is suspected, sensitisation has usually been effected by injectants (e.g. horse serum antitoxin, antibiotics) rather than by inhalants. Moreover, even inhalant antigens evoke antibodies in classes other than the IgE, when injected alone or mixed with adjuvant for hyposensitisation purposes. The blocking antibody thus produced shows the electrophoretic properties of slow γG-globulin, and there is other evidence to suggest that it is a representative of this immunoglobulin class.

An obvious implication of these observations is that IgE antibodies are produced at certain strategically situated local sites within the body, as are IgA antibodies; and, indeed, the results of recent immunofluorescence studies suggest that cells located in the nasal passages and bronchial and gastro-intestinal tracts are involved in such a process (discussed more fully in ch. 7).

Assuming, then, that sensitising antibodies of types other than IgE are implicated in certain human allergic conditions, the question of their chemical nature arises and in particular the structural characteristics which distinguish them from γE reaginic antibodies. Of the already known immunoglobulin types, a sub-class of IgG would appear to be the most likely candidate for this role because 3 out of 4 known sub-classes of this immunoglobulin are capable at least of fixing to heterologous (e.g. guinea pig) skin. In contrast, antibodies of the IgM and IgA classes produced in humans and in other species (e.g. rabbits) have consistently failed to evoke PCA reactions in guinea pigs; presumably because of some structural disability within their Fc regions (as will become apparent from the next chapter), which is possibly related to that structural characteristic which prevents them (i.e. human IgM and IgA) from getting across the placenta.

It is conceivable that isologous skin sensitising antibodies analogous to, say, the guinea pig γ_1-type (ch. 6) will prove to be operative in other species * including humans. Such antibodies would be expected to be more resistant than γE antibodies to heat and other forms of denaturation treatment; and to show distinctive sedimentation characteristics to those of reagins, although possessing similar electrophoretic properties. Carrying the analogy with the guinea pig system further, it would presumably be essential to look for a similar type of human antibody by adopting much shorter sensitisation periods than the 24–72 hr (50 hr optimum) period usually employed in the P–K assay.

Indeed, pieces of evidence are appearing from various laboratories to suggest that a second type of human sensitising antibody, with the properties outlined, is present in the sera of certain hypersensitive individuals. For instance, there are indications of the presence of a non-reaginic sensitising antibody in the sera of horse

* What appears to be a 'fast' γG1 antibody has recently been detected in immunised rabbits sera (Rodkey and Freeman 1969), but this did not show isologous skin fixing activity.

serum-sensitive individuals which is more resistant to heat treatment than reagins (which are destroyed by heating at 56° for 1 hr)[3]; and which appears to induce PCA reactions in monkeys after very short sensitisation periods (i.e. 2½ hr, Augustin 1967). Moreover, we have some preliminary evidence that the levels of this antibody in such sera do not correlate with their IgE levels as determined by the R.I.S.T. procedure. Similar kinds of observation lead one to suspect that a non-reaginic antibody of this type is also involved in certain cases of penicillin sensitivity; and in food sensitivities, where there is evidence of complement dependency (Parish 1970). Investigations now in progress are aiming to provide unequivocal evidence that such antibodies are representatives of an IgG subclass, which are capable of binding to isologous or closely related heterologous tissues in contrast to other γG antibodies produced in humans (e.g. the blocking antibodies, in response to hyposensitisation) which show a capacity to sensitise guinea pig tissues but not primate tissues.

It is not an impossibility, however, that the type of non-reaginic antibody discussed will ultimately prove to be associated with a new class of immunoglobulin. The definitive answer to this question will depend upon studies on purified material. Nevertheless, it is important to recognise that immediate hypersensitivity reactions can be mediated by more than one kind of mechanism. Hence, it is quite possible that certain types of isologous human γG antibody (with or without the aid of serum co-factors) are – like γE reagins – capable of effecting the release of vasoactive amines following combination with antigen (as will be discussed further in ch. 8, dealing with current ideas about the mechanism of allergic reactions). It will be essential to establish the clinical significance of such reactions which, I suspect, are by no means as effective biologically as those initiated by γE antibodies.

Notes

[1] Like IgA and IgM, human IgD failed to elicit reverse PCA reactions in guinea pigs; and BDB-linked aggregates of IgD proved to be incapable of inducing an increase in vascular permeability of guinea pig skin. (Henney, C.S.; Welscher, H.D.; Terry, W.D.; Rowe, D.S.; Immunochem. 1969, *6*, 445).

[2] But a later American case (Fishkin, B.G. et al., Blood 1972, *39*, 361) showed neither plasma cell leukemia nor overt Bence Jones proteinuria, and her IgE myeloma protein possessed light chains of the K-type.

[3] A time period which is dependent to some extent on the antibody concentration.

CHAPTER 5

Structural basis of reagin activity

5.1 Introduction

It is now becoming generally accepted, from an immunochemical standpoint, that immediate hypersensitivity reactions are 2-stage processes in which IgE antibodies play a central and crucial role; firstly, in the sensitisation of certain tissues and circulating cells and, subsequently, by reacting with the provoking allergen to effect the release of vasoactive amines (fig. 5.1). Any attempt to define the reactivity of reaginic antibodies in structural terms must, therefore, take into account these different but related functions.

Considering the second stage first, it now seems probable that reagins behave like other types of antibody (e.g. γG) in the manner in which they react with specific antigen (i.e. allergen). For instance, it has been shown (Ishizaka and Ishizaka 1968B) that IgE antibodies agglutinate allergen (ragweed)-coated erythrocytes, indicating that reagins are probably divalent. As was discussed earlier (ch. 3), however, it seems probable that antigens responsible for the elicitation of immediate hypersensitivity reactions are of a somewhat restricted size range; and it has yet to be demonstrated that cell-bound reagins react with specific antigen in the same manner to their mode of action in free solution.

It is, of course, their behaviour in the first stage of the immediate hypersensitivity reaction which distinguishes reagins from other types of antibody. I am referring, in particular, to their

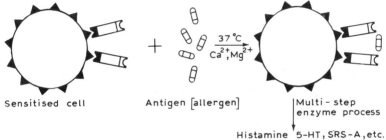

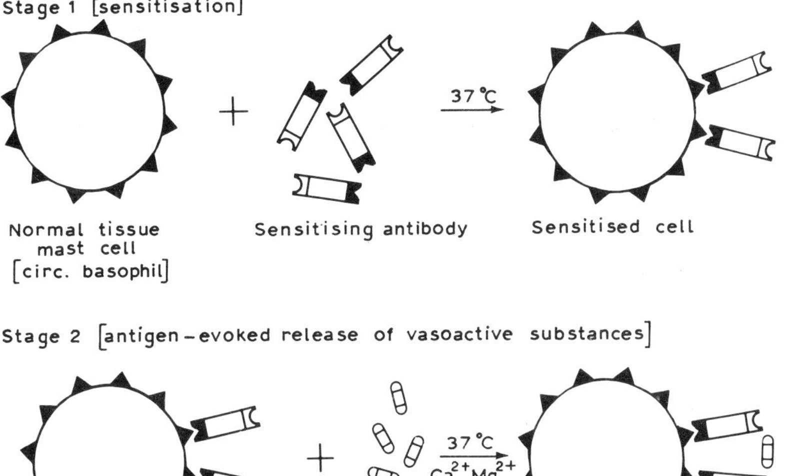

Fig. 5.1. Schematic representation of two major immunochemical stages of immediate hypersensitivity reactions (reproduced from Stanworth 1969).

ability to bind firmly to isologous and closely related heterologous primate tissues. In my experience (Stanworth and Kuhns 1965) a maximal P–K response is achieved about 50 hr after passive transfer of allergic serum (fig. 2.5); but as we, and many other investigators have demonstrated, reagins can be detected in a normal recipient's skin several weeks after transfer, and they can be shown to persist for several days in non-human primate skin (Augustin 1967), following the transfer of allergic serum. In contrast, Kuhns (1961) showed that human γG antibodies directed against diphtheria toxoid disappeared rapidly (having a half-life of 12 hr) on injection into a normal human's skin. Quantitative P–K testing, involving the pricking in of allergen solution at various points within and outside the initial transfer area (fig. 2.4, and discussed more fully in ch. 2), provided a further indication that transferred reagins become rapidly and firmly attached to isologous skin.

More convincing evidence of their strong tissue affinity is obtained, however, from in vitro studies involving the passive sensitisation of isolated human and monkey tissue preparations. For example, even after thorough washing, chopped lung fragments which have been passively sensitised by incubation with allergic serum can be provoked to liberate histamine on subsequent interaction with specific allergen (and, indeed, this procedure has become one of the most useful methods of assaying reagin activity in vitro, as is discussed in ch. 2). Normal human leucocyte suspensions can be similarly sensitised (fig. 2.15), it being assumed in this case that the reaginic antibodies become fixed to the basophils present. Until pure basophil preparations can be obtained, however, there will be uncertainty about the possible involvement of other types of cells in immediate hypersensitivity reactions. Nevertheless, recent studies (Ishizaka 1969) involving the in vitro treatment of atopic individuals' leucocytes with radio-labelled anti-IgE, have provided the first direct evidence that IgE is present on the surface of basophils. thus suggesting that the reagin–allergen interaction takes place on the surface of these histamine-rich cells. Treatment with anti-IgE effected a degranulation of the basophils, which were identified by conventional histochemical staining with Toluidine Blue and which were shown by auto-radiography to carry the labelled anti-IgE antibody. Moreover, independent evidence for the presence of γE-globulin molecules on the surface of human basophils has been obtained recently by means of a rosetting technique (Wilson et al. 1971) and by an electron microscopic procedure.[1]

The question of identification of the reagin-binding cells and location and characterisation of their reagin receptors will, however, be taken up further in later chapters. The points to be considered here are the manner in which reaginic antibodies bind to cells and the mechanism whereby their subsequent reaction with allergen at the cell surface initiates the chain of events culminating in the release of vasoactive amines. In other words, the self-appointed task is to explain the bifunctional behaviour of reagins in structural terms.

Writing in a speculative vein a few years ago (Stanworth 1965A), when most people were convinced that reagins were γA-globulins, I suggested that they might comprise a 'mixed dimer' of γA- and γG-globulin molecules (e.g. with γA Fab sites directed against the tissue and γG Fab sites directed against the antigen). This idea had the attraction of explaining not only their bifunctional nature, but also their behaviour during DEAE cellulose chromatography (which was atypical, to say the least, for γA-globulins) and their unusual sedimentation characteristics (i.e. $S^{o}_{20,w}$ = 8*S* rather than 7*S*). As far as I know, hybrid antibody molecules of this type have never been identified in nature, although there have been instances (e.g. Nisonoff and Mandy 1962; Fudenberg et al. 1964) of the production of artificial hybrid antibodies (i.e. $F(ab')_2$ sub-units) with dual antigenic specificities (by reduction of a mixture of 5*S* papain digestion fragments from 2 γG antibodies of different specificities, followed by re-oxidation of the resultant mixed univalent 3.5*S* sub-units).

As was discussed in ch. 4, however, there is now overwhelming evidence that reaginic antibodies are members of a distinctive immunoglobulin class (E), which appears to resemble other immunoglobulin classes in possessing 2 light and 2 heavy polypeptide chains. It is still conceivable, therefore, but most unlikely, that the Fab regions of monomeric IgE molecules show dual specificity i.e. one combining site directed against tissue and the other against antigen. Ignoring this type of structure, two other more plausible possibilities remain:

1) Reaginic antibodies combine to cell receptors through sites within their Fab regions, as is the case, for example, in the combination of hemolytic antibodies to erythrocytes.

2) Cell combination occurs through sites located in the Fc region of the reaginic antibody molecule, in a similar manner to the mode of binding of rabbit and human γG antibodies to heterologous (guinea pig) tissues (Ovary and Karush 1961).

If the first possibility holds, tissue sensitisation could be considered to be an autoimmune phenomenon and it would be conceivable that interaction between the Fc regions of adjacent cell bound reagin molecules might lead to complement activation culminating in cell lysis (by a process similar to that thought to be operative in the induction of hemolysis by γG antibodies). There is now ample evidence to suggest, however, that γE antibodies do not fix complement;[2] and, furthermore, in vitro studies on actively and passively sensitised human leucocytes (discussed in ch. 2) indicate that reagin-mediated histamine release does not appear to involve cell destruction but rather an active secretory process from a viable cell. On the other hand, the second possibility is much more attractive in that cell combination through sites located within the Fc regions of γE antibodies would leave receptors in the Fab regions free for subsequent combination with specific antigen (i.e. allergen responsible for provoking the second stage of the immediate hypersensitivity reaction).

As already mentioned, this type of cell–antibody interaction has been observed in another situation, involving the combination of rabbit and human γG antibodies to guinea pig tissues. It is important to recognise, however, that one is dealing here with an artificial reaction system, operating across a wide species barrier under very different conditions to those obtaining during reagin-mediated skin reactions in primate tissues. For instance, (table 6.2), the optimum period (i.e. 2–4 hr) for sensitisation of guinea pigs skin by heterologous antibody is much less than that required for maximal P–K response in humans, and complement activation could be involved in the guinea pig PCA reactions. It is reasonable to assume, therefore, that different structural characteristics form the basis of anaphylactic reactions mediated by heterologous γG antibodies; which are, after all, produced under different circumstances to the production of γE antibodies and which are presumably destined to fulfil a different role. In this connection, it is worth mentioning that the blocking antibodies produced in response to hyposensitisation of allergic individuals with allergen preparations are also capable of evoking PCA reactions in guinea pigs (Connell and Sherman 1965).

Thus, although much useful information can be obtained from the study of heterologous tissue reactions mediated by γG-type antibodies which is of relevance to a better understanding of the mode of action of reagins (as will be indicated later), it should be recognised that – unlike γE antibodies (i.e. reagins) – γG antibodies are behaving atypically in such systems. There was no reason to expect, therefore, that γE antibodies would bind to primate tissue in a similar manner to the combination of γG antibodies to guinea pig tissues.

5.2 Mode of attachment of sensitising antibody to target cell

An opportunity of making a more direct investigation of the mechanism of action of γE antibodies arose with the discovery of a myeloma form of IgE by Johansson et al. (1968) in Sweden. As mentioned in the previous chapter, not only did this protein prove to be closely related antigenically to reaginic antibody but it was also shown to possess the latter's strong affinity for isologous tissues (but without possessing its allergen-binding ability). Moreover, this myeloma form of IgE was being put out into the patient's plasma at a level of 45 mg/ml (at its peak level of production) i.e. at about 25 000 times the average level of antibody IgE encountered in the sera of allergic individuals. Here then, at last, was the key to the chemical characterisation of antibody IgE by the same token as the study of their myeloma counterparts has been responsible for the structural characterisation of the major (more abundant) classes of immunoglobulin.

From our initial studies (referred to in the previous chapter), in which were demonstrated inhibition of the P–K reaction by myeloma IgE administered prior to (i.e. 24 hr) and simultaneously with the sensitising serum, it was concluded that the myeloma protein exerted its blocking effect by preferential binding to those receptor sites in the normal recipient's skin to which reaginic antibodies bind. Hence, further inhibition tests have been carried out (Stanworth et al. 1968) with proteolytic degradation products derived from different parts of the myeloma IgE molecule (fig. 5.2), in order to locate the position of its tissue binding groups and, by inference, those of antibody IgE molecules. As before, test preparations were administered prior to and simultaneously with the sensitising serum (from our usual horse dander-sensitive donor,

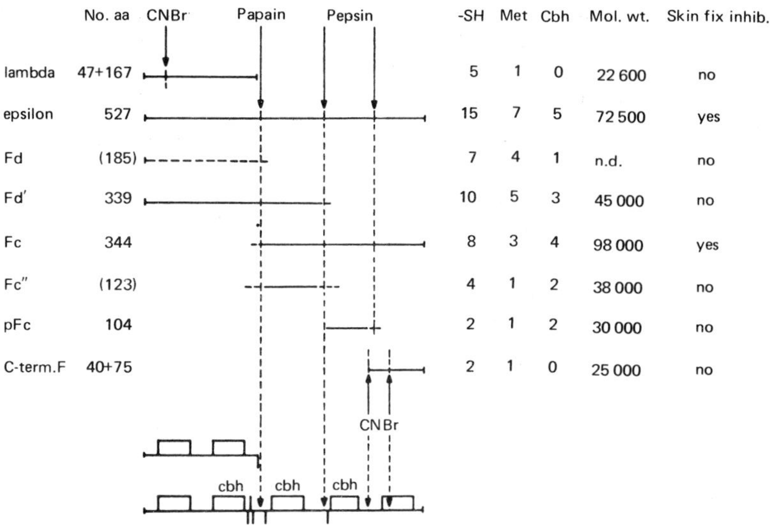

Fig. 5.2. Model of IgE structure (half molecule), showing the origin of cleavage products tested in inhibition P–K and PCA systems and the approx. positions of S–S bonds (reproduced from Bennich and Johansson, 1970, by permission of the authors). cbh: carbohydrate.

P.R.) at a standard concentration of 100 μg/ml (when pre-injected) and 50 μg/ml (when co-injected) i.e. in reasonable excess of the previously estimated minimum amount of whole myeloma IgE (i.e. between 3 and 30 μg/ml) needed to block P–K reactions induced by this particular sensitising serum (containing 615 ng antibody IgE/ml). Of all the proteolytic (papain and pepsin) digestion fragments tested, only the Fc fragment showed significant inhibitory activity (as is seen from the data given in tables 5.1 and 5.2). None of the fragments derived from the other part of the molecule (i.e. $F(ab')_2$, Fab and Fc-like) proved inhibitory; nor did whole γG myeloma proteins of human γG1 and γG2 sub-classes. Hence, it was concluded that myeloma IgE and, by inference, antibody IgE molecules bind to isologous human skin through sites within their Fc regions, thus leaving sites within their Fab regions free for subsequent interaction with allergen; and reagin combination to isolated human leucocytes and chopped lung ap-

TABLE 5.1

Results of testing myeloma IgE and various proteolytic cleavage fragments for competitive inhibition of the P–K reactions, evoked by transfer of a horse dandruff-sensitive individual's (P.R.) serum (0.05 ml) diluted with an equal volume of inhibitor solution containing 5 μg protein; allergen challenge: by pricking into the forearm sites 24 hr later.

Test substance	20′ M.W.A. (mm^2)
NaCl (control)	152 ± 17
IgE	5 ± 1
Fc	4 ± 0
$F(ab')_2$	114 ± 12
Fab	100 ± 32
Fd′	107 ± 19
λ chain	149 ± 40
IgG (normal)	121 ± 26
Allergen (direct test)	9 ± 5

peared to take place in a similar manner (Stanworth, unpublished observations).

The lack of inhibitory activity of Fc-like fragments and intermediate 7*S* 'Fc' fragments (obtained by less than 3 hr papain diges-

TABLE 5.2

Results of P–K testing at sites on a normal recipient's forearm injected 24 hr previously with myeloma IgE or a fragment. (Human IgG myeloma proteins of sub-classes 1 and 2 used as controls.)

Test substance	Dose (μg)	20′ M.W.A. (mm^2)
NaCl		57 ± 8
IgE	10	7 ± 3
Fc	5	3 ± 2
$F(ab')_2$	10	79 ± 13
Fab	5	53 ± 7
Fd′	5	47 ± 13
IgG (1)	10	47 ± 12
IgG (2)	10	65 ± 13
Allergen (direct test)		6 ± 0

tion of myeloma IgE) was disappointing, as it had been hoped to retrieve smaller sub-units than the Fc in which skin-fixing activity had survived. We have since looked into this question further, in the hope of locating the tissue-binding sites more precisely, by extending our studies to the use of non-human primates as recipients for skin testing (Stanworth et al. 1969A). We have used both rhesus monkeys and baboons for this purpose, having first demonstrated that myeloma IgE (whether pre- or co-administered) inhibits reagin-induced PCA reactions in these species at a similar dosage (e.g. 50–100 μg/ml) to that needed to block the P–K reaction in humans. A wide range of fragments of myeloma IgE have been produced by cleavage with various proteolytic enzymes, and as a result of autocatalytic changes occurring during storage, and these have been separated by gel-filtration and ion-exchange chromatography on DEAE sephadex (as previously). Duplicate competitive inhibition tests have been performed in at least 2 baboons with serum from a grass pollen-sensitive individual containing varying amounts of each fragment, to ascertain the minimum dose capable of effecting complete inhibition of reagin-induced PCA activity. A summary of the results obtained is provided in table 5.3. As will be noted, we have convincingly confirmed our previous P–K test results by demonstrating that the Fc fragment of the myeloma IgE is strongly inhibitory; whilst again failing to

TABLE 5.3
Baboon PCA-inhibition activity of proteolytic cleavage fragments of myeloma IgE.

Fragment no.	Cleavage enzyme	Characteristics of fraction	Min. inhibitory dose (μg)
II–IV (DE)	Papain	Fab + L chain	>114, >113, >111
I–II (G150)	Papain	Fc	2.3, <2.4
I–II (G150)	Papain	Fc	6.0, <2.4
I (G150)	Papain	Fc	21.6
X (DE)	Papain	Fc-like	>85.6
I (DE)	Pepsin	cont. Fc determs., carb-rich	>40
VII (DE)	Pepsin	$F(ab')_2$	>28
XI (DE)	Pepsin	cont. Fc determs.	>50
Control		whole IgND (IgE)	5–10

find evidence of tissue binding through sites located within the Fab regions of the IgE molecule (fig. 5.2). None of the other fragments in which Fc antigenic determinants were detectable (e.g. pepsin fractions I and XI and papain fraction X in table 5.3) showed convincing PCA-inhibition activity, except for certain fragments retrieved from tryptic digests in which the presence of contaminating residual IgE could not be entirely excluded.

The origin of some of the proteolytic cleavage fragments tested for PCA-inhibition activity is indicated by reference to the schematic model of the myeloma IgE (fig. 5.2). The studies of Bennich and Johansson (1970) have shown the IgE to be a compact molecule, of somewhat larger size (mol. wt. = 190 000) than γG-globulins (thus accounting for its greater sedimentation rate); which is now known to reflect the presence of an extra structural domain within the Fc region. It behaves differently from the major immunoglobulin classes (i.e. IgG, IgM and IgA) on treatment with papain and other proteolytic enzymes; cleavage processes which would be influenced by its relatively great abundance and different distribution of interchain disulphide bridges and carbohydrate prosthetic groups. Hence, some of the proteolytic cleavage fragments retrieved from digests by gel filtration and ion-exchange chromatographic procedures show different general characteristics to the classical sub-units obtained by papain and pepsin cleavage of human (and rabbit) γG-globulins. These points must be borne in mind when interpreting the data presented in table 5.3.

In this type of approach there are two requirements to be met: the isolation of cleavage products retaining the structural characteristics which they possessed in the parent immunoglobulin molecule and the location of their original position within that molecule, by antigenic and chemical analysis. The apparent lack of PCA-inhibition activity of the Fc subfractions referred to in fig. 5.2 and table 5.3 may be attributed to their lack of primary structural sequence of amino acid residues essential for tissue-binding, a possibility which can only be decided when the origin of these fragment has been fully established. On the other hand, at this stage, it is also conceivable that the proteolytic cleavage procedures adopted for the isolation of these types of fragment have caused structural alterations responsible for the destruction of the tissue-binding sites. This is always a problem to be faced in attempts to isolate biologically active polypeptide sub-units from proteins such as antibodies and enzymes, where denaturation often involves tertiary and quarternary structural changes within that part of the molecule comprising the active site(s). This then implies, of course, that the tissue-binding sites of γE antibodies are analogous to the active sites from enzymes, in comprising key amino acid residues located at widely differing positions along the ϵ chains, which are brought together into critical juxtaposition by the manner in which those chains are folded.

A similar problem has been encountered in recent attempts to isolate skin-reactive polypeptide fragments from proteolytic digests of rabbit γG-globulins. For instance, Prahl (1967) found that the products of proteolytic cleavage of the Fc sub-unit of rabbit γG-globulin were no longer able to inhibit passive cutaneous anaphylaxis induced in guinea pigs by rabbit anti-bovine serum albumin; nor were they capable of producing reverse passive cutaneous anaphylaxis reactions in the guinea pig. One of the fragments failing to show activity (namely the Pep III′, equivalent to the pF′c fragment of human γG-globulin) retains considerable structural integrity following peptic digestion, presumably because it comprises approximately half of the parent Fc sub-unit (fig. 5.3), i.e. the C-terminal 113 residue portion maintained conformationally by the presence of an intra-chain disulphide bridge. Hence, Prahl has concluded that it is likely that the site(s) responsible for skin binding activity reside predominantly or entirely in that area of the Fc sub-unit which is extensively degraded by proteolysis, namely the N-terminal 35–40 per cent of fragment Fc. This meant that alternative methods were required for recovering relatively large, intact, fragments from the N-terminal portion of the Fc region of γG-globulin molecules. Cyanogen bromide cleavage (at the methionine residues) is an obvious possibility, but this usually results in insolubilisation problems. The intermediate products produced by partial pepsin digestion of rabbit γG Fc fragment have been investigated (Goodman 1964; Paraskevas and Goodman 1965), revealing that a general decrease in PCA activity accompa-

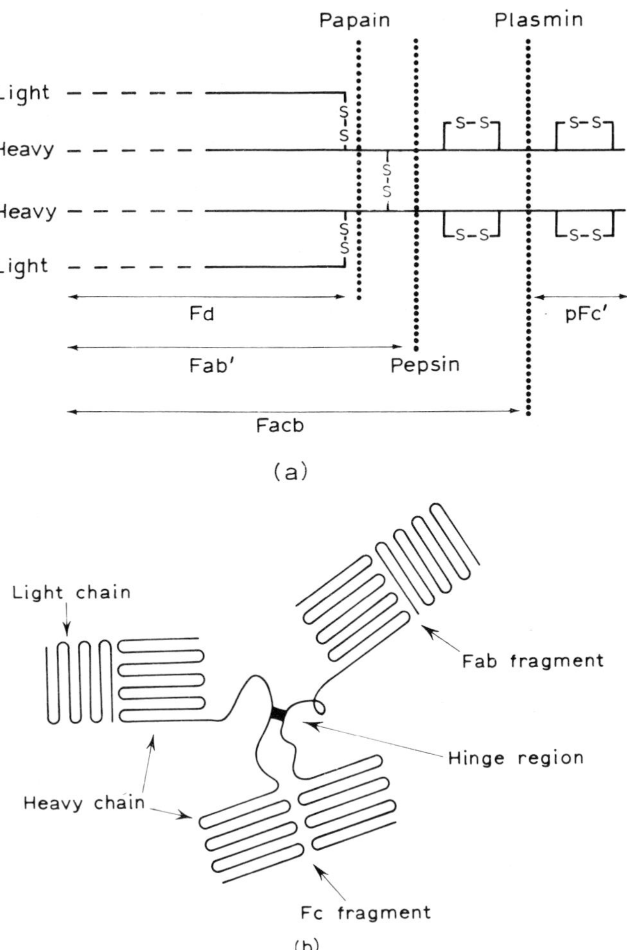

Fig. 5.3. Models of IgG structure indicating: a) points of cleavage of rabbit IgG by proteolytic enzymes; b) flexibility about the hinge region (reproduced from Noelken et al. 1964, by permission of the authors).

nies a decrease in the size of the products, which led Prahl to suggest that the enzymic degradation of rabbit γG-globulin Fc fragment occurs in stepwise fashion from the N-terminus, resulting in loss of biological activity as degradation passes through the sites responsible for PCA activity.

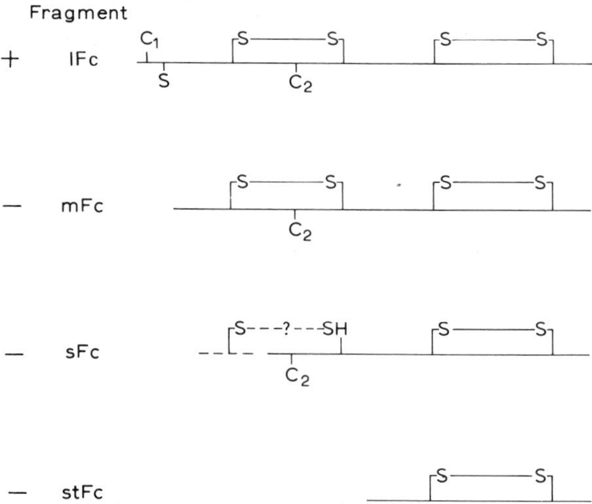

Fig. 5.4. Diagrammatic representation of the structure of various types of Fc sub-unit produced by proteolytic cleavage of rabbit IgG; showing also their reverse PCA activity in guinea pigs (reproduced from Utsumi 1969, by permission of the author).

This focuses attention on a possible role, in skin binding, of sites located within the 'hinge' region (fig. 5.3) of the γG molecule i.e. the region of relatively accessible polypeptide chain between the points of cleavage of papain and pepsin. It is interesting, therefore, that Utsumi (1969) has recently provided evidence of the importance of this part of the rabbit chain for heterologous (guinea pigs) skin-binding activity, as is illustrated schematically in fig. 5.4. He found that a papain cleavage fragment (designated 'lFc'), produced by brief digestion of rabbit IgG followed by cleavage of interchain disulphide bridges, retained a portion of the 'hinge' region and showed both skin-binding and complement-fixing activity. In contrast, another slightly smaller fragment (designated 'mFc'), produced by a more drastic digestion procedure, had lost its 'hinge' region and consequently lacked skin-binding activity (whilst retaining complement-fixing activity). Thus, it is tempting to conclude that the 'hinge' region plays an essential role in the tissue-binding of rabbit γG-globulin molecules; but, in this case, (as Utsumi points out) it is disconcerting to find that the divalent peptic $F(ab')_2$ fragment fails to give direct or reverse passive anaphylactic reactions in guinea pigs (Ovary and Taranta 1963) despite its retention of 'hinge' region at its C terminal end (Smyth and Utsumi 1967). This apparent anomaly could perhaps be due to the loss of complement binding site(s) in the $F(ab')_2$ fragment, if these prove to be essential for the elicitation of heterologous PCA reactions by γG-globulin in guinea pigs. It is possibly significant in this connection, however, that a similar situation appears to obtain with regard to the structural basis of the isologous skin-binding activity of γE antibodies where complement fixation is not involved; and, moreover, increasing evidence is appearing in the literature to suggest that complement fixation might not be necessary for γG mediated direct and reverse heterologous PCA reactions in guinea pigs. This implies that the lack of tissue-binding activity of $F(ab')_2$ fragments of rabbit IgG is attributable to a structural alteration within the 'hinge' region of the molecule, resulting from loss of the Fc region. Indeed, it is possible that the presence of the Fc region 'directs' tissue-combination via sites within the hinge region of the γG molecule. Alternatively, it is possible that whilst the tissue-binding sites are situated in the hinge region, separate 'cell-activating' sites are located further down within the N-terminal part of the Fc region; a situation which would be quite consistent with the type of triggering mechanism proposed later in this chapter, and discussed further in ch. 8. If this is the case, however, it is perhaps surprising that a newly described enzymic fragment (Facb) of rabbit antibody IgG (Connell and Porter 1971) showed only relatively weak direct and reverse PCA activity in guinea pigs (Stewart and Stanworth 1972).[3] For, as will be seen from fig. 5.3, this complement-binding fragment is produced by plasmin cleavage at a point in the Fc region between the N- and C-terminal loops (i.e. between lysine-326 and alanine-327); and would, therefore, be expected to incorporate any separate cell-activating site located within the N-terminal part of the Fc region of the molecule.

It is, of course, conceivable on the basis of present evidence that the skin binding site (or sites) in IgE antibodies are likewise located in the N terminal half of the Fc region near to the 'hinge' point. The results of the inhibition PCA testing of myeloma IgE proteolytic cleavage fragments, referred to in tables 5.1, 2 and 3, can (at this stage) be interpreted in this way. For instance, it seems possible that the unreactive carbohydrate-rich peptic fraction I (of mol. wt. = 27 000) is derived from the C-terminal half of the ϵ chain and is possibly analogous to the pF′c fragment of human IgG and the Pep III′ fragment of rabbit IgG. Consistent with this idea is our observation that a cyanogen bromide cleavage fragment (of mol. wt. = 12 000) derived from the C-terminal end of the myeloma IgG molecule appears to lack the capacity to inhibit tissue sensitisation. As stressed earlier, however, it is important to be cautious in drawing too close an analogy between the skin sensitising behaviour of isologous γE and heterologous γG antibodies, because of the difference in conditions under which the 2 types operate. Nevertheless, it seems reasonable to conclude that similar general types of conformational change are effective in both kinds of tissue reaction; which brings me to a consideration of the whole question of the importance of the tertiary and quaternary structural characteristics of tissue sensitising antibodies.

5.3 Conformational aspects of sensitising antibody activity

Much evidence is emerging to suggest that conformational factors do indeed play a critical role in immediate sensitivity reactions, both during the initial stage of binding of reaginic antibodies to tissues and sub-sequently following their combination with allergen. The unusual heat lability of reaginic antibodies even when in their native milieu of allergic serum, which cannot be attributed to the destruction of an essential complement co-factor, has always seemed to me to suggest that the biological activity of this type of antibody rests upon some fairly stringent conformational requirements; and, indeed, it is now becoming possible to define these particularly as a result of recent studies using the myeloma IgE. Earlier observations (Ishizaka et al. 1967) on the effect of heat on antibody γE-rich fractions (from ragweed-sensitive individuals' sera) had provided the first indication of the consequences of such treatment on the structure of reagin molecules. Using their radio-immunoassay procedure referred to in ch. 2, these investigators showed that the heating of antibody γE fraction at 56°C for 2–4 hr had little effect on the capacity to combine with allergen (i.e. ragweed E); but it did appear to cause a loss in specific antigenic determinants and, moreover, a loss in isologous skin sensitising activity. Johansson (1968) obtained further evidence of the heat susceptibility of the antigenic determinants of IgE, in showing that heating of the myeloma protein at 56° for 1–2 hr led to a decrease in its concentration of approximately 70 per cent as determined by immunodiffusion; whilst similar treatment of allergic sera with high IgE levels produced a 80–90 per cent decrease (Johansson and Bennich, unpublished observations).

In the light of findings from our later studies (Stanworth et al. 1968) on the mode of attachment of γE-globulins to isologous tissues, it seemed that the Fc region – in which both the tissue-binding sites and the specific antigenic determinants of IgE are located – was particularly vulnerable to heat treatment. Presumably this involves the induction of conformational changes, in which one or more of the numerous disulphide bridges located in this part of the IgE molecule (fig. 5.2) might well be implicated. This possibility has recently been investigated in studies (Stanworth et al. 1970) designed to ascertain the role of disulphide bridges in the maintenance of the tissue binding conformation of myeloma IgE. The myeloma IgE has been found to contain 21 disulphide bonds per 200 000 mol. wt., of which 9–10 are susceptible to reduction with mercaptans in aqueous solution at *p*H 8.0 (Bennich 1968). Two of these susceptible bonds link the light polypeptide chains to the heavy (ϵ) chains, and are attacked by reducing agents as rapidly as the corresponding bonds linking the light chains to the heavy (γ) chains in γG-globulins. The remaining 7–8 disulphide bonds, which react relatively slowly with mercaptans, were found to comprise inter- and intra-chain bonds characteristic of the ϵ chains. It is the effect of reduction of these which has been investigated, by treating myeloma IgE (in a 1 g per cent solution) with varying concentrations of 2-mercaptoethanol (ranging from 0.01–0.90 M) at *p*H 8.0 and 20° for 20 min fol-

TABLE 5.4
Inhibitory activity of reduced myeloma IgE preparations in reagin-mediated PCA reactions in baboons.

Preparation added to sensitising serum	SH content of reduced IgE (per mole)	Antigenicity, relative (%) to native IgE		Mean area of blueing induced in presence of 10 μg inhibitor (mm^2)	Minimum amount of IgE effecting complete inhibition (μg)
		(1)	(2)		
Saline (control)	–	–	–	98	
Normal IgG (control)	–	–	–	118	
Untreated IgE	0.0	100	100	0	(< 2)
Reduced IgE prep. 1	1.2	100	100	0	<10)
Reduced IgE prep. 2	5.2	100	100	0	3–5
Reduced IgE prep. 3	8.9	95	95	0	3–5
Reduced IgE prep. 4	10.3	90	90	0	3–5
Reduced IgE prep. 5	12.1	65	80	0	3–6
Reduced IgE prep. 6	16.0	30	75	106	20–30
Reduced IgE prep. 7	18.0	15	70	185	28

lowed by alkylation with iodoacetamide (10 per cent molar excess over reducing agent). Competitive-inhibition tests were performed in baboons with varying amounts of each reduced sample of IgE, mixed with a constant amount of sensitising serum (from an individual sensitive to grass pollen), to establish the minimum dose of each needed to block PCA activity. The types of result obtained are shown in table 5.4, where it will be noticed that cleavage of 8 or 9 of the susceptible disulphide bridges (determined by measurement of the carboxy methyl cysteine content of the reduced IgE preparations) led to a drastic reduction in PCA inhibition activity. Nevertheless, it was perhaps a little surprising to find that at least 6 of the 9 susceptible bonds could be cleaved without any apparent effect on tissue-binding activity. Presumably the other 2 bonds are essential for maintaining the tissue-binding conformation within the Fc region of the IgE molecule, and are more likely to be intra-ϵ chain disulphide bridges rather than inter-ϵ chain bridges or the 2 bonds linking the light and heavy polypeptide chains; which, as already mentioned, are readily cleaved during the initial stage of reduction of IgE (Bennich 1968) under the conditions employed.

Ishizaka and Ishizaka (1968D) also have to come to the conclusion that inter- and/or intra-ϵ chain bonds are probably necessary for maintaining the structures within the IgE molecule essential for skin fixation. This is based on the observation of a substantial loss in P–K activity of anti-ragweed γE antibodies following reduction (1 hr) with 0.1 M 2-mercaptoethanol at room temperature and alkylation with iodoacetamide, and a marked decrease (to one fifth) in the ability of pre-injected γE antibody to block passive sensitisation of humans with reaginic antibody of a heterologous system (namely against rye grass). Our findings are compatible with, but more revealing than, these in that we have investigated the effect of reducing the IgE molecule to varying extents and are able, therefore, to obtain some quantitative assessment of the number of critical disulphide bonds needed for skin attachment. On the other hand, we have restricted our attention to co-administered myeloma IgE whereas Ishizaka and Ishizaka (1968D) have looked at pre-administered antibody IgE, which has the advantage of throwing some light on the effect of reduction not only on the tissue-affinity of γE molecules but also on their overall capacity to elicit skin (i.e. P–K) reactions. The observed great decrease in P–K activity of antibody IgE following mercaptoethanol (0.1 M) treatment could be attributed at least in part, however, to a diminution in allergen-binding activity i.e. to a deleterious effect on the antigen-binding sites (located in the Fab regions, presumably) as well as on the tissue-binding sites (located within the Fc regions). In contrast, our studies on the myeloma IgE were only measuring the latter effect.

We have also studied the effect of partial reduction and alkylation on the antigenicity of myeloma IgE (Stanworth et al. 1969), as indicated by the other data contained in table 5.4. Cleavage of 2–5 of the accessible disulphide bonds was found to have no effect on the γE antigenicity as measured by single radial immunodiffusion or R.I.S.T.; but cleavage of further disulphide bonds, preferentially located within the C-terminal portion of the ϵ chains, changed drastically the antigenic characteristics of the myeloma IgE. In contrast to these findings, Ishizaka and Ishizaka (1969) have reported that reduction with 0.1 M 2-mercaptoethanol (followed by alkylation) did not impair the specific antigenicity of antibody IgE, as indicated by measurement of the minimum concentration needed to produce a precipitin line with anti-IgE in an Ouchterlony plate developed in the conventional manner or by using a radio-labelled marker IgE. A consideration of these findings in relation to our own data (table 5.4), obtained from studies of myeloma IgE reduced to varying extents, would seem to suggest that the reducing conditions employed by the Ishizakas (i.e. 0.1 M mercaptoethanol, 1 hr, room temperature) achieved cleavage of only about 3 disulphide bonds within the antibody IgE molecule and probably explains, therefore, why they failed to observe any change in antigenicity (assuming that the antibody and myeloma IgE preparations behave similarly towards such treatment). The possibility cannot yet be excluded, however, that the myeloma IgE is more resistant than the antibody IgE to treatment with mercaptans.

It seems reasonable to conclude from our own investigations that at least some of those disulphide bonds responsible for stabilising the Fc region of the IgE molecule are essential for maintaining the integrity of the tissue-binding conformation; and, as the specific γE antigenic determinants are also located in this region, it would be surprising if reductive cleavage did not also influence them. In fact, it is not impossible that tissue-binding sites and antigenic determinants will prove to occupy similar, or closely related, regions of the ϵ-chains. In this connection, it is significant that Ishizaka et al. (1967) showed that the heating of antibody IgE fractions for 2–4 hr destroyed not only skin sensitising activity but also the γE antigenic determinants (as mentioned earlier).

The recent findings which have just been discussed would also seem to explain earlier reports (Leddy et al. 1962; Rockey and Kunkel 1962; Reid et al. 1966) of the destructive effect of mercaptoethanol (0.1 M) on reaginic antibodies in pollen-sensitive individuals' sera; which needed to be interpreted with caution at the time because of the possibility that treatment of such complex protein mixtures with mercaptans could lead to spurious protein-protein interactions. It is interesting, however, that the sensitising antibodies in the serum of an individual showing sensitivity to

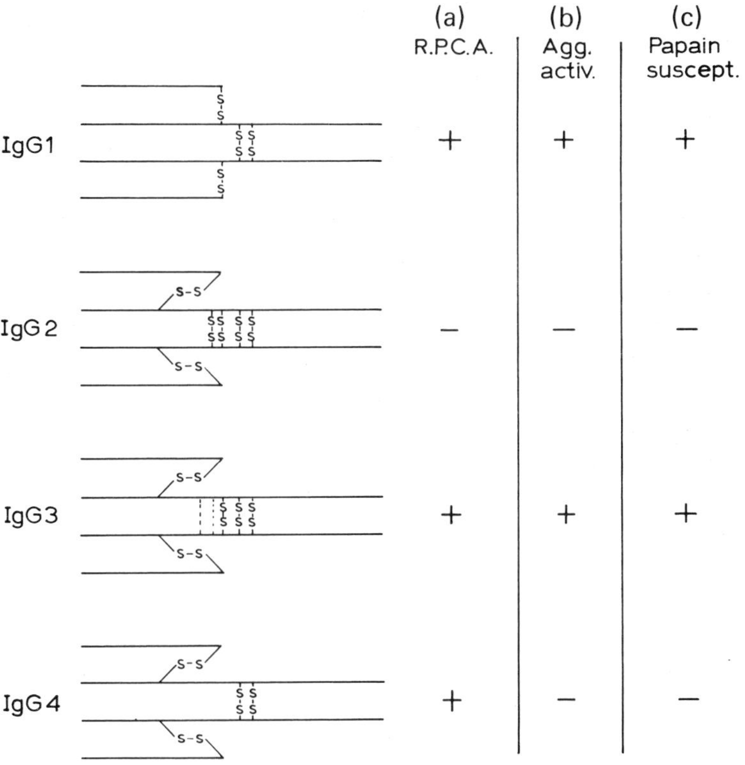

Fig. 5.5. Interchain disulphide bridge distribution of the 4 sub-classes of human IgG (from Frangione et al. 1969) compared with their: (a) skin reactivities in guinea pigs as monomers in the reverse PCA system (Terry 1965); (b) skin reactivities as aggregates (Ishizaka et al. 1967); (c) susceptibility to cleavage by papain (Jefferis et al. 1968) (reproduced from Stanworth 1970).

bovine serum albumin appeared to be much more resistant to such treatment (Reid et al. 1966); a finding which could possibly be attributed to the sensitising activity in this serum being associated with a γG-globulin (rather than IgE), as the authors suggest. In this event, it could be expected that the sensitising antibody would possess a different distribution of disulphide bonds to that encountered in γE molecules and, therefore, a different degree of susceptibility to cleavage by mercaptans. Moreover, even amongst the various human IgG sub-classes striking differences in the distribution of inter-chain disulphide bridges have been observed

(Frangione et al.1969); which could explain, for instance, the lack of heterologous PCA activity of proteins of the γG2 sub-class (Terry 1965). This is illustrated in fig. 5.5, in which is shown the arrangement of the interchain disulphide bridges within the 4 sub-classes of IgG as proposed by Frangione and his associates (1969). They have found that the amino acid sequence around the inter-heavy-chain bonds of a γG2 myeloma protein is strikingly different from that in the other 3 types, with the consequence that 4 half cysteine residues are present in a section only 8 residues long. This 'concentrated' distribution of the disulphide bonds within the 'hinge' region might also explain the outstanding resistance of IgG2 molecules to cleavage by papain (fig. 5.5) even in the presence of cysteine (Jefferis et al. 1968), as Frangione and associates (1969) have suggested. In this connection, our findings from more recent studies (Stanworth 1970) on the comparative papain susceptibility of the γG-globulins of other species would seem to be of more than a little relevance to the present discussion; for it is precisely those species (e.g. horse, cow, sheep) of IgG which are relatively resistant to cleavage by papain (in the absence of cysteine) which fail to evoke PCA reactions in guinea pigs (as will be seen from table 5.5). It seems, therefore, that these species (in contrast to humans, monkeys and rabbits) are incapable of producing γG-globulin sub-classes with the appropriate structure within their Fc regions necessary for binding to target cells; but they

TABLE 5.5
Comparison of skin reactivities of IgG of various species with their composition as reflected by their susceptibility to digestion by papain.

Species	PCA in guinea-pigs	% resistant to papain (4 hr, 37°)
Human	+	40
Monkey	+	51
Rabbit	+	66
Horse	–	95
Sheep	–	90
Cow	–	95

appear to produce, instead, γG antibodies with critical structural characteristics (particularly with regard to inter-chain disulphide bridge distribution) similar to those found in the unreactive human γG2 sub-class. In this respect they are behaving like the human in response to immunisation with pure polysaccharide antigens such as dextran, where – unlike immunisation against a wide range of protein antigens – the antiserum produced has consistently failed to evoke PCA reactions in guinea pigs. It has been shown recently (Yount et al. 1968) that such treatment leads to the production of γG antibodies confined exclusively to the γG2 subclass i.e. to the only one of the 4 human γG sub-classes which, for the reasons already outlined, possesses a structure which fails to meet the relatively exacting requirements for tissue sensitisation.

In discussing such requirements attention has been concentrated so far on the sensitising antibody structure involved in tissue binding; but it is important not to ignore the other important stage of immediate sensitivity reactions in which antibody conformation is all important, namely in relaying the effect of interaction with allergen to the appropriate activation system within the target cell. I am referring, of course, to the second major step of the sensitisation reaction depicted schematically in fig. 5.1. I have already proposed elsewhere (Stanworth 1967, 1969) that combination with specific allergen triggers off an allosteric transition within the cell-bound reaginic antibody molecules, resulting in the activation of a cell surface enzyme (or pro-enzyme) at the beginning of the chain of enzyme reactions; which, on the basis of in vitro studies discussed in ch. 8, are supposedly instrumental in the release of histamine and other vasoactive amines. The manner in which this critical reaction, involving the manifestation of the effect of reagin–allergen combination on the cell surface, might occur is indicated in diagrammatic form in fig. 5.6. Assuming a 4-chain model for the IgE molecule, analogous to that assigned originally by Porter (1959) to IgG, the antibody is depicted combining to the target cell through sites within in its Fc regions as our recent studies have demonstrated. The conformational change postulated as occurring in subsequent response to combination with allergen presupposes a high degree of flexibility about the 'hinge' region of the IgE mole-

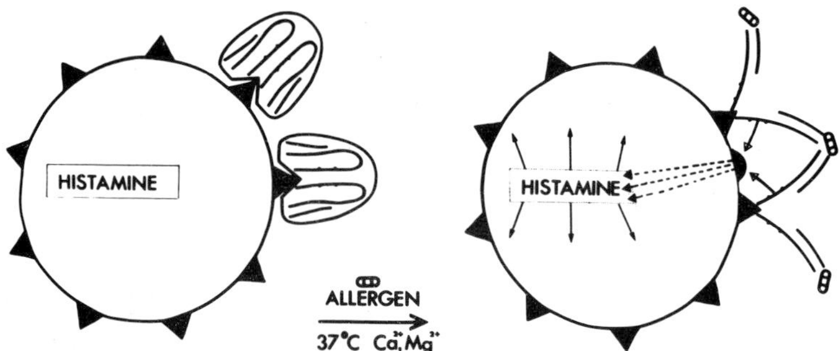

Fig. 5.6. Schematic representation of manner in which an allosteric transition induced in cell-bound anaphylactic antibody on combination with specific antigen might lead to activation of a site on the cell surface (reproduced from Stanworth 1971A).

cule. In fact I suggest that this is a critical requirement for all tissue sensitising antibodies, in addition to their capacity to fix to target cells; which is a particular attribute of γE-type (i.e. reaginic) antibodies but is also demonstrated, in a less sophisticated manner, by antibodies of certain γG sub-classes.

Taking up this question of γG sensitising antibody momentarily, it is not difficult to suppose that the presence of multiple inter-heavy-chain disulphide bridges in the human γG2 sub-class (fig. 5.5) would preclude the involvement of antibodies of this type in sensitisation reactions. By similar reasoning one might expect antibodies of the human γG3 sub-class to be likewise incapable of evoking direct PCA reactions in guinea pigs. Indeed, this might still prove to be the case because the activities of the human γG-globulin sub-classes listed in fig. 5.5 refer only to reverse passive anaphylaxis, a system in which the γG-immunoglobulin is acting as (cell bound) antigen which is provoked into inducing the release of histamine in heterologous tissue by reaction with an anti-γG-globulin antibody (fig. 5.9). In other words, the immunoglobulin structural requirements for this type of reaction (i.e. accessibility of antigenic determinants within the Fc region) need not necessarily be as demanding as those essential for direct PCA reactions, where the γG-globulin is acting as antibody; and thus – despite their possession of multiple chain disulphide bridges within their 'hinge' regions – molecules of the γG3 sub-class are at least capable of evoking reverse PCA reactions in guinea pigs. It might perhaps be anticipated, however, that a human antiserum comprising antibodies (to a particular antigen) which are confined exclusively to the γG3 sub-class would prove incapable of evoking direct PCA reactions in guinea pigs.

Returning to a consideration of the mode of action of γE antibodies it should be pointed out that there is not yet any firm evidence from direct structural studies on antibody IgE to support my suggestion of an unusual flexibility about the 'hinge' region of this molecule. In fact, in view of the large number of disulphide bridges found in myeloma IgE (as mentioned earlier) and presumably present also in antibody IgE, it might be supposed that there is much more scope for structural stabilisation by covalent cross-links in this type of immunoglobulin molecule than, say, in IgG. The distribution of the disulphide bridges is, however, a critical factor governing structural flexibility; and, although the number and location of the disulphide bonds linking the ϵ chains has yet to be fully established, the positioning of an inter-heavy-chain on the C-terminal side of the extra domain (fig. 5.2, on the basis of preliminary characterisation of enzyme digestion fragments of myeloma IgE) would be expected to have a profound and unique influence during any quaternary structural changes within the molecule. Indeed, it might be speculated that such a structure would be particularly well equiped for mediation of immediate hypersensitivity reactions by the mechanism proposed in this chapter (fig. 5.6), in that it would facilitate a buckling of the Fc region nearest to the hinge section thereby bringing an activating site into optimum juxtaposition relative to the target cell. Whereas, in contrast, γG antibody molecules lacking the extra structural domain and inter-chain disulphide bridge in this position of their Fc regions might be expected to be much less efficient at cell activation.

Nevertheless, there is now much direct experimental evidence to indicate that some γG antibodies (from species such as rabbits) undergo substantial changes following combination with specific antigen in free solution. For instance, we (Henney et al. 1965;

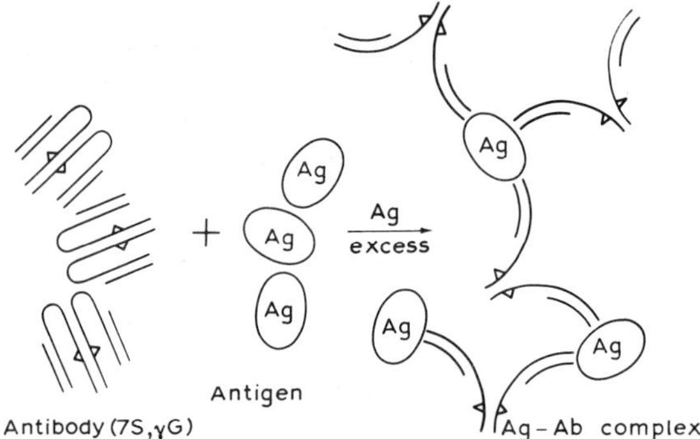

Fig. 5.7. Schematic representation of conformational change induced in γG antibody molecules as a result of combination with specific antigen (reproduced from Stanworth 1970).

Henney and Stanworth 1966) have employed chemical, physico-chemical and immunological procedures to provide convincing evidence that the formation of soluble complexes between rabbit γG antibody and bovine serum albumin (BSA), in moderate antigen excess, results in the induction of critical conformational changes within the antibody molecules with the exposure of new immunogenic determinants (fig. 5.7). Furthermore, similar studies on horse ferritin-anti-ferritin complexes revealed that a larger antigen causes greater structural deformation within complexed rabbit γG antibody molecules (optical rotation data in table 5.6), involving unfolding in both the Fd and Fc regions of the γ chains.

Evidence in support of these observations has arisen from an entirely different approach, namely electron microscopy studies of antigen (horse ferritin)–antibody complexes (Feinstein and Rowe 1965). These indicated that the cross-linking of antigenic particles causes the rabbit γG antibody molecule to 'click open' about its hinge point, thereby exposing its Fc region and (it is suggested) unmasking of the complement binding sites located there. Such a conformational change would be expected to lead also to the exposure of the heterologous skin reactive sites, which are presumed to be located in a different part of the Fc region of the rabbit γG molecule (i.e. closer to the hinge region, according to the recent findings of Utsumi 1969, discussed earlier).

TABLE 5.6
Specific optical rotation changes induced in rabbit antibody γG-globulin by combination with antigen (reproduced from Henney and Stanworth 1966).

Antigen	Specific optical rotation at 589.5 nm			
	Antigen/ antibody weight ratio	Immune complexes	Antigen-γG-globulin (non-antibody) mixture	Difference
BSA	1.9	−64.6	−58.8	+5.8
	2.4	−61.0	−59.3	+1.7
	3.2	−60.4	−59.8	+0.6
	4.5	−60.6	−60.3	+0.3
	9.1	−61.0	−61.1	−0.1
Ferritin	2.7	−40.2	−31.9	+8.3
	4.1	−35.2	−30.9	+4.3
	5.4	−33.8	−30.3	+3.5
	6.8	−30.2	−29.9	+0.3
	13.6	−28.3	−29.0	−0.7
	19.0	−28.6	−28.7	−0.1

Heat denaturation of human γG globulin (50° for 10 min) produced a rise in specific optical rotation at 589.5 nm of 9.8°.

Indeed, it is highly significant that the preliminary optical rotation studies of Ishizaka and Campbell (1959) indicated that it is these same complexes, formed in moderate antigen excess (i.e. Ag_3 Ab_2 in which structural alterations in antibody occur as manifested by an increase in laevorotation), which evoke immediate skin reactions in guinea pigs. In contrast, no evidence of a change in optical rotation is observed to accompany the formation of the biologically inactive Ag_2 Ab complexes (containing only one antibody molecule). This led Ishizaka (1963) to put forward the tentative hypothesis that antigen–antibody (γG) interaction results in the formation of toxic (i.e. skin reactive) configurations when 2 or more antibody molecules combine with one antigen molecule. As has just been indicated we and others have since obtained substantial evidence that the formation of such skin reactive complexes involves structural changes within the Fc region of the antibody molecule, i.e. the region through which attachment to guinea pig tissue occurs. The important question still to be answered, however, is whether the unfolding process exposes skin reactive sites within individual cell bound antibody Fc regions, or whether it leads to the formation of composite sites comprising determinants contributed from more than one antibody molecule. In this connection, it seems pertinent that the non-specific aggregation of γG-globulins (e.g. human and rabbit) or their Fc fragments, whether effected by heating (or some other form of denaturation treatment) or by chemical coupling with bis-diazotised benzidine (B.D.B.), also leads to the formation of soluble skin reactive (and complement fixing) aggregates (Ishizaka 1963). Moreover, recent studies (Henney and Ishizaka 1968) have shown that the new antigenic determinants exposed within the Fc regions of the antibody γG molecules as a result of such non-specific treatments are similar to the determinants revealed by specific antibody γG-antigen combination (fig. 5.7). However, the new antigenic determinants *per se* do not appear to be responsible for the biological activities shown by the aggregates, because aggregated human IgG and aggregated rabbit IgG show no cross-reactivity when tested with antisera directed against one or the other. It seems, therefore, that the appearance of these new antigenic determinants (like the appearance of -SH groups, first observed by Robert and Grabar 1957, on antigen–antibody combination) is yet another manifestation of the conformational changes undergone by γG molecules on association. Moreover, our recent studies aimed at identifying and locating the auto-antigenic determinants responsible for the rheumatoid factor-reactivity of aggregated human IgG (Matthews and Stanworth 1971), suggest that such antigenic determinants are located – like the skin-reactive and complement-fixing sites – within the N-terminal half of the Fc regions (see fig. 5.3a) of the aggregated IgG molecules; or, alternatively, require the interaction of the N- and C-terminal halves.

Thus, a comprehensive picture is beginning to emerge of the tertiary and quaternary structural changes occurring when human or rabbit γG-globulin molecules associate to form biologically active aggregates. Although the skin reactivity thereby induced is demonstrable in different species (namely guinea pigs) to those in

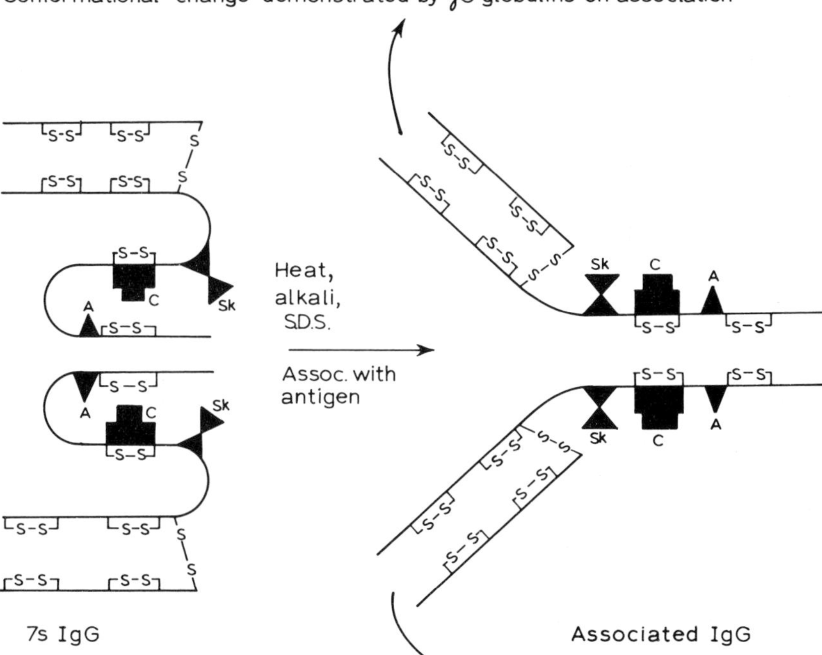

Fig. 5.8. Schematic representation of manner in which conformational changes in γG molecules resulting from specific or non-specific association could lead to the exposure of various biologically reactive groupings within the Fc regions (e.g. A=antigenic; C=complement fixing; Sk=skin reacting) (reproduced from Stanworth 1972).

which γE-mediated skin reactions are manifested (i.e. humans and monkeys), it should be apparent by now that a closer study of the manner in which these structural changes occur should throw further light on the nature of the conformational changes induced in cell-bound reaginic (γE) antibody molecules following their combination with specific allergen (fig. 5.6).

It seems probable that the association of human IgG to form large soluble aggregates (20–40 *S*), possibly as a result of intermolecular reactions through the Fab regions, is accompanied by the unfolding of the Fc regions with the 'formation' of skin reactive ('Sk') and complement fixing ('C') sites within their N-terminal halves (fig. 5.8). At the same time, the resultant association of the

C-terminal halves of the Fc regions (i.e. the pFc′ regions) of the reactive molecules leads to the appearance of antigenic ('A') determinants within these parts of the aggregated IgG. Furthermore, it appears that such structural alterations can occur when as few as 2 IgG molecules associate because 10*S* dimers separated from low temperature ethanol preparations of human IgG have been shown (Stanworth and Henney 1967) to fix complement as well as possessing new antigenic determinants not present on the monomer (Matthews and Stanworth 1972); and BDB-linked 9.5*S* complexes of rabbit IgG were found (Ishizaka and Ishizaka 1968) to evoke immediate skin reactions in guinea pigs and to fix complement in vitro.

In suggesting that a dimerisation process is sufficient to produce the biologically active sites detectable in the Fc regions of larger aggregates of human and rabbit IgG, these observations focus further attention on the question of a co-operative effect operating between determinants exposed on each of the two IgG molecules. Such a situation seems to obtain in the fixation of complement to sites on the Fc regions of hemolytic rabbit γG antibodies bound to erythrocyte surfaces through the antigen-binding sites located within their Fab regions (fig. 5.9C). For instance, electron microscopic studies (Humphrey and Dourmashkin 1965) and studies (Borsos and Rapp 1965) based on the transfer of the activated first component of complement (C1a) have indicated that a minimum of 2 molecules of hemolytic γG antibody are needed on adjacent sites on the erythrocyte surface to initiate the binding of a single molecule of C1a. Moreover, support for this idea has been recently provided by the studies of Cohen (1968), involving the reaction of untreated rabbit γG antibody in the presence of antibody whose complement fixing sites have been blocked by chemical conjugation. A quantitative study of the suppressive effect thus produced led to the conclusion that there is a requirement for 2 adjacent active γG antibody molecules acting co-operatively in the fixation of complement. It seems conceivable, therefore, that the positioning of two γG antibody molecules on adjacent receptor sites on the erythrocyte surface could lead to interaction, and quite possibly to conformational changes within the Fc regions, in

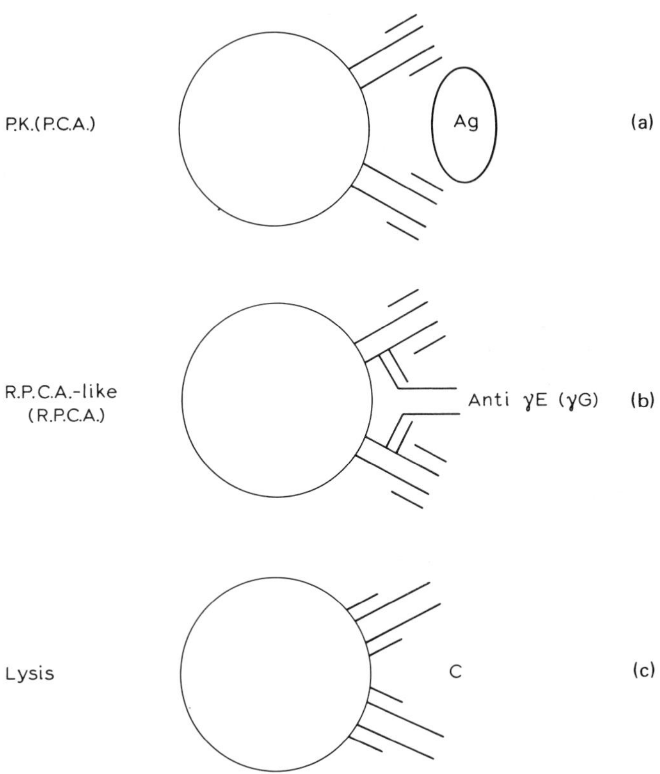

Fig. 5.9. Schematic representation of differences in the basic immunochemical mechanism of: direct (a) and reverse (b) anaphylactic reactions; and (c) lytic reactions involving complement (reproduced from Stanworth 1970).

a similar manner to that envisaged as occurring as the result of the formation of 10*S* dimer (and larger polymeric forms) of human IgG in free solution (Stanworth and Henney 1967). Furthermore, the observed ability of a single molecule of erythrocyte-bound γM antibody to initiate complement fixation could be attributed to a similar mechanism, but in this case it is postulated that an intramolecular interaction between the Fc regions of the 7*S* sub-units resulting from the unfolding of the γM antibody molecule on the cell surface is the triggering process.

The observations of Ishizaka and associates (1969) of an inhibition of complement fixation by soluble complexes of blood group A substance and γM anti-A antibody are not necessarily in conflict within this idea; because it is quite possible that the Fc regions of the γM antibody molecules comprising these complexes, formed in antigen excess, are not suitably distorted. In this connection it is of possible significance that the hinge region of μ chains has been found to be low in proline residues (Paul et al. 1971); which could be responsible for a lack of the flexibility apparent in the proline-rich hinge regions of human γG1- and rabbit γG-immunoglobulins. Moreover, it is conceivable that occupation of all the antigen-binding sites within the Fab regions of the pentameric γM antibody molecule prevents access of complement to sites within the Fc regions.

5.4 Effect of allergen combination, or artificial cross-linking agent

Increasing evidence is being obtained to indicate that a doublet of cell-bound antibody molecules is also a critical requirement for the elicitation of tissue sensitisation reactions, but in this case (as has already been discussed) the antibody molecules are bound to the cell receptors through sites within their Fc regions (leaving their Fab regions free for combination with antigen). Moreover, their dimerisation is initiated by cross-linking by antigen (fig. 5.6).

Experimental evidence in support of this idea of the bridging of adjacent cell-bound sensitising antibody molecules by antigen has been provided from studies of the valency requirements of both antigen and γG antibody in the mediation of PCA reactions. Despite some conflicting evidence (discussed earlier in ch. 3 § 3), studies with synthetic antigens such as hapten-substituted polylysines and penicillin derivatives (Levine 1965A and B; De Weck and Schneider 1969) suggest that 'allergens' require at least 2 combining groups, although the artificial antigens which have proved most effective in eliciting anaphylactic reactions in guinea pigs carry 4–5 antigenic determinants within a relatively short length of the molecule. Other evidence (fig. 3.10) for the bridging by allergen of 2 combining sites on 2 different (adjacent) antibody molecules has been provided by Ovary's (1965) observations that hybrid rabbit γG antibody molecules comprising one antibody Fab region and one non-antibody Fab region are capable of sensitising guinea pigs for passive cutaneous anaphylaxis, and by Goodman's (1965) findings that 5*S* intermediates of rabbit antibody γG, comprising an Fc region and only one Fab region, are as effective as whole 7*S* antibody γG-globulin molecules in eliciting PCA reactions. In other words, sensitising antibodies possessing a single antigen-combining site appear to be effective.

We ourselves (Stanworth et al. 1972) have recently obtained further convincing evidence in support of the bridging idea, from in vitro studies of anaphylactic reactions in the ilea of guinea pigs sensitised specifically to aggregated human IgG (ch. 3). It was found that only aggregated IgG had the capacity to evoke histamine release in the sensitised animals' tissue, but the 7*S* monomeric IgG was able to block this reaction. Thus the situation appears to be directly analogous to that involving the interaction of native and aggregated human IgG with anti- γG-globulins (such as rheumatoid factor), where the monomeric form appears to possess one binding site for the antibody whilst the aggregated form possesses several.

Assuming that the allergen does cross-link adjacent cell-bound antibody molecules, it is still necessary to establish whether this results in interaction between the 2 antibody molecules comprising the doublet as is postulated in the case of complement fixation (to different sites within the Fc regions). The crucial question is whether the allosteric effect considered to be initiated by allergen combination (fig. 5.6) is confined to individual molecules of the doublets, or whether it also involves interaction between the Fc regions of adjacent sensitising antibody molecules. The behaviour of aggregated human γG-globulin preparations on injection into guinea pigs, which have already received an intravenous injection of Evan's Blue, would seem to throw some light on these questions. As will be noted from the results (Terry 1965; Ishizaka et al. 1967) given in fig. 5.5, aggregated human γG2- and γG4-globulins fail to produce immediate blueing reactions in such animals, but monomeric γG4-globulin (unlike monomeric γG2-globulin) is capable of binding to guinea pig skin as indicated by its ability to evoke reverse passive cutaneous anaphylactic reactions. In contrast the γG1- and γG3-globulins bind to guinea pig skin when in monomeric form, and have the capacity to evoke immediate skin reactions when in aggregate form. It seems to be highly significant that the skin fixation of aggregated γG4-globulin to the guinea pig tissue is not sufificient to evoke PCA reactions and suggests (as Ishizaka et al. 1967, have pointed out) that structures other than those involved in tissue-binding need to be formed if aggregates of IgG are to prove capable of evoking immediate skin reactions. I would go further (in the light of recent studies on aggregates of myeloma IgE) in suggesting that likewise the structural basis of γE reaginic antibodies can be most readily explained by postulating the initial sensitisation step (involving the fixation of the antibodies to the tissue) is followed by a cell-activation step in which reaction with allergen initiates the formation of an activation site within a different part of the Fc region to the fixation site(s), which might comprise amino acid residues from adjacent molecules. Furthermore, this exerts its effect on the tissue without the aid of complement (in contrast to γG antibody-mediated lytic reactions, depicted schematically in fig. 5.9c).

We have recently obtained direct evidence from immediate skin testing in baboons (Stanworth et al. 1969B) that the activation sites on aggregates of myeloma IgE are located in different parts of the molecule to the skin fixing sites. Furthermore, the recent demonstration of Ishizaka (1970) that aggregated Fc fragments of myeloma IgE, as well as aggregated whole IgE, are capable of producing immediate skin reactions in humans and monkeys suggests that the tissue-activation site(s) are also located within the Fc region of the IgE molecule.

As in the case of the sensitisation of guinea pig tissue by γG antibodies, substantial evidence is accumulating in support of a bridging of adjacent cell bound γE antibody molecules by allergen. For instance, Ishizaka and Ishizaka (1968A) have observed, from studies with γE reagin–allergen (ragweed E) complexes of different compositions separated by density gradient centrifugation,

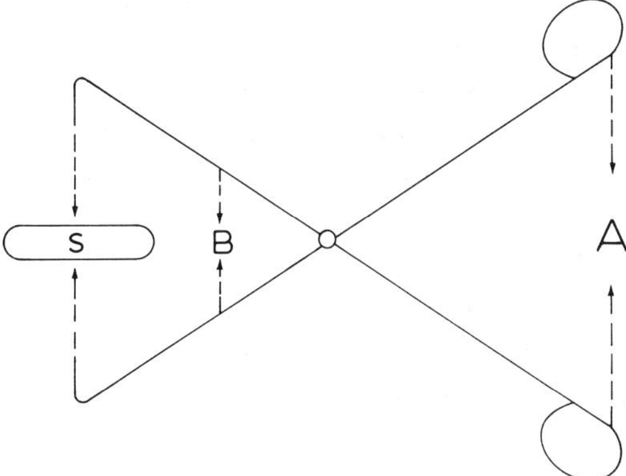

Fig. 5.10. Simple model illustrating how the concept of allosterism in enzyme molecules is also applicable to the understanding of the mode of action of artificial methods of effecting histamine release, by other agents capable of cross-linking cell-bound Ig molecules (S = site activated on target cell surface) (reproduced from Stanworth 1971).

that 2 or more γE antibody molecules are required for the formation of skin reactive complexes. Furthermore, similar immediate reactions can be effected by injection of rabbit anti-IgE, or even the $F(ab')_2$ fragment of rabbit anti-IgE which has been deprived of its complement fixing sites. This, too, is thought to effect a reaction between adjacent cell-bound γE molecules, but here the bridging presumably occurs between the Fc regions of the γE molecules i.e. closer to the cell surface (fig. 5.9). It is conceivable that such an interaction (at point B on the model depicting allosterism shown in fig. 5.10) would achieve a similar structural deformation within the Fc region to that initiated by antigen bridging between the more remote Fab regions of adjacent molecules (analogous to application of a force at point A on the model); but the latter process is the more refined one. For this reason, one might expect the size of the bridging antigen molecule to be fairly critical and, hence, it seems more than fortuitous that most inhalant allergens which have been purified and characterised to any extent have proved to possess molecular weights in the relatively narrow range of 30 000–40 000 (ch. 3).

It is also most interesting, in this connection that 'protein A', the cell wall constituent from *S. aureus* which gives pseudo-immune reactions with human and rabbit γG-globulins by cross-linking through their Fc regions (Forsgren and Sjöquist 1966), which produces anaphylactic-like cutaneous reactions in non-immunised guinea pigs (Gustafson et al. 1968) and which also effects the in vitro release of leucocyte histamine (Martin and White 1969), appears to possess a molecular weight of approximately 40 000 (Sjöquist 1971). Presumably this protein might also exert its anaphylactic-like reactivity by cross-linking tissue bound γG molecules in a similar region to that bridged by anti-γG-globulin antibody in reverse passive cutaneous anaphylactic reactions in guinea pigs (fig. 5.9) i.e. at position B in the model in fig. 5.10. It might be argued that, in contrast to the size of the protein A (acting in γG systems) and to common inhalant allergens (acting in γE systems), the antibodies which are also capable of effecting (reverse) skin reactions are of relatively larger size; but in their case the critical spacing would be the distance between the 2 Fab prongs of the γG molecule (or its $F(ab')_2$ fragment), and electron microscopic studies of antibody γG molecules suggest that these prongs are folded together prior to combination with antigen.

The implications of the mechanism of cell-bound antibody–antigen interaction proposed are obviously far reaching. For instance, as has been indicated, this does not preclude the possibility that more than one type of immunoglobulin is capable of effecting such reactions. Admittedly, with its strong tissue-affinity and presumably flexible conformation the IgE molecule appears to be particularly suited to such a role. Nevertheless, it is quite conceivable that certain γG antibodies can also mediate tissue reactions, although their weaker tissue affinity and greater structural rigidity would render them less effective. Indeed, there is already evidence of an isologous sensitising antibody of this type being produced artificially in guinea pigs and rats (ch. 6); and, as has already been mentioned, there are indications that a similar type of non-γE sensitising antibody is also produced in certain forms of human hypersensitivity (e.g. to serum protein injectants and to antibiotics). As suggested by recent observations of Morse et al. (1969), on the various modes of action of rat tissue sensitising antibodies (fig. 6.2), it is quite conceivable that different types of sensitising antibody will prove to be reacting with different target cells. Possibly a certain complementariness of structure is required between the antibody's combining groups and the cell's receptor groups, which could account for the narrow species specificity of human γE antibodies for target tissue and the inability of the IgG of some animal species to fix to guinea pig skin. This suggests that the chemical characterisation of the cell receptor groups will throw further light on the nature of the antibody's cell-binding groups and vice versa. There is also the possibility, however, that whilst possessing the ability to combine to tissues, certain immunoglobulins fail to form the appropriate activation sites; or, alternatively, these might be formed but in the wrong stereo chemical relationship to the 'substrate' on the cell surface (due, perhaps, to the target cell possessing an unsuitable spacing of charged groupings upon its surface). The extra structural domain within the Fc region of the γE-globulin molecule could be a critical factor in the meeting of these requirements (as was discussed earlier).

5.5 Nature of cell-binding groups, and target cell receptors

Little is known yet about the nature of the target cell receptors or the binding sites within the Fc regions of the tissue sensitising antibody molecules, but there is no reason to suppose that their interaction does not involve secondary valency forces (i.e. electrostatic and hydrophobic) between polar and non-polar groupings in a similar manner to antigen binding through sites located in the Fab regions of antibody molecules. The speculations of Ljaljevic et al. (1968B) based on studies involving the effect of chemical modification of the amino groups on the sensitising capacity of rabbit γG-globulins in guinea pig skin, are interesting in this connection. These investigators suggest that one or two charged ϵ ammonium groups may play a critical role in the binding of the γG-globulin molecules to receptor sites which might contain a complementary anionic carboxylate or phosphate group. If the combination between tissue receptors and sensitising antibodies is of this type, it might be expected that the antibodies would be elutable from sensitised tissues by lowering the *p*H. This treatment might lead, however, to inactivation of the relatively easily denatured γE antibodies, and failure to demonstrate their recovery.

Investigations involving the treatment of recipient tissue and cell preparations with specific enzymes would appear to offer a promising (and relatively gentle) method of characterising the cell receptor groups.[4] This approach has been used to demonstrate that the sites on guinea pig macrophages to which guinea pig γ_1-type antibodies bind are inactivated by phospholipase A but not by proteolytic enzymes such as trypsin, chymotrypsin and papain (Davey and Asherson 1967); suggesting that a phospholipid or phospholipoprotein is an important part of the macrophage receptor for cytophilic antibody. This type of cell binding, measured by the subsequent adherence of sheep erythrocytes, was unaffected by *p*H changes in the range of 5.4–9.0 or by 0.5 mM EDTA, as was also observed by other investigators (Berken and Benacerraf 1966). On the other hand, oxidising agents such as iodine, buffered periodic acid and peracetic acid destroyed receptor activity.

Chemical substitution of specific groupings is more readily applied to the cell-binding sites on the sensitising antibodies than to the receptors on the target cells themselves. It is important, however, to establish that the treatment employed has not resulted in some critical change in conformation of the sensitising antibody molecule which, as has been indicated, might well lead to loss in tissue-binding activity. This qualification must be applied to the studies of Andersen et al. (1966) of the effect of mild periodate oxidation on the skin sensitising activities of isolated fractions of rabbit γG antibodies and the human γE antibodies in allergic sera; but, in this case, there is the possibility that the observed reduction in activity was due to oxidation of amino acids (as well as carbohydrate). Furthermore, contrary to the findings of these investigators, other workers (Ljaljevic et al. 1968A) have obtained evidence that sodium metaperiodate inactivates the antigen-binding site of rabbit γG antibody; as apparently does the reagent (5 nitro-2-hydroxybenzyl bromide) used by Griffin et al. (1967) in studies claimed to indicate that the tissue (guinea pig) binding site or rabbit γG-globulin might contain tryptophane. More convincing evidence has been obtained to indicate that chemical modification of the amino groups of rabbit γG-globulins *per se* (by acetylation, carbamylation, picrylation or phthylation), rather than any gross tertiary structural change induced by such treatments, brings about loss of skin sensitising activity (Ljaljevic et al. 1968A and B). Moreover, similar reagents have been shown to diminish markedly the ability of guinea pig γ_1-globulins to fix to isologous skin; suggesting that there is some degree of homology between the tissue-binding sites of the two kinds of γ-globulin (which might, of course, extend even to γE antibodies). These workers also showed that the total removal of the neuraminic acid from rabbit γ-globulin by enzyme treatment failed to affect its skin sensitising activity; and, in studies on the effect of amidation, they obtained further evidence to suggest that complement fixation was not involved in the PCA reactions induced in guinea pigs by rabbit γG antibodies.

Thus, some headway is being made by adopting direct approaches in the characterisation of the tissue binding sites of skin sensitising antibodies. Admittedly a substantial part of this work has been carried out so far on antibodies of the γG-type operating within and across species; but (as will become apparent from the next chapter) there is growing immunochemical evidence to suggest that the mechanisms of tissue sensitisation by such antibodies are basically similar to that by γE-type antibodies. As already emphasised, one outstanding property of γE antibodies is their much stronger tissue affinity; which will quite probably prove attributable to the involvement of a greater number of amino acid side chains (located in their bulkier Fc regions) in the cell attachment process. A further characteristic of γE antibodies would appear to be a ready ability to undergo antigen-induced conformational change (for the reasons already discussed).

5.6 Summary

In summary, the structural basis of the activity shown by reaginic antibodies has been considered with regard to both cell binding and antigen combination; and an attempt has been made to outline a plausible sequence of events culminating in the triggering of the mechanism responsible for the release of the pharmacological mediators of immediate sensitivity reactions. The whole question of the nature of interaction between activator groupings on the tissue-bound antibody molecule and activation sites on the cell will be considered further in ch. 8, which deals with the various mechanisms of histamine-release effected by specific and non-specific means. Further consideration will also be given there to the key role of the allergen in the initiation of immediate hypersensitivity reactions.

Particular emphasis has been placed in this chapter on the tertiary and quaternary characteristics of the sensitising antibody, both in the initial fixation process and in the subsequent activation of the target cell. Furthermore, the molecular size of the allergen is considered to be an important factor in the latter step, involving the induction of a crucial allosteric transformation within the cell-bound antibody molecules.

It seems that there are 3 main requirements for effecting tissue sensitisation reactions of the immediate type. Firstly, the sensitising antibody must be capable of attaching to the appropriate cell receptors without undergoing any substantial change in conformation. Secondly, having done so, it must retain a sufficient degree of flexibility within its hinge region; and thirdly, its subsequent interaction with allergen must bring key amino acid residues within the correct spatial relationship to the tissue activation sites. Antibodies of the γE type would appear to meet these requirements most readily, whereas antibodies of some other classes (e.g. γM and γA) appear to lack these essential properties.

Notes

[1] See note 8, p. 126.

[2] Although evidence has recently been obtained (Ishizaka, T., Sian, C.M. and Ishizaka, K., J. Immunol. 1972, *108*, 848) to suggest that non-specifically aggregated myeloma IgE is capable of activating late components of complement through an alternative pathway.

[3] Later tests on purer Facb fragment preparations have failed to reveal any tissue-binding activity (Stewart, G., Smith, A.K. and Stanworth, D.R., to be published).

[4] This approach has recently been applied to good effect in an exhaustive study by Bach, M.K. et al. (in "Biochemistry of the Acute Allergic Reactions", 2nd Internat. Symp. Eds. Austen & Becker, Blackwell, 1972) of the influence of a wide range of enzymes on the rat mast cell receptor for IgE antibody.

CHAPTER 6

Immediate hypersensitivity in experimental animals

6.1 Introduction

Animals have been used in the study of experimental anaphylaxis ever since Portier and Richet (1902), under the patronage of the Prince of Monaco (who was no doubt a keen swimmer), employed dogs in the investigation of the toxin produced by the dreaded Portuguese man-of-war jelly fish. The guinea pig has since proved the species of choice, however, because of the ease with which it can be actively or passively hypersensitised, besides possessing other advantages as an experimental animal. Studies of anaphylactic responses in isolated guinea pig tissue preparations (chopped lung, ileum, uterus etc.), which have been passively sensitised in vitro or obtained from pre-sensitised animals, have provided a means of controlled investigation of the many factors influencing immediate hypersensitivity reactions (as will become further apparent from the following chapter). Yet it is only relatively recently, with the stimulus of the finding that similar reactions in humans are usually mediated by a unique class of immunoglobulin (E), that serious efforts have been applied to the definition of the antibodies implicated in allergic reactions in naturally and experimentally sensitised animals.

The value of experimental animal systems does not lie solely in the means they provide of isolating and characterising anaphylactic antibodies, however. Indeed, the difficulty of obtaining sufficient raw material renders this use one of their lesser attractions;

in comparison with the study of human sensitising antibodies, which has been greatly facilitated by the availability of myeloma γE-globulins (ch. 4 and 5). On the other hand, it is possible to investigate in animals the many and varied factors which influence the induction of hypersensitive (as opposed to hyperimmune) states; besides developing forms of control which could ultimately find therapeutic and prophylactic application in allergic humans.

In this chapter an attempt has been made to appraise the rapidly growing mass of data from experimental animal studies; with the purpose of assessing the value of different systems as models for the investigation of immediate hypersensitivity in humans. In particular, the new insight which the study of such systems is providing into the mode of formation and action of anaphylactic antibodies has been considered in some depth, in the light of the general picture which has been built up in other chapters of the immunochemical basis of allergic reactions.

6.2 Nature of the antibodies responsible for the mediation of experimental hypersensitivity

Despite certain species peculiarities, the overall pattern which is emerging is noticeably similar from one mammalian species to another. In particular, physico-chemical and immunological approaches similar to those employed in the identification and characterisation of human reaginic antibodies (ch. 4) have revealed the presence of γE-type antibodies in the sera of a whole range of animal species. Furthermore, such antibodies are seen in spontaneously sensitised dogs, with clinical manifestations of pollinosis similar to those shown by allergic humans (Patterson and Sparks 1962), and in monkeys with naturally acquired sensitivity to *Ascaris* (Weiszer et al. 1968); as well as in monkeys, dogs, rabbits, rats, mice, guinea pigs and sheep in which a state of immediate hypersensitivity has been induced experimentally to hapten, protein antigen or infecting parasite (by the procedures to be discussed further in § 6.4).

In general, although in most cases reaginic type antibodies have not yet been isolated in pure form, preparations obtained under fractionation conditions comparable to those employed in the isolation of human γE antibodies have shown similar characteristics. Experimentally induced antibody shows a similar heat lability (at 56°), has a relatively long period of sensitisation (e.g. 48–72 hr) and persists at isologous-tissue sensitisation sites for many days. It is not associated with the major classes of immunoglobulin, moves in the fast γ region on electrophoresis (at *p*H 8.6) and is distinguished by a slightly faster sedimentation rate (and greater molecular weight) than the more common 7*S* antibodies (as is apparent from table 6.1). Furthermore there is direct serologic evidence that rabbit (Zvaifler and Robinson 1969) and rat (Kanyerezi et al.

TABLE 6.1
Sedimentation characteristics of reaginic antibodies observed in various mammalian species.

Species	Mode of antibody formation	Sensitisation period	Sedimentation coefficient (S^0)	Reference proteins	Authors
Human	Spontaneous	50 hr (opt.)	7.4*S* – 7.9*S*	Human γG-globulin (6.8*S*) Aldolase (7.8*S*) Catalase (11.9*S*) Thyroglobulin (18.6*S*)	Andersen and Vannier (1964), J. Exp. Med. *120*, 31
Dog	Spontaneous	48 hr	6.8*S* – 10.1*S*	Canine γG-globulin (6.8*S*), Canine γA myeloma glolin (10.1*S*, 1.5 mg/ml)	Rockey and Schwartzman (1967), J. Immunol. *98*, 1143
Rat	Induced by antigen inj. (eg. DNP-B.G.G. + *B. pertussis*)	16 hr (opt.)	>7*S*, <<19*S*	G. pig anti-ovalbumin antibody (7*S*) Rabbit anti-sheep rbc antibody (7*S*) Rheumatoid factor (19*S*)	Binaghi et al. (1964), J. Immunol. *92*, 927
Rabbit	Induced by antigen inj. (eg. B.G.G. or DNP-B.G.G. + complete adjuv.)	60–84 hr (opt.)	>7*S*, <<19*S*	Rabbit anti-sheep rbc (7*S*)	Zvaifler and Becker (1966 J. Exp. Med. *123*, 953

1971) γE-globulin are related to human γE-globulin, and that rabbit and monkey γE-globulins also share antigenic determinants (Ishizaka et al. 1969); observations which are not entirely unexpected in view of the known inter-species structural homology between the heavy polypeptide chains of other immunoglobulins, notably IgG. There could, however, prove to be individual species variation in some of the biological properties exhibited by γE-globulins. For instance, reaginic antibody activity has been detected in the sera of rabbits newly born to experimentally sensitised mothers (Lindqvist 1968); suggesting that, unlike human γE antibodies, rabbit reagins are able to get across the placenta.

There is also some preliminary evidence, put forward on the somewhat insubstantial basis of a differing susceptibility to the effect of relatively long periods of heat treatment at 50°, of a heterogeneity within the γE class of rabbit anaphylactic antibodies (Strejan and Campbell 1971); a situation which it is suspected obtains, too, with regard to human IgE (ch. 4), and which could reflect structural differences within the Fc regions of the molecules which have no influence on their tissue sensitising ability. There is need for caution, however, in drawing too close analogies between species; particularly in the case of the rabbit (Keogh and Stanworth 1972), which seems to be unusual in that it appears to lack the ability to produce sub-classes in a similar manner to all other mammalian species whose γG-globulins have been studied in any detail (i.e. human, baboon, rat, mouse, guinea pig, horse, etc.).

A somewhat surprising finding resulting from the study of experimentally induced hypersensitivity in animals has been the identification of non-reaginic types of sensitising antibody; which whilst also possessing the ability to mediate anaphylactic reactions in normal isologous tissue or cell systems, differ fundamentally from γE antibodies both with regard to their structure and mode of action. Of these, the guinea-pig γ_1-type antibody (Benaceraff et al. 1963) is the prototype, and it has become the practice, therefore, to refer to physico-chemically similar non-reaginic antibodies produced experimentally in other species such as the mouse (Nussenzweig et al. 1964) in like manner. It seemed until recently that a similar type of antibody was produced in experimentally

TABLE 6.2
Proposed classification of 3 major types of anaphylactic antibody observed in various mammalian species (reproduced from Stanworth 1970).

Property	Reagin-like	G-pig γ_1 type	G-pig γ_2 type
Tissue sensitised	Isol.	Isol.	Heterol.
Optimum sens. time	50–80 hr	2–4 hr	2–4 hr
Persistence in skin	> 4 weeks	1–2 days	1–2 days
Min. sens. dose (μg)	10^{-5}	10^{-2}	10^{-2}
Ag-coated rbc agglut.	+	+	+
Complement fixability	–	–	+
Heat (56°, 30′)	Labile	Stable	Stable
Placental transmission	–	+	+
Elect. mobility	γ_1	γ_1	γ_2
Sedimentation rate	8*S*	7*S*	7*S*

sensitised rats too, which prompted the proposed general classification of anaphylactic antibodies along the lines indicated in table 6.2. But it now seems likely that the non-reaginic, homologous tissue sensitising antibody produced in this species (Orange et al. 1970) – like that seen in the sera of hyperimmunised rabbits (Henson and Cochrane 1969) – is both physico-chemically and biologically different to guinea-pig and mouse γ_1-type anaphylactic antibody. Perhaps, therefore, it would be more appropriate to refer to anaphylactic antibodies comprising this group as the γG-homoreactive type.

As will be noted, the third class included in table 6.2 comprises anaphylactic antibodies which are only capable of inducing immediate sensitivity reactions in heterologous species. Again taking the guinea pig as the prototype, these are conveniently referred to as the γ_2-type; because, although they are antigenically related to the electrophoretically fast γ_1-type (both being sub-classes of guinea pig IgG), they move in the slow region on electrophoresis at *p*H 8.6 (as is seen from the immunoelectrophoresis patterns in fig. 6.1). Members of the γ_2-type would be correctly termed 'pseudo-anaphylactic' antibodies, however; because as Benacerraf (1967) has pointed out, their activity probably reflects a chance complementariness between a structural site within their mole-

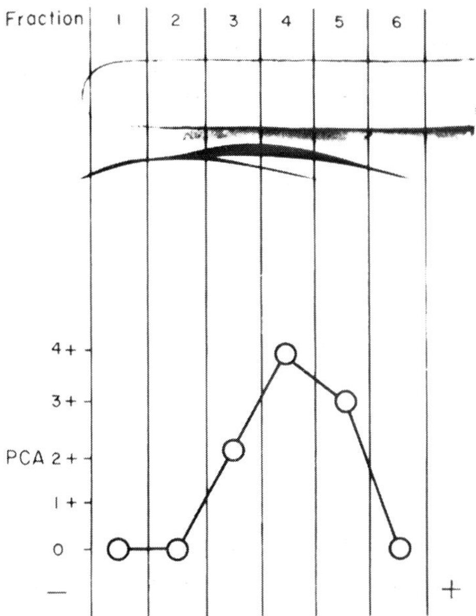

Fig. 6.1. Immunoelectrophoretic demonstration of two types of 7*S* guinea pig γG-globulin; with isologous PCA activity confined to the faster component, as revealed by testing of fractions separated in agar. Antiserum: rabbit anti-guinea-pig γG-globulin (reproduced from Benaceraff et al. 1963, by permission of the authors).

cules (in the Fc region) and receptors on guinea pig mast cells (or on the mast cells of other heterologous species used in detecting their anaphylactic activity). This does not mean, however, that antibodies within this class do not fulfil other important cell-binding functions; to take one example, their cytophilic activity for macrophages has been shown to be an essential part of their opsonizing property (Berken and Benaceraff 1966). Furthermore, as will be discussed in the next section, cross-inhibition studies and comparisons of the heterologous tissue sensitising activity of γ_2-type antibodies in various species, are throwing new light on the nature of the cellular interactions involving reaginic and γ_1-type anaphylactic antibodies.

It is interesting that despite the use of the guinea pig as a model for anaphylaxis over a considerable number of years, it has only been realised recently that in some experimental situations – such as in vivo or in vitro passive sensitisation with hyperimmune rabbit antiserum– γ_2-type antibody has been involved; whereas, local and systemic anaphylactic reactions in actively sensitised guinea pigs (or their tissues) would have been mediated by antibodies of a different (γ_1-type) and even (in some cases) by a γE reaginic type of antibody. For recent studies have shown that γE-type (and γ_1-type) antibody is produced by guinea pigs immunised with repeated doses of a hapten (BPO)–protein conjugate in alumina gel (Levine et al. 1971); as well as by guinea pigs infected with parasites such as *Trichinella spiralis* (Catty 1969) and *Ascaris suum* (Dobson et al. 1971).

At first sight, recent reports (Strejan and Campbell 1967; 1968) of the identification, in the sera of guinea pigs hyperimmunised with *A. suum* extracts and keyhole limpet hemocyanin, of a 7*S* γ_2 antibody capable of eliciting local anaphylactic reactions in the skin of normal guinea pigs would seem to conflict with the classification of anaphylactic antibodies proposed in table 6.2. For, although the antibody responsible was found to be very electrophoretically heterogeneous, substantial evidence has been presented to suggest that preparations are not contaminated with γ_1-type anaphylactic antibody. But as PCA reactions elicited by this γ_2-type antibody (which might prove to be a sub-class of the guinea pig γG2-globulin) do not appear until 45–60 min after antigen challenge and are not fully developed before 2 hr, they would not seem to qualify as true immediate-type hypersensitivity reactions according to the criteria adopted throughout this work.

The various types of anaphylactic antibody which have been identified in mammalian species are listed in table 6.3. It is obviously dangerous to draw too rigid analogy between the immunoglobulin classes of one species and another. Nevertheless the identification of a second, non-reaginic, anaphylactic antibody in certain animal species might encourage further attempts to demonstrate that a similar type of immunoglobulin is operative in some human allergic situations; particularly as there is already circumstantial evidence (mentioned in earlier chapters) of the involvement of non-γE antibodies in some cases of sensitivity to drugs and other sensitogens. It might also prove fruitful to attempt the

TABLE 6.3
Types of anaphylactic antibodies identified in those mammalian species which have been studied in any detail. (The earlier terminology is included in brackets)

Species	γ_1-type	γ_2-type (pseudo-anaphylactic)	γE-type
Guinea pig	IgG1 (γ_1)*	IgG2 (γ_2)	IgE
Mouse	IgG1 (γ_1)	IgG2a (γ_{2a})	IgE
Rat	IgGa (γ_1)	IgG2 (γ_2)	IgE
Rabbit		IgG2 (γ_2)	IgE
Dog		IgG2	IgE
Monkey		IgG2	IgE
Human		IgG1, IgG3, IgG4	IgE (reagin)

* Two different forms of γ_1-type antibody have now been identified.

experimental production of such antibodies in more convenient species than the guinea pig and the mouse. With this objective in mind we have made a rigorous investigation in my own laboratory (Keogh and Stanworth 1972) into the possibility of inducing the production of γ_1-type anaphylactic antibodies in the rabbit. This formed part of a broader study designed to demonstrate the existence of rabbit γG-globulin sub-classes in which the expression of antibody activity depended upon the charge properties of the antigen used for immunisation. Although 2 populations of rabbit IgG were demonstrated by papain susceptibility testing, and shown to vary in proportion in isolated antibody preparations according to the charge of the immunogen, neither of these proved capable of eliciting passive cutaneous anaphylactic reactions in normal rabbits. In the event of such an effect being demonstrable, it was hoped that it might have been possible to establish that a property located within the Fc region of the molecule (namely isologous tissue binding activity) was – like the antigen binding activity located in the Fab region – also subject to the influence of the structural characteristics of the immunogen. The finding that immunochemically pure *7S* γ_1 (IgG), isolated from the sera of rabbits after primary and secondary immunisation with ovalbumin in complete Freund's adjuvant, did not behave as a homocytotropic antibody (Faulk et al. 1969) is supported by our own observations.

6.3 Mode of action of artificially-induced anaphylactic antibodies

The study of anaphylactic reactions mediated by artificially-induced antibodies has, of course, greatly contributed to present knowledge of the mechanism of immediate hypersensitivity processes. This will become apparent from ch. 8, which indicates that a substantial amount of evidence about the nature of the processes involved in the triggering of release of vasoactive amines has been obtained from studies on rat mast cells, guinea pig organ preparations and other suitable in vitro systems.

The aim here is to consider briefly the sites of action of the anaphylactic antibodies referred to in the previous section; and, in particular, to draw attention to mechanisms involving cell-antibody interactions which diverge from the basic γE-mast cell system.

6.3.1 Role of various antibody types

It seems reasonable to assume that the mechanism of interaction of γE antibodies will prove to be essentially similar, irrespective of the species of origin. Evidence has already been obtained that the mast cells of the rat (Mota 1964; Binaghi and Benaceraff 1964) and the mouse (Vaz and Prouvost-Danon 1969), as well as the rabbit basophil (Greaves 1968), are primary targets in γE-mediated anaphylactic reactions. Despite the technical difficulties encountered in the passive sensitisation of such cells in vitro, they obviously provide a valuable alternative to the use of human anaphylactic systems (i.e. chopped lung or heterogeneous leucocyte suspensions). Peritoneal mast cell suspensions are readily obtainable from rats and mice; and basophils are ten times more plentiful in rabbit than in human blood. Furthermore, the recent chemical induction of a basophil leukaemia in rats (Lennard 1971) offers prospects of even richer sources of these target cells; and mastocytomas are being profitably used to provide an abundant supply of dog mast cells. Yet another possibility is the culture of human mast cells, which is now being actively investigated in some laboratories.

It is important to recognise, however, that there are certain species peculiarities which might preclude the use of some target cells on both practical and academic grounds. For instance, mouse mast cells are much more fragile than rat mast cells; and appear to respond differently to both non-specific histamine releasers like compound 48/80 (in which property they resembly guinea pig mast cells) and to specific stimulation by divalent haptens (Vaz and Prouvost-Danon 1969). The latter finding has been attributed to the relatively low binding affinity of the mouse anaphylactic antibody for the hapten (Hurlimann and Ovary 1965); but, as Vaz and Prouvost-Danon have noted, this fails to explain the inability of rabbit antibodies to mediate PCA reactions with divalent haptens in mice whilst proving effective in guinea pigs. Possibly the strength of binding of the heterologous rabbit antibodies for the mouse mast cell receptor sites was too low; implying, perhaps, that the degree of complementariness between the rabbit antibody binding site and the mouse target cell receptor was less than that towards guinea pig mast cell receptors.

The identification of the non-reaginic sensitising antibodies referred to in table 6.3 has raised the interesting possibility that target cells other than mast cells might be involved, releasing pharmacological mediators other than histamine (e.g. serotonin, SRS-A, bradykinin). Unfortunately, the unavailability of guinea pig mast cells is an obstacle to obtaining definitive information about the role of γ_1-type antibodies, in this respect. Nevertheless, indirect evidence has been obtained from studies using chopped lung preparations (Stechschulte et al. 1967) to suggest that guinea pig $7S$ γ_1 antibodies (in contrast to γ_2-type antibodies) sensitise the mast cell for the release of SRS-A and histamine; processes which have been observed to run parallel (Austen and Brocklehurst 1961). But, as Stechshulte and his associates admit, it is possible that both mediators are liberated by the union of antigen with γ_1 antibodies on the surface of different cells. Obviously, therefore, this system needs further investigation; particularly as the production of a γE reaginic type of antibody by the guinea pig has now been confirmed. Indeed, some investigators are of the opinion that the effects attributed in earlier studies to γGl-type antibodies were mediated by a contaminant; a role which would be most readily attributable to a guinea pig γE antibody. To counteract this claim, further evidence has been recently presented in support of the involvement of γ_1-type antibody in the mediation of anaphylactic reactions in the guinea pig (Nussenzweig et al. 1969). But this work has been criticised (Pondman, 1971) on the grounds that the specific rabbit anti-guinea pig γ_1-globulin used was prepared by absorption with a γ_1-globulin preparation which could itself have been contaminated with γE-type antibody.

Studies on the mouse system are somewhat more straight forward in that the production of both reaginic and γ_1-type anaphylactic antibodies in this species is now well established, and peritoneal mast cell suspensions are readily obtainable. It seems that, whereas the γE antibody behaves true to form for this type and binds firmly to mast cells, the mouse γG1 antibodies are incapable of binding to any extent; a single saline washing of sensitised mast cells being sufficient to abolish γG1-sensitisation (Vaz and Prouvost-Danon 1969). In other words, a firm prior attachment of antibody to the target cell is not essential in anaphylactic reactions mediated by mouse γG1 antibodies; which instead appear to be induced by active antibody–antigen complexes independently of any complement involvement. Moreover, there is some preliminary evidence to suggest that such complexes might also contain γG2 antibodies, which can interfere with anaphylactic reactions in the mouse mediated by γG1-type antibodies; a situation which Davies (1971) feels obtains, also, in anaphylactic reactions in guinea pigs.

Present knowledge about the role of anaphylactic antibodies in the rat has resulted mainly from the studies of Austen and his associates, and is based almost entirely on experiments in which both the initial sensitisation process and subsequent antigen challenge is effected in vivo (intraperitoneally). These have pointed to a distinctive mechanism of interaction of the γE and γGa antibodies, involving different target cells (fig. 6.2). There has been some uncertainty, however, about the process responsible for the release of one of the pharmacological mediators, SRS-A. It was concluded from initial studies (Morse et al. 1969) that antigen-

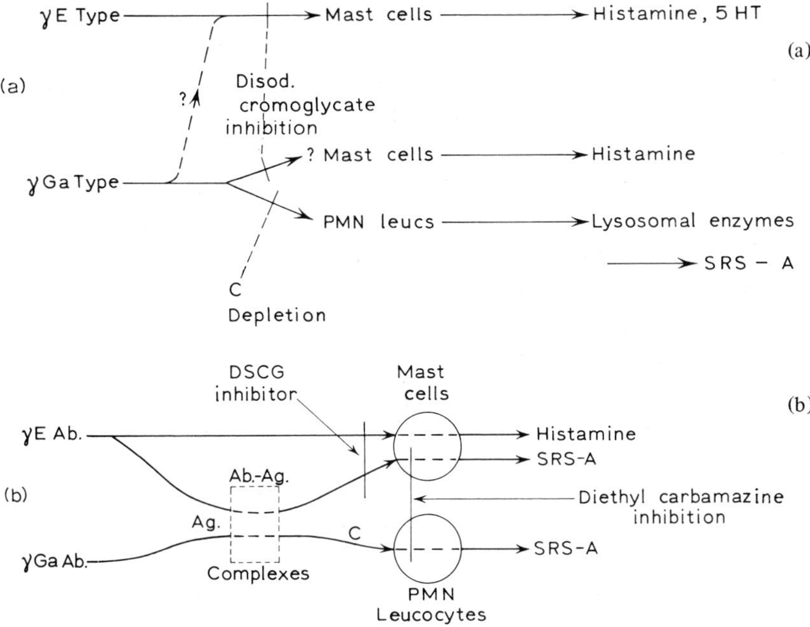

Fig. 6.2. Supposed modes of action of rat anaphylactic antibodies: (a) based on original data of Morse et al. 1969; (b) revised according to the more recent findings of Orange et al. 1970.

induced release of SRS-A in animals sensitised with homologous or heterologous antisera differed from that of histamine release in requiring the presence of polymorphonuclear (PMN) leucocytes rather than mast cells (fig. 6.2a). But, although more recent investigations from the same group (Orange et al. 1970) have confirmed that PMN leucocytes are a pre-requisite for antigen-induced release of SRS-A by hyperimmune sera containing γGa antibodies, they have now shown that SRS-A release can also be mediated by γE-type antibodies quite independently of any PMN leucocyte involvement. This form of SRS-A release was apparently missed in previous experiments because of the adoption of too long a latent period for intra-peritoneal antigen challenge.

A revised picture of the various mechanisms thought to be responsible for mediation of anaphylactic reactions in the rat, based on these new findings, is shown in fig. 6.2b. The current idea is that the heat stable γGa antibody in hyperimmune rat sera operates in the form of an antibody-antigen complex, which activates the complement system and results in interaction with PMN leucocytes as well as in the elaboration of various chemotactic factors. Furthermore it is assumed that, in contrast to histamine release effected by cell-bound γE antibody in the conventional manner, SRS-A release from rat mast cells is mediated by a non-complement activating γE antibody–antigen complex; which might be capable of identifying a different target cell from the PMN leucocyte triggered by the γGa antibody–antigen complex.

This idea is entirely consistent with the triggering mechanisms discussed in ch. 5 and 8. For according to the mode of action of γE antibodies proposed there, combination with antigen either on or off the target cell leads to the formation of cell-activation sites distinct from the cell binding sites. Moreover, it is quite conceivable that antibody of a different immunoglobulin class (i.e. γG) would form structurally different activating sites, with reactivity for a different type of target cell. In similar vein, it is reasonable to suppose that other such sites would be responsible for the mobilisation of chemotactic factors. Because studies on the structural basis of biological activities associated with human and rabbit γG-globulins (Stanworth 1972) have shown that the combination of antibody with specific antigen leads to the formation of a wide variety of active sites within different parts of the Fc region of the same molecule.

In this connection, it seems to be particularly pertinent to the present discussion that a recent study (Kay et al. 1971) has shown that γG1 antibodies of the guinea pig, but not those of the γG2-type, prepare guinea pig lung for the antigen-induced release of an eosinophil leucocyte chemotactic factor of anaphylaxis. Moreover, this appears to be quite independent of the eosinophil chemotactic factor generated from whole serum by the action of antigen–antibody complexes comprising either guinea pig γG1- or γG2-globulins (Kay 1970); which has been identified with the complement component C5a and is thought to be associated with the moderate accumulation of eosinophils observed in Arthus reactions. The implication of the more recent observation of Kay is that the eosinophilia associated with immediate hypersensitivity reactions is, however, independent of the complement system. It will obviously be important, therefore, to ascertain whether γ_1-type anaphylactic antibody is similarly responsible for the induction of the eosinophilia often shown by hypersensitive humans.

Thus, largely as a result of the study of anaphylaxis in animals, and particularly so far in the rat, it is becoming possible for the first time to start to form a comprehensive picture of the varied and complex pathways set in train by sensitising antibody–antigen (allergen) combination. It is becoming increasingly apparent that tissue mast cells and circulating basophils are only two of several cell types involved, either directly or indirectly; although they do appear to be the primary seat of reaction of γE-type antibodies. Non-reaginic antibodies, on the other hand, seem to be often concerned with the incrimination of other cell types; and prior binding to the target cell is not necessarily a prerequisite for the expression of their activity. To mention one further example, there is evidence of the involvement of both neutrophils and platelets in the complement-dependent anaphylactic activity of a rabbit γG-type antibody (Henson and Cochrane 1969). It seems likely, too, that in certain circumstances the products of reaction of one cell type can effect the release of vasoactive amines from another. Mast-cell rupturing factor, a basic polypeptide isolated from PMN leucocytes (ch. 8), comes into mind in this connection. But this substance does not seem to have played any role in the release of SRS-A induced by γGa antibody in the studies summarised in fig. 6.2, because the process was found to occur even in the absence of peritoneal mast cells.

6.3.2 Nature of the binding of γ-globulins to target tissues

As already indicated, the study of the uptake of homologous and heterologous γG-globulins to animal tissues in vivo (in PCA systems) and in vitro (to isolated cell and tissue preparations) is contributing indirectly to the elucidation of the nature of the anaphylaxis target cell receptor sites. This applies even to studies employing the pseudo-anaphylactic γG2-type antibodies which, in addition to effecting PCA reactions in appropriate heterologous species, are also often capable of blocking sensitisation by γ_1-type anaphylactic antibodies of isologous or heterologous species.

In some cases, such as inhibition of sensitisation of guinea pig skin or other tissue preparations by γG1-type guinea pig antibodies, high concentrations (e.g. 100-fold excess) of homologous γG2 antibodies (of similar antigen specificity) are needed to block the reaction; in contrast to the high efficiency of guinea pig γG1 antibodies of different antigen-specificity (Ovary et al. 1963). This apparent inhibition by the γ_2-type antibodies can be attributed however, to their competition with the γ_1-type antibody for antigen (Bloch 1967); because γG2 guinea pig antibodies can be shown to be incapable of fixing to isologous tissue. On the other hand, there has been a claim that mast cells possess 'receptors' for mouse γG2-globulins as well as for the anaphylactic γG1-type mouse antibodies. This would seem, at first sight, to be in contradiction with my early suggestion that mouse γ_1 anaphylactic antibodies might well prove to react with the target cell whilst complexed to specific antigen. It should be pointed out, however, that the claim is based on observations of mast cell binding (Tigelaar et al. 1971) obtained by use of an indirect rosette technique; in which the mouse mast cells were incubated with sheep erythrocytes coated with the antigen ($DNP_{37}BSA$) which has already been reacted with the test (anti-DNP) antibody. Nevertheless, it is interesting to note that mouse γG1, γG2a and γG2b myeloma proteins but not those of the γA or γM class have been found to inhibit mice PCA reactions mediated by γG1 antibodies (Ovary et al. 1971). It is of some significance, too, that guinea pig γG2 antibodies have also proved capable of binding to mouse mast cells (Tigelaar et al. 1971) despite their inability to mediate anaphylactic reactions in the mouse. This observation is consistent with the general rule that only antibodies of the γG2 class are capable of eliciting PCA reactions in heterologous species. But it is in direct contrast to the findings of White and his associates (Todorov et al. 1968) who used an immunofluorescence technique to show that guinea pig γG1- but not γ2-type antibodies react with mast cells in mouse tongue and mesenteric preparations. As, however, a lack of correlation was observed between the in vitro fixation of some guinea pig γ1 antibodies to mouse tongue mast cells and their ability to induce PCA reactions in the mouse, the immunofluorescence approach adopted by these investigators would seem to be of dubious value in the context of the present discussion.

Another indirect approach to the characterisation of target cell receptors involves comparative PCA (or in vitro) testing in a whole range of species, to ascertain whether there are underlying relationships connecting the reactors and the non-reactors. It is also interesting to compare the species whose γG2-globulins are capable of inducing PCA reactions (e.g. in guinea pigs) with those whose γG2-globulins are unreactive (ch. 5; table 5.5). It is possibly of some significance that those species which produce pseudo-anaphylactic γ_2-type antibodies (e.g. human, monkey and rabbit) have been reported to lack Forsmann antigen on their erythrocytes, in contrast to those species (e.g. horse, sheep, etc.) whose γG-globulins are unable to evoke PCA reactions in guinea pigs. The behaviour of the γG-globulins of some other species such as the guinea pig, would seem to be consistent with the relationship apparent from table 5.5; although there is some evidence (Kabat and Mayer 1961) that Forsmann antigen is present in guinea pig capillary endothelium but not in its smooth muscle fibres. The mouse, on the other hand, seems to be the striking exception to the rule in that its erythrocytes possess Forsmann antigen and its γGa-globulin sub-class (but not the γG2b sub-class) is capable of sensitising guinea pig tissue for reverse PCA (Bloch 1967). Nevertheless, it would seem to be worthwhile looking for other correlations of this type which might throw further light on the nature of anaphylactic antibody receptor sites.

As already mentioned, in the previous section, antibodies of the γ_1-type appear to have the capacity (albeit after combination with antigen) to react with various cell types including neutrophils and eosinophils; and γ_2-type antibodies have been shown to sensitise the macrophage in preparation for phagacytosis (Berken and Benacerraf 1966). There is, however, no firm evidence available yet to undermine the assumption that the location of γE antibody binding sites are restricted to mast cells and basophils. Although it should be mentioned that there has been a recent startling claim (Hubscher et al. 1970), made on the basis of immunofluorescence studies, that a non-reaginic ragweed binding antibody not belonging to any of the major immunoglobulin classes is (like γE-type antibody) capable of fixing to monkey skin mast cells.

6.4 Factors influencing the experimental induction of reaginic antibody formation

Another major contribution of studies of experimental anaphylaxis systems in animals has been the considerable illumination of the many factors influencing reaginic antibody formation, as well as those governing the initial induction of a hypersensitive state.

In preliminary investigations in rats (Binaghi et al. 1964) and rabbits (Zvaifler and Becker 1966) involving sensitisation with relatively high doses of protein or hapten-protein conjugates, together with adjuvants such as *Bordetella pertussis* or complete Freund's adjuvant, the early reaginic antibody response induced was usually of a transitory nature (like that seen in human cases of serum sickness); and could not be recalled by secondary stimulation. More marked and persistent reagin responses have been achieved, however, in certain species such as the rat by repeated infection with the nematode parasite *Nippostrongylus brasiliensis* (Wilson and Bloch 1967; Ogilvie 1967), and secondary responses have been observed on re-infection. These findings suggested that perhaps the form as well as the route of administration of the nematode allergenic stimulus was important; but a more recent observation (Orr and Blair 1969), that a subsequent (10 days later) infection with parasite could potentiate the reaginic antibody response of rats to unrelated protein antigens (ovalbumin and conalbumin), indicated that the parasite might exert a non-specific stimulus on the reagin-producing system. Later investigations (Orr et al. 1971) have shown the time-course of this potentiated reagin response to be transient; and it is suggested that a sustained high serum reagin titre is dependent upon live forms of parasite being present.

On the other hand, persistent γE(reaginic) responses have been induced in rabbits by immunisation with relatively large doses of tetanus toxoid (Lindquist 1968), ascaris extract (Strejan and Campbell 1970) and even isolated proteins like ovalbumin (Richerson et al. 1968). Furthermore, an amnestic response to each of these sensitogens was observed; but the most significant point to emerge, in my opinion, from this work is that in every case the protein administered was adsorbed to a precipitated aluminium salt, $Al(OH)_3$ or Al_3PO_4. Moreover, other studies in rabbits have specifically demonstrated the superiority of this form of adjuvant in the production of reaginic antibodies against DNP-bovine γG-globulin conjugate (Revoltella and Ovary 1969) and bovine serum albumin (Freeman et al. 1969).

Hence it is particularly interesting to note that, in recent demonstrations of the production of a persistent and boostable high titre reagin response in guinea pigs (Levine et al. 1971) and mice (Vaz et al. 1971) following repeated injections (i.p.) of minute amounts (0.1–1.0 μg) of protein, $Al(OH)_3$ gel has again proved a very effective adjuvant. Indeed, a single injection of only 0.1 μg of ovalbumin in $Al(OH)_3$ gel was sufficient to induce an intense and persistent reagin formation in mice; whereas other immunogens (e.g. BPO-ovalbumin) failed to induce a primary reaginic antibody response at such small dose levels.

Apart from providing a striking example of the efficiency of this form of adjuvant in reagin production, this experiment underlines the sensitogenic potency of ovalbumin; a conclusion which has been drawn by many investigators working in the field of experimental hypersensitivity. This is perhaps surprising in view of the findings (§ 3.3.4) that ovomucoid was the constituent of egg white which proved particularly allergenic in egg-sensitive humans. It is possible, however, that the structural requirements for sensitogenicity in experimental animals are somewhat different to those obtaining in humans; assuming that the observed hypersensitivity responses in animals are not due to contaminants of the commercial preparations which are usually employed in such studies. But, in any case, the ovalbumin molecule would appear to possess the appropriate size and charge characteristics of an allergen; according to the criteria discussed in § 3.4.

The suggested influence of the adjuvant on the reaginic response of various animals to experimental sensitisation is not unique. For, there have been various reports that this factor can influence γG antibody responses, too. For example, immunisation of guinea pigs with protein antigens in the absence of mycobacteria was found to induce largely γ_1-type antibody; whereas mycobacteria appeared to act as a stimulus specifically for biosynthesis of antibody of the γ_2-type (Askonas et al. 1965). An essentially similar type of conclusion was reached from a parallel study in mice (Coe 1966), which indicated that a primary response to 5 μg of ovalbumin comprised only 7*S* γ_1 antibody. Apart from this adjuvant effect, three other factors were found to influence the production of γ_1- and γ_2-type antibodies; the nature of the antigen, the strain of the mouse and previous exposure to the antigen.

It is beginning to look as if all of these factors have a critical influence on the production of γE-type antibodies too; as has been indicated by the example quoted and by the results of recent studies of the genetic control of reagin production. Of these, the most exciting are some studies recently undertaken in the dog (Schwarzman et al. 1971); the only species other than primates in which the spontaneous production of γE reaginic antibodies has been observed,* and one which experiences a seasonal disease similar to that endured by human hay fever sufferers. A high incidence of spontaneous hypersensitivity was found in the progeny of atopic dogs, as is illustrated in fig. 6.3. Furthermore, evidence was also obtained of the inheritance of an autosomal gene mutation controlling histamine release, which (by analogy) might explain why only certain human individuals' leucocytes are suitable for use in passive sensitisation testing (ch. 2).

Another fascinating and highly significant observation resulting from this work was that a spontaneously ragweed-sensitive dog produced anti-DNP γE-type reaginic antibody following a single injection of a dinitrophenylated ragweed pollen, whereas repeated

* Excluding the responses of parasite-infected monkeys referred to earlier (p. 250).

Atopic sire and atopic dam

Atopic sire and normal dam

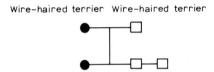

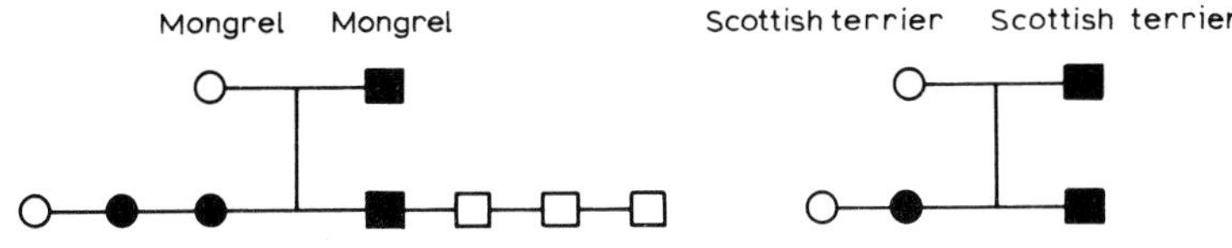

Normal sire and atopic dam

Wire-haired terrier Wire-haired terrier

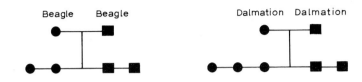

Fig. 6.3. Development of atopic hypersensitivity in the progeny of atopic dogs after a natural exposure to environmental allergenic material (reproduced from Schwartman et al. 1971, by permission of the authors).

exposure to DNP-canine serum albumin by nebulisation had failed to do so. It was concluded, therefore, that the nature of the carrier of the haptenic determinant, or an adjuvant effect of materials contained in the crude ragweed pollen, could be of prior importance in the γE antibody response; and that prior spontaneous sensitisation of the atopic dog to ragweed pollen may have promoted the observed reaginic anti-DNP antibody response following sensitisation with DNP ragweed pollen antigens. These observations would seem to support the idea, discussed in ch. 3, that certain structural characteristics differentiate allergens (and sensitogens) from ordinary antigens (and immunogens). The switch from the use of canine serum albumin to a pollen constituent as hapten-carrier would be a favourable one as far as molecular size is concerned; whilst the substitution of lysyl residues of ragweed pollen allergen with DNP groups would tend to render it more acidic, and possibly therefore more effective in the induction of reagin formation. But a possible effect of the change of route of administration cannot be ignored. Obviously further experiments along these lines are needed to define more clearly the structural requirements for sensitogenicity; preferably in genetically predisposed dogs (and, better still, monkeys) who have not become spontaneously hypersensitised to the test protein.

Other species, notably the mouse, offer obvious advantages in the study of the genetic control of reaginic antibody formation. Thus, it has been revealed that an ability to respond to a low dose of antigen (0.1 μg ovalbumin) is related to the histocompatability antigen H-2 (Vaz and Levine 1970). But this genetic control can be overcome by strong immunogenic stimuli, as mice from all strains responded to a secondary injection of ovalbumin in $Al(OH)_3$. The pattern of reagin formation then observed is similar to that induced by relatively large doses of other antigens in rats and rabbits as well as guinea pigs; where early and transient peaks of reagin formation were accompanied by longer periods of γG1-type antibody formation. Other studies in mice (Prouvost-Danon et al. 1971) have shown that animals genetically selected into high and low responding lines on the basis of the magnitude of their agglutinin response to sheep red cells were also selected for reagin and γ_1-type antibody production against ovalbumin (administered as a single large sub-cutaneous dose).

It is, however, the low dose antigen (allergen) system which seems to be the most appropriate model, resembling in many ways the immune responsiveness and reagin production shown by human atopic individuals. Studies of the effect of a combination of inbred strain and antigen (hapten–bovine γG-globulin or hapten–ovomucoid conjugate) dose on the responsiveness of mice (Levine and Vaz 1970), suggest that atopy consists in part of a genetically controlled[1] capacity to respond immunologically to minute doses of antigen; rather than consisting of a unique ability to synthesise reagins.

It seems that reagin production constitutes a prominent part of any response of experimental animals to minute doses of antigen. The reason for this finding is not yet clear; but it is possible, of course, that hypersensitisation of suitably predisposed humans occurs by a similar process involving regular exposure to small doses of pollen (or some other inhalant). One possible explanation (Vaz et al. 1971) is that reaginic antibodies have a higher avidity for antigen than antibodies of other immunoglobulin classes, with the result that a precursor reagin-forming cell population would be expected to respond to lower concentrations of antigens whilst becoming tolerised to higher doses. Another factor to be considered is that higher doses of antigen would induce the formation of antibodies of other classes, which could suppress reagin formation. It seems significant, in this connection, that evidence from recent experimental sensitisation studies suggest that γG-type antibodies exert a feed-back regulatory mechanism on reagin formation in rabbits and rats (discussed further in the next chapter in dealing with the biosynthesis of IgE). A similar effect operating in the human atopic individual would obviously have important prophylactic possibilities.

Adrenal function is another factor which has been shown, from studies of artificially induced reagin formation (in rats), to exert some influence on immediate sensitivity responses. For instance, adrenalectomy was found to potentiate reagin production against ovalbumin, when *B. pertussis* vaccine is used as adjuvant (Crunkhorn and Meacock 1971). This has prompted the interesting speculation that exposure of humans to allergens during a period of adrenal insufficiency – such as would follow severe stress occurring in a bacterial illness – might increase the likelihood of sensitisation. In preliminary support of this idea is the recent report of 2 cases of Addison's disease with bronchial asthma (Green and Lim 1971), suggesting that an asthmatic tendency had been uncovered by deteriorating adrenal function.

Summarising the main observations discussed in this section, it is apparent that reagin production in appropriate genetically-predisposed animals can be most effectively achieved by sub-cutaneous injection of low doses of protein antigen (notably ovalbumin) adsorbed to an aluminium salt; and that this process can be influenced by antibodies of other immunoglobulin classes. It remains to be demonstrated that other routes of administration of allergen, such as the intra-nasal one, are more effective. It is, however, worth mentioning in this connection that the intra-nasal administration of aerosilized protein was found to induce weal and erythema reactivity in atopic, as opposed to normal individuals (Salvaggio et al. 1964). It will also be important to confirm by animal experimentation (preferably in primates) that the structure of the sensitogen is of some consequence in the induction of reagin formation.

Other aspects of this subject will be considered in the following chapter; which is concerned particularly with cellular aspects of γE antibody synthesis and catabolism, and which will include further reference to the prominent efficacy of parasitic infections in the induction of localised anaphylactic reactions.

Note

[1] Evidence has since been obtained (Levine, B.B., Montreal Allergy Meeting, 1972) of two different kinds of genetic control of reagin production in the mouse:

[a] Operating on antigen recognition is expressed largely in T lymphocyte function and involves a single (Ir) gene within the H-2 histocompatability region;

[b] Operating on reagin production "per se" rather than on immune responsiveness generally.

CHAPTER 7

Cellular aspects of reagin formation and disappearance

7.1 Introduction

Of all aspects of immediate hypersensitivity so far considered, least is known about the mode of synthesis and subsequent fate of anaphylactic antibodies. In view of their involvement in sensitising, as opposed to immunising, responses the question arises as to whether the biosynthesis and catabolism of reagins are distinguished by unusual features; or do they behave like the more common classes of immunoglobulin in these respects? Furthermore, are there situations where anaphylactic antibodies, too, can operate in a protective capacity?

A means of answering fundamental questions of this type has arisen with the emergence of the experimental animal systems described in ch. 6; which, as will have been noted, appear to be valid models for the study of reagin antibody formation in general. Moreover, the availability now of specific antisera against human IgE is permitting the direct location of this immunoglobulin in the tissues of spontaneously and artificially sensitised primate hosts. Consequently it is becoming possible to identify the sites of γE-globulin synthesis, as well as to investigate more directly those cellular processes in which reaginic antibodies are specifically involved.

7.2 Sites of synthesis of γE antibodies

7.2.1 Role of lymphoid cells

Until recently there was only indirect evidence, based largely on limited observations of immediate hypersensitivity in hypogammaglobulinaemic patients (Stanworth 1963), to suggest that reagins – like antibodies of other immunoglobulin classes – were synthesised by lymphoid cells.

Justification for this conclusion has now been provided, however, by immunofluorescence studies of the tissues and circulating cells of allergic individuals and experimentally sensitised subhuman primates. Thus, it has been demonstrated that IgE-forming plasma cells are prominent in respiratory and gastro-intestinal mucosa and in regional lymph nodes; in contrast to spleen and sub-cutaneous lymph nodes (Tada and Ishizaka 1970). These observations, and the finding that tonsils and adenoids removed after recurrent infection possessed the greatest number of plasma cells stainable by labelled anti-IgE antibody, are consistent with the growing view that reaginic antibodies are synthesised at local tissue sites. This is also suggested from indirect studies, involving the measurement of the levels of IgE in various secretions (i.e. colostrum) of normal and allergic individuals (Bennich and Johansson 1971). The findings from the R.I.S.T. measurement of IgE in the nasal polyp fluid and serum of allergic and normal individuals (Donovan et al. 1970) are particularly interesting in this respect. An earlier observation, based on P–K testing (Berdal 1952) of a heightened reagin level in allergic polyp fluid compared with the serum level was substantiated and this was shown to be in excess of that explicable in terms of filtration; but relatively high levels of IgE were also seen in the polyp fluids of individuals without clinical symptoms, and shown to correlate with a tendency of the patient to sneeze.

It seems, therefore, that the local production of IgE can occur in non-allergic individuals; but is greatly potentiated in atopics who are subjected to an appropriate allergenic stimulus. In its sites of production it appears to resemble IgA, which originates from cells of the gut, respiratory tract and exocrine glands; and which, of course, has an important function in external secretions. In this case, too, the route of administration of antigen is a decisive factor influencing local synthesis of γA antibody, as has been revealed by experiments in which the oral and nasal routes have been adopted. For instance, studies involving the administration of virus via the respiratory route in mice (Blandford 1970) have indicated that localisation of antigen on the mucous membranes is a pre-requisite for local γA antibody production; and immunofluorescence studies (Brandtzaeg et al. 1967) have revealed a predominance of γA-producing plasma cells near the glandular areas and secretory ducts, in contrast to γG-producing cells which occur in the stroma between the glands and the surface epithelium. On the other hand, if the antigen reaches the alveoli of the mice, the stimulus is likely to be similar to that evoked by systemic administration (Blandford 1970). This has led to a consideration of the possible clinical potential of immunisation by aerosol against pathogenic organisms of the respiratory tract. But there is some recent evidence (Waldman 1971) to suggest that γA antibodies produced locally in this manner are not as specific as systemically produced γG antibodies. Another potential difficulty might be that this route of administration would favour γE production in certain individuals; in view of the observation (e.g. Salvaggio et al. 1964; and others) mentioned earlier that the intra-nasal route of presentation of an aerosolized protein (such as ribonuclease) was found sufficient to sensitise atopic as opposed to normal individuals. This was attributed to the atopics' mucosal membranes having greater permeability than those of normal individuals, thus permitting greater absorption of the aerosolized antigen across the upper respiratory tract. But other studies revealed that atopics had a greater tendency to develop immediate skin reactivity following a single sub-cutaneous injection of emulsified pollen allergen, to which they had not shown previous sensitivity (Sparks et al. 1962; Feinberg et al. 1962) and to ascaris antigen (Fisherman 1962); suggesting that there is a difference in the capacity of atopics and non-atopics to respond to parenterally administered antigen. In line with these observations is a recent suggestion (Tada and Okumura 1971A) that the prolonged state of sensitisation and sustained reagin production which occurs in the allergic individual might be attributable to a disturbance in the mechanisms regulating formation of this antibody. This, it is suggested, might result from a functional weakness of the thymus-dependent lymphoid system; or from the production of γG antibodies, which (as will be discussed further later) appear to play a role in the regulation of γE antibody formation. The suggestion that a cellular imbalance obtains in the lymphoid system of atopics has been prompted by the finding that adult splenectomy and thymectomy greatly enhanced and prolonged reaginic antibody formation in the rat as did X-irradiation (Tada and Okumura 1971B and C); and by the lone observation that the number of γE-forming cells was normal (or somewhat elevated) in a single case of dysgammaglobulinaemia.

Further studies of the various factors governing the local production of γE antibodies in suitable animal species are obviously needed to define the precise role of cells of the lymphoid system.[1] It is encouraging, in this respect, that there has been a recent report (Strannegård 1971) of the successful induction of reaginic antibody formation in rabbits as a result of the oral and nasal administration of soluble and particulate antigens. But sub-human primates and dogs would seem to be more appropriate experimental animals for this purpose (ch. 6), particularly as a valuable model has been provided by the thorough studies of Heremans and his associates (Vaerman and Heremans 1969; 1970) on the origin of γA antibodies in the latter species. It will also be important to consider a possible inter-relationship between γE and γA antibody production, in view of the finding of an intimate relationship between these 2 classes of immunoglobulin in patients with ataxia-telangiectasia (Ammann et al. 1969); which has led to the interesting suggestion that possibly γE antibodies act as a reserve line of local defence in situations of IgA deficiency. In this connection it could be of some relevance that recent immunofluorescence studies (Callerame et al. 1971) revealed more IgE-containing cells in tissue from patients with acute or chronic bronchitis or bronchiectasis than in that from asthmatics or control subjects.

At the free cellular level there have been reports (e.g. Zeitz et al.

1966; Girard et al. 1967) of the induction of blastogenesis in the washed peripheral lymphocytes of pollen-sensitive individuals following stimulation with specific allergen; the transformed cells being observed to contain a large amount of vacuolated cytoplasm. As there is no evidence that leucocytes other than basophils take up γE antibody, it is assumed that these findings reflect a primary immune response of some sort; which, it has been suggested (Zeitz et al. 1966), might represent a vestige of a development stage in the sequence of immune responsiveness. This, it is thought, could be related to a delayed-type of sensitivity response; which would be anticipated in allergic patients whose lymphocytes show significant blast cell transformation and which has been observed occasionally in atopic individuals (Brostoff et al. 1969), although antibody production does not of course occur under these circumstances.

The production of antibody by the peripheral lymphocytes of atopic individuals was suggested by the detection of free reaginic antibody in the culture medium. More direct evidence has come from specific immunofluorescence studies, which have revealed that the small proportion of lymphocytes transformed in response to specific grass pollen allergen contained IgE; and, in general, similar numbers of cells stained specifically for IgE, light polypeptide chain and pollen-binding antibody (Brostoff et al. 1969). It will be important to substantiate these findings, however, by more definitive evidence of reaginic antibody synthesis by peripheral lymphocytes; such as the demonstration of incorporation of labelled amino acids into specific γE antibody as suggested by Zeitz and his associates. In this connection, it is encouraging to note that it has proved possible to maintain in culture a line of lymphoid cells taken from the original Swedish IgE myeloma patient (N.D.) which are synthesising γE-globulin (Nilsson 1971). The potential value of such a system in the further elucidation of cellular processes involved in reagin production needs little emphasis.

Although the full sequence of antibody formation in immediate hypersensitivity responses has yet to be described, it has been shown that IgE production occurs very early after the initial stimulation of experimental animals. Furthermore, as mentioned earlier, there is evidence that antibodies of other classes exert some control on γE antibody formation; an effect which is not unique to immunoglobulins of the γE class. Indeed, recent studies (Pernis et al. 1970) suggest that chain receptors on the lymphocyte control the switching on of antibodies of other classes. Nevertheless, it is possibly of some significance in this connection that the administration of γM antibodies a day before or a day after antigenic stimulus resulted in the enhancement of formation of reaginic antibody in the rabbit (Strannegård and Belin 1971). Conversely, reagin synthesis in the rabbit (Strannegård and Belin 1970) and rat (Tada and Okumura 1971A) is suppressed by passive administration of the γG fraction of hyperimmune sera. It is interesting to note that the administration to monkeys of the γG-globulin fraction of rabbit antiserum directed against human lymphocytes (i.e. ALG) has been found to lead to a small but significant increase in serum IgE level (Hawker et al. 1971); but similar treatment with normal rabbit IgG appeared to produce the same effect.

It will obviously be important to extend this type of investigation to the study of isolated cell systems, in an endeavour to obtain further evidence of a negative feed-back regulation of γE antibody formation. The suggestion (Tada and Okumura 1971) that immunocompetent cells responsible for γE antibody production are more susceptible to immunosuppression than cells involved in the production of immunoglobulins of other classes is of obvious relevance here.

Lymphoid cells have been considered, so far; but there is also a need to establish the nature of the contribution of other types of cell in the stimulation of anaphylactic antibody formation. Presumably macrophages 'process' sensitogens, in an analogous manner to their handling of immunogens; but it is conceivable that the distinctive physico-chemical properties of natural sensitogens (ch. 3) constitute an influence which directs towards a γE-type response. In this connection, the effect of adjuvant would also be of some consequence; whether it be natural (e.g. a constituent of nematodes, pollen etc.) or artificial (*B. pertussis,* aluminium precipitates etc.). For example, some evidence has been obtained

(Tada and Okumura 1971B) to suggest that the efficiency of *B. pertussis* vaccine in this respect can be attributed to a lymphocytosis-promoting factor (Morse and Bray 1969), which has been isolated from culture media and shown to enhance reagin formation in rats. Furthermore, the marked lymphocytosis which it promoted, mainly involving small lymphocytes, was characterised by a suppression of γM and γG antibody formation. But, as will have become apparent from ch. 6, *B. pertussis* vaccine is by no means unique in its adjuvant effect on reagin formation in experimental animals; aluminium salts having proved particularly effective in many studies, presumably through their capacity to activate macrophages.

7.2.2 Role of mast cells

No discussion of the cellular aspects of immediate hypersensitivity responses would be complete, of course, without considering the unique role of the tissue mast cells and circulating basophils. There is now substantial evidence from the application of immunofluorescence (Hubscher et al. 1970), auto-radiographic (Ishizaka and Ishizaka 1971) and rosetting (Wilson et al. 1971) techniques to indicate that γE-globulin is located on the surface of such cells; and, as has been assumed throughout earlier chapters, that the mast cells are at the seat of immediate sensitivity reactions as a result of their ready capacity for uptake of γE antibody, which is presumably synthesised in a similar manner to immunoglobulin of other classes. But could these cells have other functions perhaps in reagin production, besides being targets for reagin–allergen interaction? In this connection, it is most interesting to note that a proliferation of mast cells has been observed in the regional draining lymph nodes of mice following a primary antigenic (BSA, ferritin, etc.) stimulus (Roberts 1970). Active proliferation depended upon the strength and quality of the antigenic stimulus, and was very rapid; large clusters of mast cells appearing at the peak of the response in the interfollicular cortex and medullary regions. But no degranulation of the mast cells was observed, indicating the absence of cytophilic antibodies on their surfaces at this stage; nor was there evidence of incorporation of tritiated thymidine into the nucleus. It seems unlikely, therefore, that mast cells *per se* are capable of synthesising antibody; despite recent claims (Ginsburg and Lagunoff 1967) of the in vitro differentiation of mast cells from lymph node and thoracic duct cells of hyperimmunised mice, when cultured on embryo monolayers in the presence of the (protein) antigen (i.e. ovalbumin). Both histochemical and ultrastructural analyses were able to distinguish numerous clones of mast cells from the phagocytic histocytes, which usually arise in abundance from non-immunised mouse cells cultured in the absence of antigen.

The possibility cannot be ruled out, however, that mast cells – which are long-lived and stable on once reaching maturity – act in a 'helper' capacity in reagin formation. Could it be that interaction of mast cells with allergen 'turns on' neighbouring lymphocytes in a similar manner to the action of the factor supposedly released from the lysosomes of macrophages following antigen-activation in immune responses?

It seems more than fortuitous, in this respect, that there appears to be basic similarities between the supposed mode of action of cytophilic antibody on macrophage surfaces and that of reaginic antibodies on mast cells (ch. 5). In each case, it seems reasonable to suppose that combination with specific antigen leads to the formation of activation sites within the Fc regions of the antibody molecules; which trigger the release of active substances from macrophage lysosomes or mast cell granules. Moreover, as Greaves (1972) has recently pointed out, both of these systems have features in common with antigen-activation of receptor immunoglobulin on the surface of lymphocytes. It is not impossible that the mechanism responsible for antigen-induced blast formation is triggered by allosteric changes within the receptor immunoglobulin resembling those postulated to operate in allergen-induced histamine release (ch. 5 and 8), as I have already suggested elsewhere (Stanworth 1971).

An important implication of this analogy is that mast cells might perform similar functions in hypersensitivity responses to those engaged in by macrophages in immune ones; whilst lacking the ability to synthesise antibodies themselves. It might also follow that the relationship between basophils and mast cells is not unlike that between monocytes and macrophages, representing different stages of maturation of a single cell line. This would mean that anaphylactic antibody (γE- or γ_1-type) fulfils a similar role to that of cytophilic antibody (γ_2-type) in the uptake of antigen on the cell surface; and, that cells from untreated donors can be artificially sensitised or 'allergized' (to use a Coombs expression) by pretreatment with anaphylactic antibody in vitro or in vivo under appropriate conditions (ch. 2).

7.3 Fate of immunoglobulin E

The ready uptake of γE-globulin on to tissue mast cells has most probably constituted a serious source of error in turn-over studies of this immunoglobulin in man and other primates.

Measurement of the turn-over of ^{125}I-labelled myeloma IgE in the myeloma patient himself and in other patients (Bennich and Johansson 1971), as well as in normal humans (Waldmann 1969), revealed values ranging from as low as 0.7–4.4 days, compared with a value of 25 days for the half-life of human IgG. Moreover, the extremely rapid decrease in intravascular labelled IgE was matched by a correspondingly high increase in the urinary level. But the use of relatively high doses (i.e. 2 mg) of labelled protein could have been a complicating factor here; as was suggested by the observations in my own laboratory (McLaughlan and Stanworth 1972) of the lack of excretion of a substantial proportion (of order of 60 per cent) of the labelled material following the systemic administration to baboons of much lower doses (e.g. 10 μg) of ^{125}I-labelled myeloma IgE, which nevertheless disappeared from the circulation at an extremely rapid rate.

On the other hand, the half-time of disappearance of radiolabelled IgE (1.0–2.5 μg) following injection into human or monkey skin sites, as revealed by local monitoring, was of the order of 8–14 days (Ishizaka and Ishizaka 1971). This is comparable to the half-life of persistence of reaginic antibodies in P–K sites (Stanworth and Kuhns 1965; Gass and Anderson 1968). In contrast, locally administered radio-labelled human IgG was found to have a half-life of approximately 2 days (Ishizaka and Ishizaka 1971) and human γG anti-diphtheria toxoid antibodies of approximately 12 hr (Kuhns 1961); again pointing to the preferential uptake of γE-globulins by tissue mast cells at the local injection sites.

The short half-lives revealed by the IgE turnover studies just referred to have been taken to indicate that γE antibodies are being formed continuously in atopic individuals, and that the production is greater than would be expected from the observed levels of antibody in the serum. It is significant, in this respect, that the high levels of IgE seen in the urine of healthy individuals (Turner et al. 1970)* are also thought to be attributable to local production of this immunoglobulin, somewhere in the urinary tract. This, it has been speculated (Bennich and Johansson 1971), is more likely to be a normal function than the reflection of a local urinary reagin-mediated disorder. But, a recent report (Gerber et al. 1971) of the localisation of IgE in the kidneys of 13 patients with nephrotic syndrome suggests that there could be renal conditions in which γE antibodies are operating deleteriously.

It is hoped that studies now in progress in my own and other laboratories on the metabolism of radio-labelled IgE in sub-human primates, will provide more definitive information about the fate of γE antibodies. With this objective in mind, direct autoradiographic examination of autopsy tissue and organ specimens from injected animals is being undertaken.

7.4 Alternative functions of γE antibodies

Finally, it would seem to be appropriate, in a chapter concerned with the origin and fate of γE antibodies to consider roles other than those concerned with the mediation of adverse anaphylactic reactions. Are there, for instance, other situations where antibodies of this class act in a protective capacity? Such an idea would obviously prove attractive, on teleological grounds, to those

* But it now seems likely (Turner, M.W.; personal communication) that fragments of IgE were being measured in these studies.

who consider that antibody formation – irrespective of immunoglobulin class – is destined to benefit the host.

It is conceivable that substances released as a result of allergen-induced disruption of mast cell granules would fulfil similar roles to the enzymes and other constituents released from the lysosomes of polymorphonuclear leucocytes during phagocytosis. In particular there have been suggestions that the release of vasoactive substances like histamine can sometimes have a protective function; for example, by increasing vascular permeability and thus forming part of a local defence mechanism against bacterial infection (Bloch 1967). The strongest claim for assigning a role of this type to anaphylactic antibodies has come, however, from studies of parasite-infected animals: from which evidence has been put forward to suggest that a local reagin-mediated immediate sensitivity reaction in the gut plays a crucial part in the subsequent expulsion of the offending helminth by producing an environment unfavourable for its survival. Although this so-called 'self cure' process was initially studied in sheep injected with *Haemonchus contortus* and *Trichostrongylus colubriformis* (Stewart 1955), it has been more recently studied in considerable detail in rats infected with the nematode *Nippostrongylus brasiliensis.* Intravenous injection of normal antigen will evoke a localised anaphylactic reaction in the intestinal mucosae of animals previously injected by sub-cutaneous injection of larvae (Urquhart et al. 1965). The infective organisms remain localised in the lumen and do not multiply within the rest of the body, so that the infections can be carefully controlled and their immunological effects measured in a quantitative and accurate manner. This type of approach has offered a means of studying the role of mast cells in immunological reactions within a mucous membrane, namely the jejunal mucosae, with reference to the structural and functional changes thereby produced.

Evidence was obtained (Mulligan et al. 1965) that adult worms transplanted into susceptible rats were subsequently expelled by the development of an immunological reaction, the time of onset of which could be shortened by the passive transfer of hyperimmune rat sera. Furthermore, the pretreatment of recipient rats with a heterologous protein antigen (ovalbumin) and *B. pertussis* adjuvant, which is known to favour reagin production, was found to accelerate the self-cure process (Barth et al. 1966). This suggested that an intestinal anaphylactic reaction, albeit involving a heterologous non-worm allergen, can facilitate the passage of anti-worm antibody into the intestinal lumen. Moreover, the exponential expulsion of the nematodes from the infected rat is associated with a sharp burst of intestinal mast cell activity and enhanced permeability of the bowel wall to macromolecules as revealed by studies with labelled polyvinyl pyrollidone (PVP) and electron microscopic examination using protein enzyme tracers (Murray et al. 1971A). Observations such as these have encouraged the idea that a stimulus from the infecting parasite induces the synchronous development of a population of mast cells, as well as IgE-producing plasma cells and plasma cells producing antibodies of other classes with anti-worm activity. The mast cells are supposedly triggered to release their pharmacological mediators by a reagin–allergen (nematode) interaction, which could result in the opening up of a pathway through the intestinal mucosa permitting the transfer of neutralising antibody which potentiates the expulsion of the parasites. Furthermore, other evidence of a link between amine release and self-cure has been obtained from investigations in which it has been shown that the daily administration of inhibitors of histamine and 5-hydroxytryptamine (5-HT) to rats infected with *N. brasiliensis* prevented the onset of the rapid phase of worm expulsion (Murray et al. 1971B); and that a rise in 5-HT levels in the bowel wall was associated with a marked episode of mast cell activity and worm expulsion (Murray et al. 1971C).

But there are other reasons for supposing that a local anaphylaxis might not play a direct role in worm expulsion. For instance, the possibility has yet to be excluded that a mast cell degranulating factor secreted by *N. brasiliensis* (Keller 1971) is directly responsible for producing a subepithelial vascular leak, without any requirement for reagin-allergen induced release. Besides, evidence has been recently reported, from a study of the sequence of events involved in worm expulsion from the infected rat intestine (Jones and Ogilvie 1971), which indicates that if local anaphylaxis is involved it acts subsequent to antibody-mediated damage to worms; which, it is claimed, is not caused by reaginic antibodies. This secondary action, it is suggested, could take the form of a direct effect by amines (liberated from mast cells) on the metabolism of the damaged worms; thus causing their ultimate expulsion. It refutes, therefore, the idea of Jarrett and his associates, that a gut lesion induced by a reagin-mediated anaphylactic reaction is an early crucial step in worm expulsion.

Be as this may, the work of the Jarrett group has thrown important new light on the nature of the mast cell response to local antigenic (i.e. parasite) stimulus. Of particular interest in this respect, and in relation to the earlier discussion of mast cell function, is the observation that under the stimulation of a worm infection lymphoblast-like cells appear in the *lamina propria*, multiply exponentially and differentiate into mast cells (Jarrett et al. 1969). This process, it has been suggested, might be initiated by a factor produced by helminths which stimulates the production of mastoblasts which – like large lymphocytes of the thoracic duct – home on the intestinal *lamina propria*. Incidentally, a similar stimulation of lymphoblast-like cells might possibly account for the observed ability of infective helminths to potentiate reagin-formation to an unrelated protein antigen such as ovalbumin (ch. 6).

Other cell transformations seen in experimental parasitic infections in rats and other mammalian species involve the controversial globular leucocyte; which, it is claimed (Murray et al. 1968) derives from the subepithelial mast cell and which seems to differ in several ways from classical mature connective tissue mast cells. For instance, it contains large acidophilic globules rather than the characteristic basophilic granules; which supposedly results from an alteration in the relationship between the constituent acid mucopolysaccharide and basic protein. It will be important to establish whether such cells, whose peak of production occurs apparently at the commencement of worm expulsion, play any role in classical immediate hypersensitivity reactions. Indeed, it is to be hoped that the studies which have been undertaken on mast cell changes in the jejunal mucosal membranes of parasite-infected rats will be extended to include investigations of the possibility of similar cellular changes occurring at the sites (e.g. nasal linings, lungs etc.) of true immediate sensitivity reactions in primates (i.e. rhesus monkeys, baboons etc.).

Finally, although discussion so far has centred on processes mediated by vasoactive amines, a possible protective role of other substances released from mast cells during reagin-mediated anaphylactic reactions cannot be ignored. Of these, apart from proteases, heparin seems to be a likely candidate in view of its observed ability to inhibit the injurious effects of certain viruses, snake venom and microbial metabolites (Higginbotham and Karnella 1971). It is possible that polyanions of this type play an essential defensive role in the neutralisation of quick-acting polycationic substances, such as the melittin of bee venom, which are themselves not noticeably immunogenic and consequently not prone to destruction by immune mechanisms. In this connection, it seems particularly significant that local tissue mast cells in the mouse were found to secrete their heparin-containing granules rapidly in a dose-related response to subcutaneous injection of relatively small amounts of bee venom; and that the shed granules were observed to form complexes with cationic protein in vivo, which were subsequently ingested by adjacent mononuclear cells (Higginbotham and Karnella 1971). Hence, it has been suggested that mast cell granules may, during transfer from mast cell to phagocytic cell, sequester noxious cationic proteins of bee venom (and presumably those from other sources); and that dermal mast cells may, therefore, be strategically situated and uniquely adapted to serve as a local means of resistance to bee and other stings. Likewise it is thought that secretion of heparin containing granules from mast cells may provide a local means of sequestration of potentially injurious lysosomal proteins released from PMN leucocytes, for subsequent ingestion by connective tissue cells (Clark and Higginbotham 1968).

As Bloch (1967) has pointed out, the wide distribution of tissue mast cells, particularly in those areas of the body which are most frequently in contact with external agents, and their notable stability, is consistent with their involvement in a protective capacity in reagin-mediated anaphylactic reactions. But the studies outlined above have indicated that there are other situations where mast cell responses are not initiated directly by immunological processes.

Note

[1] Recent observations (Ishizaka, K. and Kishimoto, T., Montreal Allergy Meeting, 1972) have indicated that both carrier-specific helper (T) cells and hapten-specific (B) memory cells participate in the in vitro formation of IgE antibody against hapten-protein conjugate; whilst in vivo evidence has been obtained (Tada, T. et al., Montreal Allergy Meeting, 1972) of independent antibody mediated and T cell-mediated mechanisms regulating reagin formation in the rat.

CHAPTER 8

Mechanism of release of mediators of immediate hypersensitivity

8.1 Introduction

The elucidation of the mechanism of release of the amine mediators is being pursued with increasing vigour in many laboratories now that a distinctive type of immunoglobulin (γE) is known to play an active role in classical immediate hypersensitivity reactions. As mentioned earlier, in vitro studies based on the use of sensitised human leucocytes and tissue preparations from artificially sensitised animals have suggested that the interaction between antibody and antigen on the cell surface sets in train a multi-step, energy requiring, enzyme process. But the mechanism of the crucial triggering process responsible for this, and the nature and sequence of the events which follow, have yet to be depicted in biochemical terms.

Obviously before such a mammoth task is ultimately accomplished it will be necessary to obtain far more information about the structure and function of the target cells involved (i.e. mast cells and basophils); and, in particular, of their cytoplasmic and granular membranes. Even at this stage, however, it is felt that a discussion and appraisal of various possible release mechanisms might fulfil a useful purpose; if only to stimulate further investigation.

Apart from those observations which have been made directly on γE-mediated anaphylactic reactions in primate cell and tissue systems, important clues about the nature of the triggering mechanism can be gleaned from a consideration of other areas of investigation. These include: a) anaphylactic reactions mediated in actively and passively sensitised animal tissues by γE-like antibodies; and even by γG-type sensitising antibodies because (as already mentioned in ch. 5) there is reason to suppose that they behave essentially similarly to γE antibodies; b) artificial, immunological and non-immunological, methods of inducing the release of vasoacamines from mast cells and basophils; c) other types of release process, such as complement-mediated hemolysis, which are also initiated by antibody–antigen reaction at the cell surface.

It is worth noting that for some time before the role of γE antibodies had been established, investigators of mechanisms of anaphylaxis in experimental animal systems had been suggesting that histamine release is initiated by the combination of cell-bound antibody with specific antigen; which brings about the transient activation of an intracellular enzyme system (as discussed, for example, by Mongar and Schild 1962). This is an attractive idea, which is rapidly gaining in plausibility, although the enzyme (or enzymes) involved has not yet been identified.

Before considering the claims of possible candidates for this role, it seems reasonable to rule out the participation of any extra-cellular enzyme, such as serum C1a esterase, because there is no firm evidence that complement or any other serum factors are essential for γE *antibody-mediated* histamine release. Artificial histamine release, induced in rat mast cells by treatment with rabbit anti-rat mast cell antiserum does, on the other hand, rely upon an esterase of this type (Austen and Valentine 1968). But this is a cytotoxic process, which is fundamentally different from that in which γE antibody 'passively' bound to the target cell (through Fc groups) reacts with specific antigen (ch. 5, and fig. 5.9).

8.2 Intracellular enzyme systems possibly involved in anaphylactic histamine release

8.2.1 Proteases

It is quite conceivable that intracellular esterases are implicated in some way, in true anaphylactic reactions. In this connection, it is interesting to note that evidence has been obtained of the activation of a rat mast cell esterase during histamine release effected by treatment with a rabbit anti-rat γG-globulin (Austen and Valentine 1968). But even in this type of reaction system, which can be likened to reverse passive anaphylaxis (fig. 5.9), there is a dependence on certain complement components (C1–C6). Moreover, there is evidence that the response (like that effected with anti-mast cell antiserum, as mentioned above) is cytotoxic. In this case, however, it is thought that a precursor form of the mast cell esterase is activated on interaction of the target cell with the serum complement components. This, then, relegates the cell-bound rat (γG) antibody to a secondary role in the triggering of histamine release; the complement system being activated by the antibody's subsequent interaction (as antigen) with the rabbit

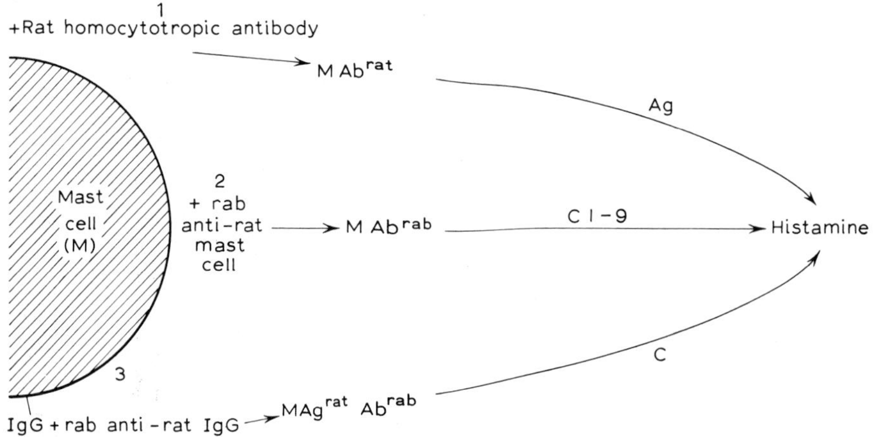

Fig. 8.1. Schematic representation of various immunological pathways leading to histamine release from rat peritoneal mast cells in vitro (reproduced from Austen and Valentine 1968, by permission of the authors).

anti-rat γG antibody (fig. 8.1). Such a process need not be considered further, however, because of its basic difference to a γE antibody–antigen triggered response.

Precursor esterases appear to be involved in other types of cell triggering processes, such as the chemotactic stimulus of neutrophils (Ward and Becker 1970). But here, too, certain complement components (i.e. C5, 6, 7) are implicated. Nevertheless, Becker (1968) has gone so far as to suggest that a similar type of enzyme reaction, namely the activation of a cell bound serine esterase, working through the same common pathway, comprises a general trigger mechanism operative in all exoplasmotic responses; including histamine release from rat peritoneal mast cells mediated by homocytotropic antibody or Compound 48/80.

This idea is quite contrary to the thesis which has been developed throughout this monograph, that γE-mediated cell lysis is accomplished by a unique form of triggering process because of the manner in which the antibody is bound to the target cell prior to interaction with specific antigen. In contrast, it has been suggested that processes mediated by other types of antibody (e.g. γG), bound to the target cells in other ways (as mentioned above), are less efficient relying upon the agency of co-factors such as components of the complement system.

No convincing evidence has been presented which indicates that a mast cell(or basophil)-bound serine precursor esterase, of the type just discussed, comprises the primary trigger site of γE antibody-mediated histamine release; possibly because of the complications which have arisen in the use of phosphonate ester inhibitors in the human leucocyte assay (§ 2.3.3). For instance, it has been observed that sensitised human leucocytes which have been treated with appropriate concentrations of di-isopropyl phosphofluoridate (DFP) and then washed are unable to release histamine, even on challenge with high doses of specific antigen (Lichenstein and Osler 1966). But this seems to be due to the blockage of a general metabolic pathway, rather than one which is essential for histamine release (Lichenstein 1968). In this type of approach, it is, of course, essential to demonstrate that an inhibitor blocks histamine release at the time of reaction of antigen (allergen) with the antibody-sensitised cells, if a case is to be made for the activation of a particular cellular enzyme.

It is quite conceivable, however, that other types of protease are involved at the γE antibody–antigen trigger site. Of these α-chymotrypsin has received most attention, in attempts to effect histamine release by direct treatment of rat mast cells with enzyme. Treatment with this enzyme has been shown to produce cellular damage, but only at relatively high concentrations (Keller 1961). There is need for .caution, however, in interpreting the results of this sort of experiment. because it is possible that the same enzyme would behave differently when acting sequentially in a highly organised system within the target cell. Indeed, it is probably significant in this connection that chymotrypsin acting in conjunction with phospholipase A proved capable of inducing substantial (i.e. 80 per cent) histamine release from isolated rat peritoneal mast cells, in contrast to the relatively low release (25 per cent) it effected when acting alone (Amundsen et al. 1969).

Microscopic (light and EM) studies, using radio-labelled inhibitors, have provided evidence of a chymotrypsin-like enzyme in rat mast cells located within the granules (Darzynkiewicz and Barnard 1967; Budd et al. 1967). It is possible, however, that this protease is involved in some secondary release mechanism; unless the primary activation site is on the granules, which seems unlikely from present evidence. * Incidentally, in this connection it is interesting to note that there is evidence (Budd et al. 1967) that a chymotrypsin-like enzyme is held in inactive form in mast cell granules as a result of its combination with heparin; where presumably it could be involved in loss of histamine.

It seems more reasonable to suppose, however, that the initial triggering process occurs on the cytoplasmic membrane: in (or on) which it might be anticipated that certain functional enzymes will be sited, fulfilling similar roles to the enzymes now known to be located in the membranes of other types of cells. Taking erythrocyte membrane composition as an example, it is interesting to

* Although Killingback and Orr (personal communication) have recently observed the specific staining of mast granules of sensitised rats by fluorescent labelled allergen.

note that there is thought to be a fair measure of independence in the organisation of the protein and lipid moieties (Green 1971); with the protein molecules being anchored firmly in the membrane, but being at the same time free to rotate and diffuse in the plane of the membrane where restriction from polar interactions does not occur. Microscopic studies (e.g. da Silva and Branton 1970) have revealed that proteins tend usually to protrude from one or other surface of cell membrane rather than stretch right through. Phospholipids, on the other hand, are not readily accessible on the outer surface of erythrocyte membranes; possibly because of screening by the membrane proteins or because they are built predominantly into the inner surface (Bretscher 1971). This does not necessarily mean, however, that enzyme reactions involving the lipid moieties of mast cell membranes are unlikely to play any part in histamine release processes; as should become apparent.

8.2.2 Phospholipases

This leads to the consideration of the possible role of phospholipases in γE antibody–antigen induced histamine release. Of these, the phospholipases A and C have received particular attention, because hydrolysis of those phospholipids which are known to be essential for the functional integrity of the cell membrane would seem to provide a relatively simple and effective method of achieving lysis. It has been postulated, therefore, that both specific antibody–antigen reaction and non-specific histamine liberators (such as Compound 48/80) effect disruption of rat mast cells by activation of a phospholipase normally present in inactive form on their surface (Högberg and Uvnäs 1957).

Early studies (discussed by Mongar and Schild 1962), based on the use of various metabolic inhibitors and antagonists, indicated that the disruption of rat mast cells effected by treatment with phospholipase A resembled in many ways that induced by antibody–antigen reaction or by treatment with Compound 48/80. More recent studies have indicated that the phospholipase preparations (isolated from snake and bee venom) used in the early investigations were contaminated with potent histamine liberators such as melittin. Nevertheless, as already mentioned, it is possibly of some significance that phospholipase A has been found (Amundsen et al. 1969) to cause substantial release of histamine from isolated rat mast cells when acting synergistically with chymotrypsin (or kallikrein).

Attempts in my own laboratory to obtain direct evidence of phospholipid hydrolysis during γE-mediated histamine release, from passively sensitised chopped human lung or monkey skin suspensions, have failed to provide clear-cut results. These experiments (performed in conjunction with a lipid chemist, Dr. V. Long) involved the inclusion of ^{14}C-labelled lecithin in the tissue-suspending fluid at the time of allergen challenge, followed by thin layer chromatographic analysis of the concentrated fluid after the histamine release reaction was complete. It is possible, however, that the number of cells involved in the anaphylactic reaction were too small to yield sufficient phospholipid degradation products for ready detection by the technique adopted. A similar explanation has been put forward by Finke and his associates (1966) to account for their failure to detect any change in the total lipid composition of the leucocytes of ragweed-sensitive individuals following allergen-induced histamine release.

In considering the potential role of phospholipase A it is important, of course, to take into account the possible releasing action of lysolecithin (lysophosphatidyl choline); which is one of the main products of phospholipid hydrolysis by phospholipase A and noted for its powerful lytic action. Moreover, this substance was thought to be formed in the serum during complement-binding antibody–antigen reactions (Fischer 1964), where it supposedly contributed to cell injuring processes. Results of studies of the possible role of lysolecithin in the induction of immune cellular injury to isolated rat mast cells (Keller 1964) seemed, however, to rule out any significant cytotoxic effect; besides suggesting that it was unlikely to be involved in localised complement-mediated cellular injury. Furthermore, in studies on systems more pertinent to the present discussion, it has been observed (Finke et al. 1966) that conditions (e.g. absence of Ca^{2+} ions) which influence antigen-induced histamine release from human leucocytes had little effect on lysolecithin-induced release. This was disappointing because, as Keller (1966) suggested, it seemed reasonable to suppose that lysolecithin released within the target cell might play some secondary role in the mediation of anaphylactic reactions. Nevertheless, it is conceivable that it contributes to the fusion of the granular and cellular membranes of mast cells; because there is evidence (Poole et al. 1970) that lysolecithin facilitates erythrocyte membrane fusion, by promoting a transition from a bimolecular lipid leaflet to an arrangement of radially oriented molecules.

It might prove possible to obtain more direct evidence of the involvement of phospholipid hydrolysis in histamine release processes by the use of artificial phospholipid spherules (liposomes). In this connection, it is interesting to note that liposomes made from sheep erythrocyte lipid have been shown (Humphrey 1973) to release constituent glucose on treatment with anti-Forsmann antibody together with the appropriate complement components (C5–9); but there was no evidence of action of phospholipase A or lysolecithin, nor was it possible to demonstrate changes in the composition of lipid extracted from the surface. On the other hand, in a similar type of study, Lachmann and associates (1970) have observed that small amounts of diglyceride and fatty acid are produced; and this effect seems to be independent as to whether the system is a lytic one or not.

It would be interesting to see whether liposomes containing histamine or, better still, isolated rat mast cell granules could be prepared; and whether any significant changes, including histamine release, could be effected by treatment with sensitising antibody followed by challenge with specific antigen. This presupposes, of course, that the antibody can be persuaded to bind to the liposome surface in the first place. Possibly this problem could be ultimately solved by the use of mast cell membrane lipid for preparation of liposomes, when it becomes possible to isolate such material in sufficient yield. It would also be interesting, however, to determine whether preformed γE antibody–antigen complexes or aggregated γE myeloma protein possessed any ability to induce histamine release from this type of artificial system.

8.2.3 Adenyl cyclase

No discussion of enzymes which possibly operate at the trigger site of γE antibody–antigen-induced anaphylactic reactions would be complete without consideration of the adenyl cyclase system. Indeed, even if it proves to play no role, its supposed mode of action would seem to offer a model worth studying in some detail. For this enzyme system is now known to be located on the inner surface of many types of cell, where it acts as the trigger site for a whole range of different hormones (including histamine itself). By catalysing the formation of cyclic adenyl monophosphate (AMP)

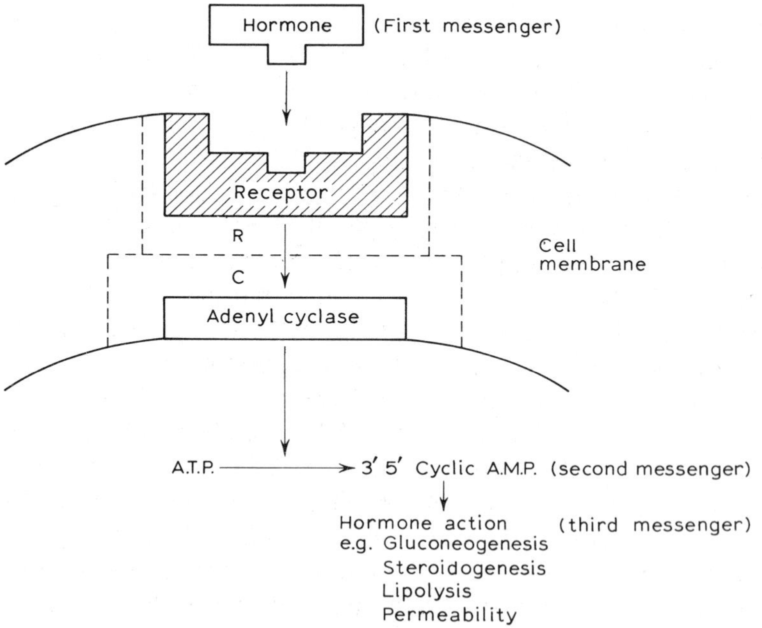

Fig. 8.2. Proposed mode of action of hormones on the adenyl cyclase system (modified from Catt 1970, by permission of the author). R and C refer respectively to the regulatory and catalytic regions of a regulatory enzyme (following the suggestion of Robison et al. 1967).

from adenyl triphosphate (ATP) it is considered to play a crucial role in the conveyance of information to within the cells, the cyclic nucleotide thus formed functioning as a 'second messenger' in acting on the appropriate intracellular site for that particular hormone activity (Catt 1970). Alternatively, this process can lead to the synthesis and secretion of other hormones (e.g. steroids) which act as 'third messengers' (fig. 8.2).

It is tempting to suggest that histamine release might be triggered in an analogous manner. In other words, might not the active site supposedly formed in the ϵ-chains of mast cell-bound γE antibodies, as a result of combination with specific allergen (in the manner postulated in ch. 5), act directly upon a similar receptor site within the target cell membrane (fig. 8.3a)? The immediate histamine releasing activity of γE antibody–antigen complexes and aggregated γE myeloma protein might then be attributed to the pre-formation of a similar activating site by association of the immunoglobulin in free solution (fig. 8.3b). Moreover, as will be discussed further later, it is not impossible that certain artificial histamine liberators (such as basic polypeptides) act upon a similar cell membrane receptor site. A common outcome of each of these triggering actions would then be the formation of cyclic AMP, which perhaps acts subsequently on the mast granule membrane to initiate exoplasmosis and the release of histamine and other vasoactive amines ('third messengers' in fig. 8.2). For, amongst the wide variety of cellular activities in which this cyclic nucleotide has been implicated are mitosis (Rixon et al. 1970) and phagocytosis (Weissmann et al. 1971).

It would seem to be worth while, therefore, to look a little more closely at the present knowledge of the role of cyclic AMP in hormone action (see also recent articles by Butcher et al. 1968; Robison et al. 1968). Its level at any given instant depends upon the activities of at least 2 enzymes; adenyl cyclase, which catalysis its formation from ATP in a reaction requiring Mg^{2+} ions; and a specific phosphodiesterase, which inactivates it by catalysing its hydrolysis to 5′ AMP (fig. 8.4). Furthermore, there is evidence of a requirement for Ca^{2+} and Mg^{2+} – the 2 divalent cations which have been found to be necessary for γE antibody–allergen in-

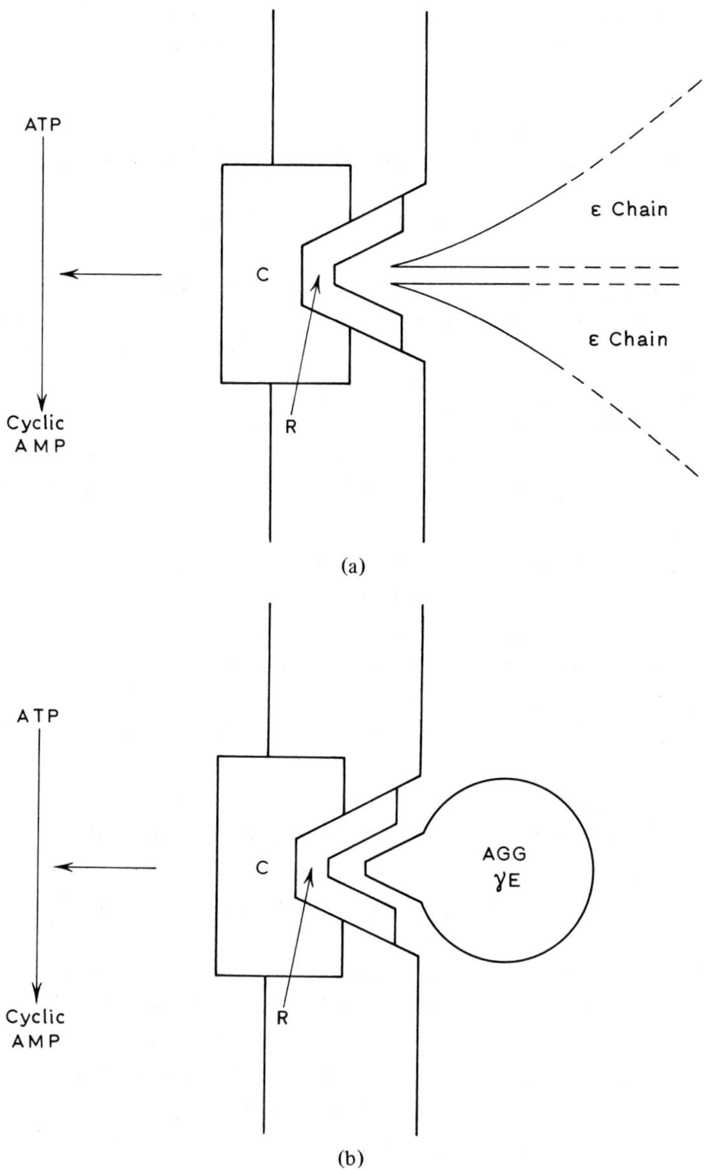

Fig. 8.3. (a) Possible nature of trigger action of cell-bound γE antibody initiated by combination with specific allergen. (b) Possible mode of action of pre-formed aggregated γE-globulin (or γE antibody–allergen complex).

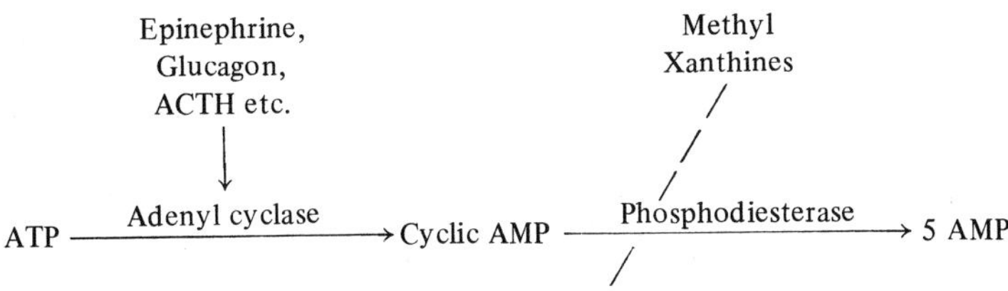

Fig. 8.4. Adenyl cyclase enzyme system.

duced histamine release – at the stage of reaction of cyclic AMP.

The different physiological effects which cyclic AMP initiates (e.g. glucose oxidation, lipolysis, increase in membrane permeability, release of enzymes and hormones etc.) can be attributed to the different characteristics of the cells within which it is produced. This does not explain, however, the apparent hormone-specificity of the adenyl cyclase at the trigger site. It has been suggested (Robison and associates 1967), therefore, that the adenyl cyclase located within the membrane of the target cell is a regulatory enzyme (fig. 8.2); not unlike aspartate transcarbamylate, for example, which is comprised of 2 sub-units involved in distinct regulatory and catalytic functions. According to this idea, the hormone receptor would form part of the regulatory sub-unit, which would differ from one type of target cell to another; whereas the catalytic sub-unit would be common to all adenyl cyclases. It might be expected, therefore, that mast cells would possess adenyl cyclase in their cytoplasmic membranes with a different regulatory sub-unit to that, say, in the adenyl cyclase on the surface of the B cells of the islets of Langerhans responsible for the production of insulin.

To explain the mechanism of the initial triggering process it has been suggested (Schimmer et al. 1968) that the action of hormone on the surface receptor of the target cell brings about a conformational change within the cell membrane which activates the adenyl cyclase; either directly, by influencing the catalytic sub-unit, or indirectly by altering the permeability of the membrane. The idea of a single protein extending from one side of a cell membrane to another is not incompatible with current concepts of cell membrane structure but, as mentioned earlier, negative staining has revealed many examples of proteins that project from one surface of the cell membrane or another but rarely any that stretch right through (da Silva and Branton 1970). As will be indicated later, however, this is not necessarily a prerequisite for the postulated role of adenyl cyclase as a hormone receptor or, indeed, for the mast cell membrane site supposedly activated by γE antibody–allergen combination.

Another interesting suggestion (Robison et al. 1967) which has been put forward recently proposes that the α and β adrenergic receptors are in fact regulatory sub-units of adenyl cyclase, thus offering an explanation of the puzzling observation that stimulation of α or β receptors leads to the same response. It is significant, therefore, that β stimulants such as epinephrine and isoproterenol, as well as theophylline, have been shown to prevent allergen-induced histamine release from γE-sensitised leucocytes (Lichenstein and Margolis 1968); and that these, and other catecholamines, have been shown to inhibit also allergen-induced histamine release from sensitised human lung (Assem and Schild 1969). These findings, as well as the rank order of the inhibitory activity of the different sympathomimetic amines in the anaphylactic release of histamine in the lung system, have been taken to indicate that the catecholamines are exerting their effect by stimulating adrenergic receptors. Furthermore, essentially similar findings have recently been reported from a study (Ishizaka et al. 1971) based on the use of monkey lung sensitised with human γE antibodies, where isoproterenol and epinephrine were found to inhibit the allergen-induced release of both histamine and slow reacting substance (SRS-A).

The inference from all of these observations is that the intracellular accumulation of cyclic AMP is responsible for the inhibition of release of histamine and other mediators of anaphylaxis; and it has been suggested, therefore, that it is acting in a regulatory capacity in immediate hypersensitivity reactions. This is also concluded from the observation (Ishizaka et al. 1971) that diethyl carbamazine (hetrazan) inhibits the release of both histamine and SRS-A when present on allergen challenge of γE-sensitised monkey lung tissue; and from the similar inhibition by N^6–2′-*O*-dibutyryl cyclic AMP, a derivative which has been found to mimic the effects of hormones in situations where cyclic AMP itself is ineffective (Butcher et al. 1968).

As Johnson and Moran (1970) point out, however, none of these studies provide any evidence that catacholamines activate adenyl cyclase in mast cells; nor do they offer any direct evidence for the involvement of cyclic AMP in the release of histamine and SRS-A. Indeed, these authors conclude that the observation that both agonists and antagonists of α and β adrenergic receptors inhibit release excludes the association of known adrenergic mechanisms with selective amine release reactions in rat mast cells. They also suggest that the lack of specificity of inhibition of histamine release by a given class of antagonists and agonists, and the high concentration of drugs needed to inhibit release, indicates that the blockage of specific receptors involved in the initial steps of histamine release is unlikely. Presumably, however, this does not exclude the possibility that the adenyl cyclase system is involved in some secondary role in the histamine release process.

Obviously it will be important to perform further, more direct studies to investigate this point. In this connection, it is worth noting that Butcher and his associates (1968) have specified that positive findings in 3 types of experiment are necessary before it is reasonable to conclude that cyclic AMP is involved in a particular hormone action. Included in these is the measurement of intracellular cyclic AMP levels in intact cell preparations and measurement of the physiological response simultaneously; an approach which would seem to be necessary in mast cell studies before an essential role can be unequivocally assigned to this cyclic nucleotide[1].

Despite these reservations, however, the supposed mode of action of various hormones, involving the activation of adenyl cyclases sited within the target cell membranes, would seem to offer a useful model and stimulus to current attempts to obtain more definitive information about the nature of the γE antibody–allergen-triggered activation site on mast cells and basophils. For it seems reasonable to suppose, at this stage, that a similar type of triggering mechanism is involved. Many enzymes besides adenyl cyclase (e.g. phosphatases, phosphodiesterases, etc) are known to fulfil essential functions in cell membranes (as is discussed, for example, by Dowben 1969); and it would seem quite possible that at least some of these would be influenced by antibody–antigen reactions occurring on the cell surface. To take an example, a magnesium-requiring sodium, potassium-activated adenyl triphosphatase (Skou 1967) has been found widely in erythrocyte ghosts and other membranes. Moreover, it appears to be orientated across the cell membrane with the sodium site facing the exterior and the potassium site facing the interior. It is also interesting to note that included amongst the inhibitors of this enzyme are basic proteins, such as protamines, histones and polylysine (Schwartz 1945; Yoshida et al. 1965); which are, of course, potent histamine liberators.

It is quite conceivable that an enzyme such as this (which is reputed by Tanaka and Strickland 1965, to be a lipoprotein), capable of exerting a directional action within the membrane, is implicated in the primary trigger site of mast cells and basophils undergoing anaphylactic reaction. The attempted identification and isolation of such an enzyme, which might also prove to be activated by γE antibody–allergen complex in free-solution, presents one of the next major tasks in the elucidation of the mechanism of immediate hypersensitivity reactions. In the meantime, can anything significant be learned about the nature of the complex processes involved from the multitude of studies which have already been performed on the in vitro release of histamine from isolated rat mast cells?

8.3 Mode of action of artificial liberators

At first sight the propensity of data yielded by such studies, which have been based largely on the use of artificial liberators, is bewildering; and one is inclined to the impression that practically any form of treatment will persuade mast cells to part with their granules and their histamine. But, as a result of increasing information about the manner in which various types of reagent react with cell membrane phospholipid and protein, together with the availability of more detailed observations on the morphological and biochemical changes thus induced, it is possible to begin to form a comprehensive picture of the various ways in which mast cell degranulation can occur. Such an exercise seems to be justified, because it has been noted that the morphological changes induced in rat mast cells by artificial agents such as Compound 48/80 (in relatively low doses) are very similar to those mediated by homocytotropic antibody; and, furthermore, many of the factors which influence antibody-mediated histamine release (table 8.1) are also effective in certain artificial release systems.

An attempt has been made in table 8.2, to classify the various agents which have been employed to effect histamine release. Functionally, these can be divided into non-selective and selective reagents; which, as is indicated, can also be loosely distinguished as lipid reactants or protein reactants respectively. The former tend to produce more drastic general effects upon the cell and cytoplasmic membranes; which ultimately result in granule release by deterioration of the cell and granule-containing compartments, in contrast to the dynamic expulsion of these structures promoted by the selective reagents (Bloom and Haegerman 1967). The cytotoxic effects of the non-selective agents such as aliphatic amines (e.g. ocytyl amine) and other types of detergents (e.g. Triton X-100) can be attributed to their surface active properties, which can also lead to complete disorganisation of the granular structure (Mota 1959). Moreover, it is also possible for some of the less potent histamine releasers to act similarly as non-selective surfactants when tested at sufficiently high doses. This could account for the apparent conflict of opinion over the mode of action of melittin; for, whereas Uvnäs (1968) has stated that melittin differs in action from other artificial releasers (such as Compound 48/80 and basic polypeptides) in causing damage to the mast cell membrane, Bloom and Haegermark (1967) claim that bee venom (whose main histamine-liberating constituent is melittin) releases the vasoactive amine in a very similar manner to that effected by Compound 48/80. In this connection, it is interesting to note that liposome studies (Sessa et al. 1969) have revealed melittin to possess an extraordinary affinity for lipid membranes which causes their disruption; because of a polar association between the acyl

TA

Factors influencing th

This table is not meant to provide an exhaustive survey of the subject, but rather an indication o complex processes which contribute to both anaphyl

Agent	Anaphylactic release (by antigen)		
	System	Effect	Reference
Fluoride	Human leucocytes	Inhibition	Lichenstein (1968)
2-Deoxy glucose	Human leucocytes	Inhibition	Russo and Lichenstein (19
Glucose	Rat mast cells	Inhibition by glucose lack	Perera and Mongar (1965)
ATP	Human leucocytes	Potentiation	Lichenstein (1968)
2-4-Dinitro phenol	Guinea pig lung Human leucocytes	No inhibition No inhibition	Mongar and Schild (1962) Lichenstein (1968)
Sodium cyanide	Guinea pig lung Human leucocytes	Inhibition No inhibition	Mongar and Schild (1962) Lichenstein (1968)
Diisopropyl phosphofluoridate (DFP)	Human leucocytes	Inhibition	Osler et al. (1968)
Amino acid esters	Guinea pig lung	Inhibition	Austen and Brocklehurst (1961)
Phenol	Guinea pig lung	Reversible inhibition	Mongar and Schild (1957)
Di basic acids (e.g. succinate, malonate)	Guinea pig lung	Potentiation	Austen and Brocklehurst (1961); Austen (1968)
Oxygen	Rat mast cells Guinea pig lung	Inhibition by profound O_2 lack Inhibition by O_2 lack	Perera and Mongar (1965); Mongar and Schild (1957)
Thiols (e.g. thioglycollate)	Guinea pig lung Rat mast cells	Potentiation (at 10 mM) Inhibition (at 50–100 mM)	Schild (1968)
-SH-blockers (e.g. *N*-ethyl maleimide, *p*-chloro mercuribenzoate, iodoacetate)	+Guinea pig lung	Inhibition	Edman et al. (1964)

release of histamine.

of studies being undertaken with various cell systems to permit a picture to be formed of the rtificially-induced histamine release in vitro.

cial release (by Compound 48/80)			Inference
m	Effect	Reference	
nast cells	No inhibition	Högberg and Uvnäs (1960)	
nast cells	Inhibition		Glycolytic pathway critical (for anaphylactic release)
nast cells	Inhibition by glucose lack	Perera and Mongar (1965)	
			Energy requiring process occurring at cell membrane
nast cells	*Inhibition	Högberg and Uvnäs (1960)	
ung	Inhibition	Diamant and Uvnäs (1961)	Oxidative phosphorylation not involved in anaphylactic release
nast cells	Inhibition	Högberg and Uvnäs (1960)	
nast cells	No inhibition	Moran et al. (1962)	
			Due to alteration of cell homeostasis
			Inhibition of an esterase
			?Inhibition of essential enzyme step
ea pig lung	No effect	Moussatche and Danon (1957)	Succinate effect probably not on tricarboxylic acid cycle
nast cells	Inhibition by O_2 lack	Perera and Mongar (1965)	?Due to reduction of S–S bonds
ea pig lung	Potentiation by O_2 lack	Mongar and Schild (1957)	
ea pig lung	Similar to effect on anaphylactic release,	Perera and Mongar (1965)	-SH-activated enzyme involved
nast cells	but not as marked		S–S bonds in Ab or trigger site disrupted
nast cells	Inhibition	Högberg and Uvnäs (1960)	-SH-activated enzyme involved

TABL

Agent	Anaphylactic release (by antigen)		
	System	Effect	Reference
Protein denaturants (e.g. EtOH, urea)	+Guinea pig lung	Potentiation (by low concentrations); inhibition (by high concentrations)	Edman et al. (1964)
Temperature change (from physiological)	+Guinea pig lung	Potentiation by increase to 41°	Edman et al. (1964)
	Human leucocytes	Decrease with decreasing temperature (complete inhibition at 20°)	Osler et al. (1968)
	Rat mast cells	Irreversible inhibition at 5°	Johnson and Moran (197
*p*H change (from physiological)	Human leucocytes	Sharp decrease with rise or fall in *p*H	Osler et al. (1968)
Divalent cations (EDTA)	Human leucocytes Rabbit basophils Rat mast cells Guinea pig lung	Ca^{2+} essential Mg^{2+} essential in leucocyte system, cannot be excluded in lung system	Lichenstein and Osler (19 Schild (1968); Osler et al. (1968)
Colchicine	Human leucocytes	Inhibition (enhanced by cold)	Levy and Carlton (1969)
Catecholamine (e.g. epinephrine, isoproterenol)	Human leucocytes Human lung Monkey lung Rat mast cells	Inhibition Inhibition Inhibition Inhibition	Lichenstein and Margolis (1968); Assem and Schild (1969); Ishizaka et al. (1971); Johnson and Moran (197
Theophylline	Human leucocytes	Inhibition	Lichenstein and Margolis (1968)
Dibutyryl cyclic AMP	Human leucocytes	Inhibition	Lichenstein and Margolis (1968)
Disodium cromoglycate (Intal)	Human lung Human leucocytes Rat mast cells	Inhibition No effect Inhibition (of IgGa mediated resp.)	Sheard and Blair (1970); Stanworth (1971C); Morse et al. (1969)

+ Tissue pre-treated with agent.

* But finding that DNP-blocked oxidative phosphorylation was counteracted by glucose suggested this agent also inhibits glycolytic pathway.

tinued)

icial release (by Compound 48/80)			Inference
em	Effect	Reference	
ung	Inhibition by high concentrations of EtOH	Chakravarty (1960)	?Due to freeing of -SH groups ?Due to irreversible denaturation of sensitising Ab
			?Due to freeing of -SH groups
			High temperature coefficient for one or more of reaction steps
mast cells	Reversible inhibition at 5°	Johnson and Moran (1970)	?Irreversible denaturation of cell-bound antibody
mast cells	Sharp decrease with rise or fall in *p*H (from 7.4)	Högberg and Uvnäs (1960)	Enzyme reactions involved
mast cells lung, guinea ung	Ca^{2+} essential Ca^{2+} essential	Högberg and Uvnäs (1960) Chakravarty (1960)	?Direct effect on phospholipid in cell membrane
mast cells	Partial inhibition	Gillepsie et al. (1968)	Effect exerted on cytoplasmic microtubules
mast cells	Inhibition (but not by isoproterenol)	Johnson and Moran (1970)	Cyclic AMP system involved in regulation of biochemical pathways
mast cells	Inhibition	Orr et al. (1971)	?Stabilizes cell membrane, blocking of triggering action

TABLE 8.2
Proposed classification of agents capable of initiating histamine release.

Non-selective (cytotoxic) agents		Selective (protein) reactants	
General surfactants	Phospholipid reactants	Direct (?v membrane enzyme)	Indirect (v membrane-bound Ig)
Aliphatic amines (e.g. octylamine, decylamine) Triton X-100	Lysolecithin	Sensitising Ab + Ag Aggregated Ig	Anti-Ig Protein A
Antibody v cell surface antigens	Melittin ←– – – – –→	Bee venom (Melittin)	Denaturing agents (e.g. EtOH, urea)
		Compound 48/80	
Hypotonic solutions		Basic polypeptides * e.g. polymyxin B colistin gramicidin Corticotrophin polypeptides αMSH 'Mast cell rupturing factor'	
Polycations ←– – – – – – – – – – – – – – – – – – –	– – –→	Polycations (e.g. poly-Lys, protamine) Stilbamidine d-Tubocurarine morphine	

* It is interesting to note that anaphylatoxins, the low mol. wt. fragments (C3a and C5a) derived from complement components C3 and C5, are also basic polypeptides.

chains of the phospholipid and the hydrophobic portions of the polypeptide chain which are situated in a separate sequence (i.e. residues 1–20) to that containing the hydrophilic residues (i.e. residues 21–26). I suppose it is possible, however, that at lower doses this polypeptide reacts with protein structures in the target cell membrane.

Lysolecithin, as already mentioned, appears to act by decreasing the stability of phospholipids within the mast cell membranes; and antiserum directed against cell surface antigenic determinants (i.e. anti-mast cell antibody) would also be expected to cause substantial membrane disruption.

In contrast, it is likely that the selective releasing agents act, in one way or another, with non-lipid constituents of the membrane. Here too, however, if sufficiently low concentrations are not employed more general cellular changes are induced. This is perhaps not surprising as far as the use of strong basic releasers such as polycationic acids is concerned, because these readily react with the polyanionic groupings (e.g. carboxyl groups of sialic acid) on cell membranes. It seems highly significant, however, that basic low molecular weight substances (such as Compound 48/80 and polymyxin B) act as selective histamine liberators (Ellis et al. 1970); inducing in rat mast cells essentially similar morphological changes to those seen in γE antibody–antigen-mediated histamine release from sensitised human basophils (Hastie 1971).

Apparent differences between the mode of action of reaginic antibody–antigen combination and Compound 48/80 have been revealed by studies (Johnson and Moran 1970) performed with rat mast cells at low temperature (5°). For instance, whereas the lowering of the reaction temperature to this degree reversibly inhibited the release of histamine induced by the artificial inhibitor, it appeared to inhibit irreversibly release from sensitised mast cells in response to challenge with specific antigen. On the other hand, the low temperature had no effect on non-selective release brought about by a powerful detergent such as Triton X-100.

But, it seems to me that these apparently divergent behaviours of the different releasing agents can be satisfactorily explained without the need to conclude that the stimuli effected by the artificial liberator and the antibody–antigen reaction are of a fundamentally different nature. The effect of the reduced temperature on Compound 48/80 induced release can probably be attributed to the phase transition which membrane lipids have been found, by X-ray diffraction analysis (Engelman 1971), to undergo as the surrounding temperature is lowered; resulting in the very much restricted movement of the lipid molecules as the side chains become packed together in regular arrays, which presumably could restrict access of the artificial liberator to a membrane enzyme in the trigger site. In contrast, the more drastic (non-selective) detergent action of Triton X-100 would not be expected to be influenced in the same way by changes in lipid conformation brought about by the reduced temperature. The situation with regard to antibody–antigen-induced histamine release is presumably different, however, because of the influence of the lowered temperature on the interaction of the challenging antigen with cell-bound antibody. The effect might be one of an irreversible structural change within the antibody molecule which damps down its capacity to undergo an allosteric transformation as a result of combination with antigen at physiological temperature (ch. 5). This could account for the observation that on rewarming the mast cells are unresponsive to antigen, but still capable of releasing histamine in response to stimulation by Compound 48/80.

The artificial selective releasing agents behave like γE antibody–antigen interaction, in producing morphological changes which reflect a disturbed balance between cytoplasmic and granular compartments. For instance, one of the first steps in rat mast cell degranulation induced by Compound 48/80 involves fusion of the granular membranes with each other and with the surface membrane (Horsfield 1965); a process which presumably utilises a high proportion of the energy known to be required for degranulation and histamine release (Uvnäs 1967). This seems to lead to the formation of 'pores' within the cell membrane; and it is presumably as a result of a widening of these pores that the granules now lacking their membranes (i.e. residual granular material) move freely to the exterior of the cell (fig. 8.5a). According to an alternative idea (Padawer 1970) the mast cell granules are topographi-

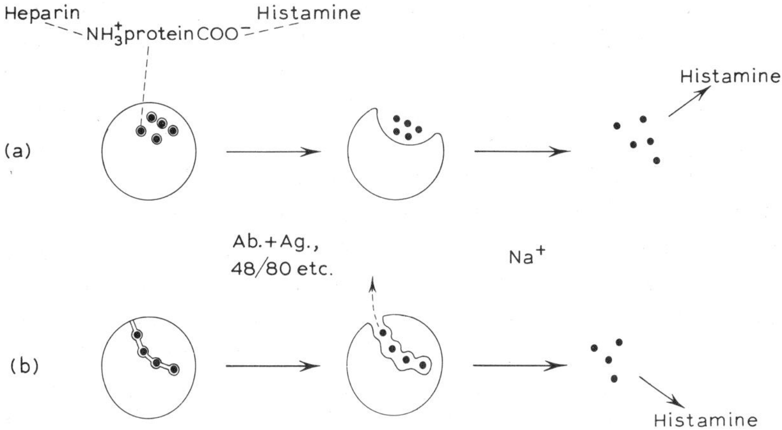

Fig. 8.5. Schematic representation of 2 possible mechanisms of rat mast cell degranulation: (a) modified from Thon and Uvnäs, 1967; (b) based on a hypothesis of Padawer 1970.

cally outside the cell, whilst being held intimately within extensive folds and recesses. This implies that the cellular and granular membranes are contiguous in the untreated cell (fig. 8.5b), but their connecting channels are so small that they are not observed in EM sections. I suppose this sort of arrangement might account for the claim (e.g. Ritzen 1966) that membrane delineated granules can shed their amine (i.e. 5-HT) whilst still in pores within the mast cell; due, perhaps, to an influx of cations.

The morphological changes occurring on degranulation of human atopic individuals' basophils on challenge with specific allergen (described in considerable detail by Hastie 1971) have been observed to be fundamentally comparable to the changes induced in rat mast cells by Compound 48/80, although the phase-dark structures seem remaining in the transformed basophil granules are larger and can often be seen being discharged from the cell. Here too, however, coalescence of phase-pale vesicles (i.e. vacuolated granules) is thought to result probably from fusion of their bounding membranes; and disappearance of the vesicles probably occurs when their membranes fuse with the plasma membranes, whereupon the contents are discharged from the cell.

These, then, are much more refined processes than the cruder cytotoxic effects initiated by the non-selective releasing agents referred to earlier. In view, however, of the evidence that mast cell degranulation and histamine release are 2 consecutive steps in response to treatment with Compound 48/80 (Thon and Uvnäs 1967; Nosal et al. 1970), it is conceivable that the only selective stimulus necessary for initiating the whole process is the triggering of an energy-releasing enzyme system which promotes fusion of the cellular and granular membranes. This would result in passage of the residual granular material into the medium, where exchange with extracellular cations (i.e. Na^+) leads to dissociation of their heparin–histamine–protein complex (fig. 8.5a). Furthermore, it is conceivable that any derangement of the cell membrane resulting from bound antibody–antigen interaction would enhance its permeability; directly or, possibly, by activation of the sodium pump ATPase. This might be expected to facilitate an influx of cations and the premature release of histamine, whilst the granules are still within the 'pores' of the cell. Moreover, this secondary effect could be of a co-operative nature, possibly explaining why antigen applied locally to sensitised mast cells seems to induce only gradual morphological changes (Kruger et al. 1970).

A puzzling question is how the apparently diverse collection of reagents listed in the 'selective reactants' column in table 8.2 are able to trigger an essentially similar response within the target cell. It seems highly significant, however, that they are all basic in nature. It is conceivable, of course, that strongly basic substances such as polylysine act by producing electrostatic changes in the mast cell surface (as suggested by Thon and Uvnäs 1967); and in this connection it is possibly significant that the exclusion of the acidic residues in the terminal part (residues 25–39) of the polypeptide chain of native ACTH, omitted from the considerably more basic synthetic β^{1-24} corticotrophin hormone (Synacthen), leads to a substantial increase in histamine-liberating activity (fig. 8.6). It seems to me to be possible, however, that the mechanism of the releasing action of the low molecular weight basic reagents is more subtle (as will now be discussed).

β^{1-39}ACTH

Ser–Tyr–Ser–Met–Glu–His–Phe–Arg–Trp–Gly–Lys–Pro–Val–

Gly–Lys–Lys(16)–Arg–Arg–Pro–Val–Lys–Val–Tyr–Pro(24)–

Asp–Glu–Ala–Glu–Asp–Glu–Leu–Ala–Glu–Ala–Phe–Pro–Leu–Glu–Phe(39)

Fig. 8.6a. Primary structure of β^{1-39} ACTH, indicating the C terminal sequence omitted from the synthetic β^{1-24} polypeptide (Synacthen).

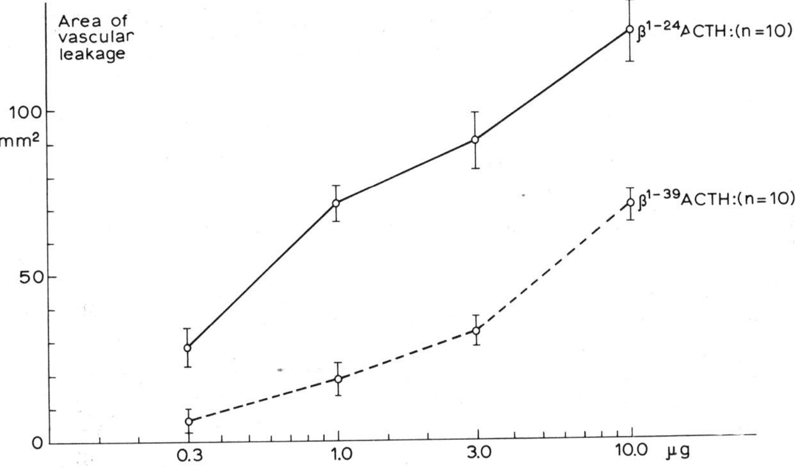

Fig. 8.6b. Comparison of the increase in vascular permeability induced in rat skin by β^{1-24} and β^{1-39} ACTH (reproduced from Jaques 1965, by permission of the author).

8.4 Possible mechanisms of antibody-mediated histamine release

A common denominator of these artificial histamine liberators appears to be the possession of at least one aromatic residue and at least one basic nitrogen-containing residue (Ellis et al. 1970; Rothschild 1966); it has also been suggested some time ago (Paton 1958) that any molecule in which 2 basic groups are separated by an aliphatic chain of 5 carbon atoms or more, or by some corresponding aromatic skeleton, is likely to be a noticeable histamine liberator. It is possible that structures of this type act directly upon an enzyme located in the trigger site of mast cells and basophils. Indeed, I would go further to suggest that a grouping of amino acid residues showing similar structural characteristics might form the activating site within the Fc region of the sensitising antibody, which (as suggested earlier) is formed following combination with specific antigen. In other words, it is suggested that basic polypeptides and other basic low molecular weight histamine liberators are capable of 'short circuiting' antibody-mediated histamine release, because of their structural similarity to the antibody activating site. In a sense, therefore, they could be likened to haptenic groups which cross-react with antibody directed against a structurally related grouping on a complete antigen.

The implications of this proposal, which should be verifiable by appropriate experimentation, are far reaching. For instance, identification of the precise amino acid residues of basic polypeptides responsible for histamine releasing activity (such as Synacthen and polymyxin B) might permit the prediction of the likely sequence within the antibody activating site responsible for triggering the target cell. It might also be expected that a similar grouping of amino acid residues would constitute the activating site preformed in aggregated myeloma IgE (fig. 8.4); and in cell-bound IgE cross-linked by appropriate reagents such as anti-IgE antibody and protein A, or by denaturation in situ by reagents such as dilute ethanol or urea solutions (table 8.1) which have been shown (Edman et al. 1964) to produce an irreversible activation of the anaphylactic reaction in chopped guinea pig lung. It is interesting, therefore, to attempt (fig. 8.7) to collate possible active sequences in various polypeptide histamine liberators; and to see whether a similar sequence appears in that region of the heavy polypeptide chains of skin-reactive immunoglobulins which would be expected to contain the active site on the basis of tests on Fc sub-fragments (ch. 5). The main ϵ-chain sequence is not available yet; but (fig. 8.6) it is possible to find potentially reactive sequences in the heavy chain of human γG1-globulin, which is capable of evoking reverse passive cutaneous reactions in guinea pigs following reaction with rabbit anti-human IgG1.

As is indicated in fig. 8.7, the residues in the region 243–248

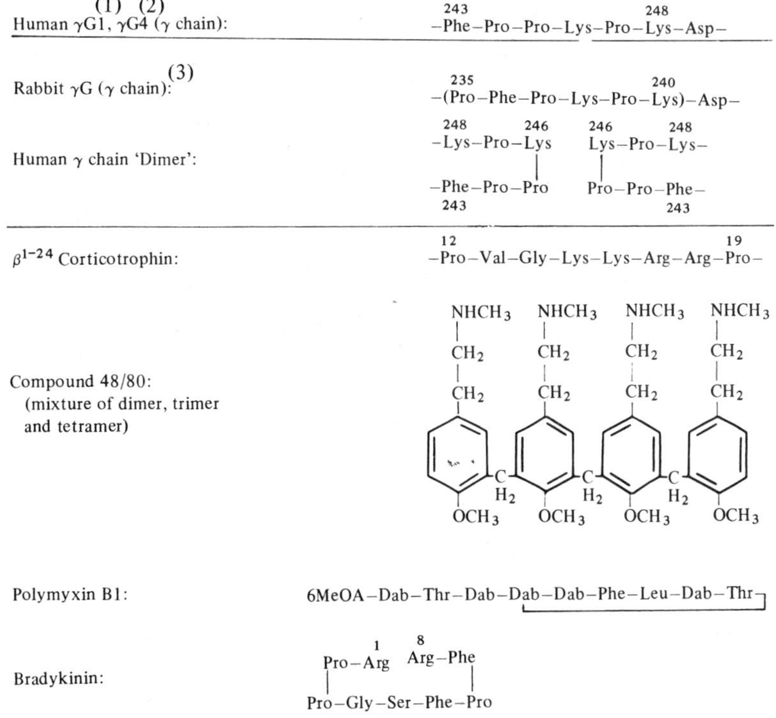

Fig. 8.7. Comparison of potentially active structural regions of various artificial histamine liberators, and bradykinin, with potentially active regions of human and rabbit γG-globulin heavy chain sequences. Dab = diamino butyric acid. Refs: (1) Edelman, G.-M. et al. Proc. Nat. Acad. Sci.; 1969, *63*, 78. (2) Hill, R.L. et al. Proc. Roy. Soc. B. 1966, *166*, 159. (3) Frangione et al.; Nature 1969, *221*, 145.

(i.e. Phe. Pro. Pro. Lys. Pro. Lys) of the human γG1-globulin heavy chain, and a similar sequence in the 235–240 region of rabbit γ chains, might prove to be directly involved in the triggering of histamine release.[2] Moreover, if these come together in dimer form (ch. 5) as might occur in a co-operative site comprised of polypeptide chains from similar regions of adjacent cell-bound antibody, a paring of basic (lysine) residues might occur which would resemble those seen in many artificial polypeptide histamine liberators (the sequences of some of which are also illustrated in fig. 8.7). This would then point to the lysine residue in position 246 of human γG1 heavy chain being crucial to the cell triggering process; but it is also conceivable that the adjacent proline residues would be necessary to provide a substantial degree of polypeptide chain folding at that point; a requirement which, incidentally, might prove to be essential if protruding parts of the unfolded polypeptide chains are to activate a membrane enzyme in the manner depicted schematically in fig. 8.3.

It is interesting to note that this amino acid sequence is located in that part of the γG-globulin Fc region in which (ch. 5) the tissue-binding sites are thought to be located. As mentioned earlier, however, there is reason to suppose that the position of the target-cell-activating site is distinct from the binding sites (fig. 8.8). Furthermore, if there is any substance in the idea proposed that the activation site comprises certain types of amino acid residues common to all polypeptide histamine liberators, it would not be expected to show the species specificity shown by the cell binding site. This might well account for the recent claims (of Korotzer et al. 1971) that human γE antibodies react with rat mast cells following their interaction with reaginic antibody or anti-human γE antibody; as this might merely reflect the direct action of basic amino acid residues (formed on γE-globulin–anti-γE-globulin interaction) with the same activation site (on the heterologous rat mast cell) that is triggered by artificial histamine liberators such as basic polypeptides and Compound 48/80. On the other hand, there is no firm evidence that human γE antibodies bind to rat tissue in vivo or in vitro; and even heterologous-tissue sensitising γG antibodies show clear-cut specificity with regard to the species or tissue to which they will bind (as revealed by PCA and RPCA testing, and indicated by table 5.5).

If the cell-activating sites of sensitising antibodies (both γE and γG) are comprised of amino acid residues of the type suggested, it might be expected that it would be possible to isolate small basic peptide fragments, from their proteolytic digests, which would show immediate histamine releasing activity (e.g. in a normal guinea pig ileum preparation). Attempts in my laboratory to separate such fragments by ion-exchange chromatography of peptic digests of human IgG, have produced a basic fraction with only very weak histamine liberating activity. The low activity is possibly due, however, to the presence of neutralising contaminants. It is also conceivable that essential peptide bonds in a histamine liberating sequence were sacrificed during enzymatic cleavage of the parent immunoglobulin. Perhaps the use of γE-globulin in this type of study would provide more active fragments but, so far, no fragment smaller than the Fc fragment has been reported to possess immediate skin reactivity. Moreover, this was only after aggregation (Ishizaka and Ishizaka 1970); suggesting that there were certain conformational requirements for this form of activity, as already discussed in ch. 5.

Another possibility must be considered, however, namely that residues sited close to the basic residues in artificial polypeptide liberators and in the unfolded ϵ chains of tissue-bound antibodies are more directly involved in the activation of sites on the cell membrane; the nearby basic residues merely playing a secondary role. In this connection, it is interesting to note that the enhancement of hydrolysis of erythrocyte ghosts by phospholipase A caused by synthetic (e.g. poly-Lys-Leu) and natural basic polypeptides has been attributed (Klibansky et al. 1968) to the promotion of electrostatic attraction of the enzyme for the negatively charged membrane. But the mere attachment of the polypeptide to the membrane does not appear to be sufficient; an additional role being ascribed to lipophilic side chains, which supposedly facilitate (by their phospholipid penetrating ability) the approach of the enzyme to the membrane substrate. It is conceivable that lipophilic residues adjacent to the basic residues in histamine-releasing structures play a similar role in the activation of the appropriate site on the target cell membrane. This is also suggested by the observations of Jacques and Brugger (1969), who found that the histamine liberating activity of synthetic β^{1-24} corticotrophin (Synacthen) could be greatly enhanced by the addition of an aliphatic (e.g. *n*-hexadecylamide) chain; which confers on it certain physico-chemical properties closely resembling those of melittin.

It is also important to consider the possibility that the basic histamine liberators operate merely in a relatively non-specific physico-chemical manner, by interaction with opposite charges in the target cell surface (as already mentioned). This idea has certain attractions, particularly as a possible explanation of the mode of action of non-polypeptide basic substances (e.g. Compound 48/80) and of dipeptides (e.g. Lys-Leu). The effect of such substances might be likened, perhaps, to antigen-latticing on the lymphocyte receptor surface; which some investigators (e.g. Greaves 1973) suggest could be the process responsible for the triggering of blast formation and antibody production by increasing the number of antigen receptors bound per unit area, per unit time. By analogy, a certain number of negatively charged groupings (possibly the carboxyl groups of sialic acid) on the target mast cell surface would need to be spanned by an optimum sized cluster of reactant groups (of artificial histamine liberator or anaphylactic antibody activating sites) before the cell is triggered into degranulation. This hypothesis has the attraction of possibly explaining why the basophils of normal individuals appear to carry a certain number of γE molecules on their surface without triggering into histamine release on contact with suitable antigen. Presumably they would not possess the requisite intensity of distribution (mosaic) of γE antibody molecules.[3] Moreover, this mosaic would have to comprise antibody molecules of the same antigen-specificity; because it is apparently possible to 'fire off' a reaction to one allergen on sensitised rat mast cells without influencing subsequent reactivity to another (Orr et al. 1970). This assumes, however, that antibodies of both specificities are carried on the same mast cell.

In considering the feasibility of this idea it has to be recognised, however, that many artificial releasing agents are small basic molecules; and although it is possible that they 'line up' on appropriate oppositely charged groups on the cell surface, the ability of low doses to release histamine in a highly selective manner without disruption of the cell membrane (as indicated, for example, by a lack of release of cytoplasmic lactic dehydrogenase) is in sharp contrast to the action of detergent such as Triton X-100. It is conceivable, of course, that the low molecular weight histamine liberators find their way into the cell; and, possibly, even act directly upon the granular membranes (or, on their contents) by displacing histamine from the heparin-histamine-protein complex. This is a question which could be answered by following the fate of radio-labelled releasing substances in rat mast cells. In this event, it might be expected that a cell membrane protease would be responsible for releasing a structurally similar portion of basic polypeptide chain from the region of the 'activating site' of sensitising antibody supposedly formed as a result of combination with specific allergen (in the manner already postulated, fig. 8.8); and that this fragment then finds its way into the granules. It might then be expected that it should be possible to isolate low molecular weight basic peptides with immediate histamine liberating activity; but, as mentioned earlier, attempts to accomplish this have not met with much success yet. Nevertheless, it is interesting to note in this connection that a relatively low molecular weight (1200–2400) arginine-rich (approximately 30 per cent) cationic peptide with potent mast cell rupturing activity can be isolated from the lysosomes of rabbit polymorphonuclear leucocytes (Seegers and Janoff 1966). It is tempting to suggest that this might offer a means of 'cross-over' into the type of mast cell histamine liberating system which I have been discussing, consequent to a different activation process occurring in another cell type.

Finally, it is perhaps worth considering briefly the role of antibody prosthetic groups in the triggering of histamine release. There does not appear to be any evidence that carbohydrate groups are active in this respect, but possibly one of the groups known to be sited in the Fc region of γE-globulin molecules will prove to be involved in some way in the activation process. There is, on the other hand, evidence that -SH-blockers such as *N*-ethylmaleimide (NEM) and *p*-chloro-mercuribenzoate (at doses of 1 mM) almost completely inhibit antigen-induced histamine release from chopped sensitised guinea pig lung (Edman et al. 1964) to take just one example; which raises the question of the possibility of activation of an -SH-dependent enzyme within the target cell membrane, by -SH groups occurring in the cell-bound antibody on combination with antigen. For, -SH groups have been shown to appear as a result of soluble antibody(γG)–antigen complex formation or non-specific aggregation of γG-globulin (Henney 1965); and it seems significant that NEM treated anaphylactic antibody or antigen, in contrast to NEM treated lung, remained fully effective in mediating histamine release.

8.5 Concluding comments

It will have become apparent that the evidence available at present about the mode of release of mediators of immediate hypersensitivity is mainly of an indirect nature. Despite this, I am finally going to attempt to formulate a basic mechanism (see fig. 8.8) which takes into account the apparently diverse immunological and non-immunological initiation processes which I have discussed in this and earlier chapters.

As already mentioned, more than once, the first requirement in true anaphylactic reactions is the relatively firm binding of the sensitising antibody to the target cell, through sites located within

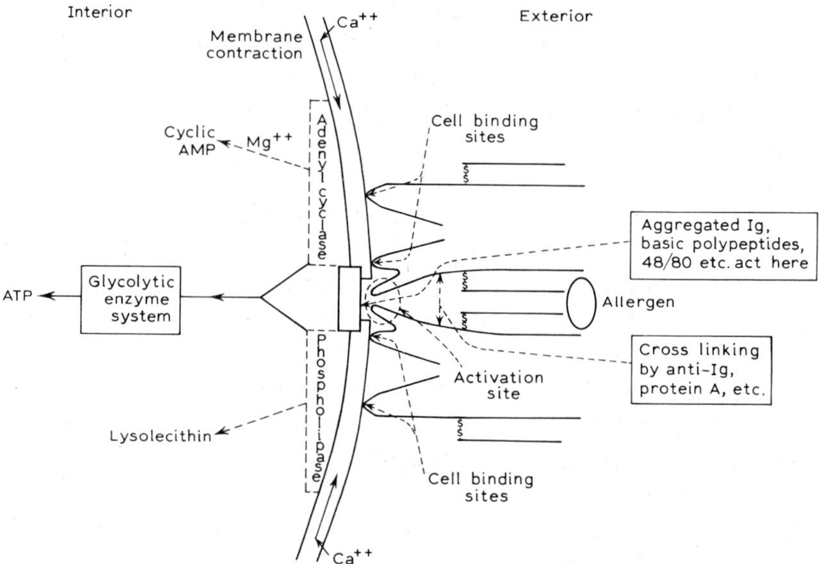

Fig. 8.8. Summary diagram, comparing suggested mechanism of trigger action resulting from cell bound antibody–allergen combination with that supposedly effected by various artificial means.

its Fc region. This, according to findings from studies of the inhibition of binding of rabbit γG antibody to chopped guinea pig lung by non-antibody IgG (Mongar and Winne 1966), could involve 2-point attachment to appropriate receptors; but the possibility of other forms of attachment cannot (according to Colquhoun 1968) be excluded. Furthermore, sensitisation, which requires only minute amounts of antibody, is not a simple adsorption process; although little seems to be known yet about the nature of the forces involved. The preliminary inhibition studies mentioned in ch. 5 suggested amino groups (presumably lysyl), within the Fc region, form electrostatic bonds with carboxyl groups on the target cell surface. But there have been claims (e.g. King and Francis 1967) that covalent bonds play a major role in the fixation of γG-globulins to heterologous guinea pig tissue. There does, nevertheless, seem to be a certain degree of specificity involved; because, as already mentioned, only the γG-globulins of certain species are capable of binding to heterologous guinea pig tissue. Moreover, it is also probable that sensitising antibodies show intra-species 'tissue' specificity as well; because γE antibodies, for example, seem to bind only to mast cells and basophils but not to other types of cell (which presumably lack the appropriate receptors).

As suggested earlier (ch. 5) the subsequent bridging of adjacent cell-bound antibody molecules by specific allergen initiates an allosteric transition, which brings specific amino acid residues (some of a basic nature) in the unfolded antibody polypeptide chain into precisely the correct juxtaposition with respect to an activation site on the target cell membrane; which is probably distinct from the antibody-binding sites. The adoption of this new conformational form might be facilitated in γE antibody molecules by the possession of the extra structural domain within the Fc region. On the basis of the evidence discussed earlier, it can be expected that the activating group will include lysine or arginine residues suitably spaced by other residues (e.g. proline) to permit adequate chain bending. Furthermore, it is quite possible that corresponding residues of this type act co-operatively within antibody molecules 'dimerised' on the cell surface as a result of bridging by specific antigen.

It is suggested that the active site thus formed then triggers a regulatory enzyme located within the target cell membrane (fig. 8.8). This, in turn, might well initiate other systems including glycolytic enzymes which provide the ATP needed to promote cell-granule membrane fusion; a process which could be aided by ancillary agents, such as lysolecithin formed as a result of membrane phospholipid hydrolysis and cyclic AMP resulting from concomitant activation of adenyl cyclase. Other agents, such as calcium ions,[4] might be expected to act by influencing the spacing of the bimolecular phospholipid layer; thus enhancing the derangement of the membrane caused by antigen-bridging of tightly bound antibody molecules and thereby facilitating access to enzymes sited beneath it. The neutralising effect of newly exposed basic groups, on the anionic groupings on the cell surface, would also facilitate access to membrane enzyme.

There does not seem to be any objection to supposing that more than one type of enzyme system is involved, possibly coupled in some as yet undefined way. Furthermore, it seems a useful working hypothesis at present to assume that artificial liberators (such as basic polypeptides) act directly upon the same membrane activation sites that are triggered by the antibody–antigen reaction; and that structurally similar activating sites are produced in cell-bound antibody which has been cross-linked by artificial means or by pre-aggregation in free solution. If this is the case, it is perhaps surprising to find that disodium cromoglycate inhibits immediate skin reactions induced in baboons by aggregated IgE, but not those induced by a basic polypeptide (β^{1-24} corticotrophin)[5] or protein A (Stanworth, unpublished data). This apparent paradox might, however, be due to a highly selective inhibitory effect of this drug; which it has been suggested (Stanworth 1971) might be attributed to a capacity, because of its bifunctional nature, to chelate across co-operative 'histamine liberating sites' formed in the pre-aggregated IgE.

We are now undertaking more direct, kinetic, studies in my own laboratory; in an attempt to ascertain whether artificial histamine

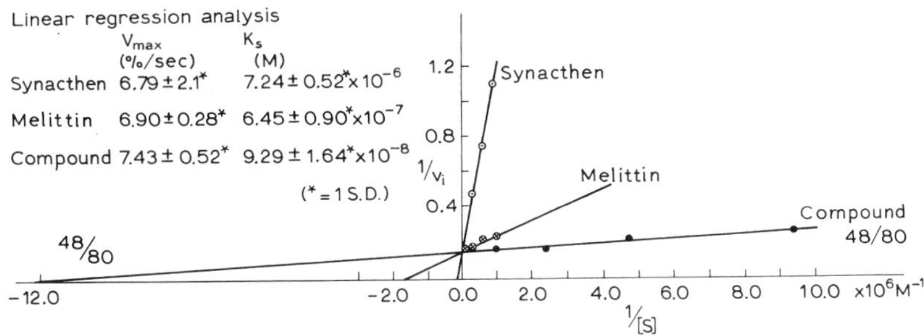

Fig. 8.9. Lineweaver–Burk plot of histamine release data from comparative studies on Synacthen, melittin and Compound 48/80 using an in vitro rat peritoneal mast cell system (in presence of 35 μg/ml heparin as anti-coagulant).

liberators (such as Synacthen, melittin and Compound 48/80) trigger those same sites which are activated by cell bound reagin–allergen interaction and by pre-aggregated IgE. Preliminary results (Jasani and Stanworth 1971) are promising in as much as the time-course of the artificially mediated histamine release from rat peritoneal mast cells at 25° has been found to resemble that of an enzyme catalysed reaction. This is consistent with the idea, discussed earlier, that basic polypeptides and Compound 48/80 behave like immunological triggers in exerting their effect selectively through a substrate-enzyme type of reaction. Furthermore, it can be concluded from the constant maximum rate of release revealed by a Lineweaver–Burk plot of our data (fig. 8.9) that the overall mode of release is the same for each of the 3 artificial liberators so far studied in this manner.

It is hoped, also, to follow the fate of radio-labelled basic polypeptides and peptides, to establish whether they reach the mast granules or merely remain at a surface activation site.

It is important to recognise when interpreting results obtained from model systems of this type that the activating action of the combination of anaphylactic antibody with specific antigen will probably not be mimicked completely. For example, the effects of the assumption of a more rigid conformation by the antibody on combination with antigen might be expected to be transmitted to the cell membrane to which the antibody was already bound; thus producing a structural re-arrangement (or rigidification, as Levine 1965, has termed it). Moreover, such an effect would obviously be more pronounced if the antibody was initially bound to the target cells through covalent bonds (a possiblity which was discussed earlier). Another point to consider is the scope for involvement of more than one type of activation site formed as a result of the unfolding of the relatively large antibody polypeptide chains on the cell surface. In contrast, the artificial histamine liberators would be expected to be more limited in the extent of their effect, acting directly upon the trigger site. But even amongst these substances, some differences in the mode of cell activation can be expected for the reasons already discussed. (To take one example, a cyclic basic polypeptide such as polymyxin B would possess a more rigid structure than other basic polypeptides lacking an intra-chain loop.)

Throughout this chapter I have deliberately avoided making any distinction between the mechanism of classical anaphylactic reactions mediated by γE antibodies and artificial heterologous sensitising systems involving, for instance, the sensitisation of guinea pig tissue by γG antibodies. Because, as already discussed in ch. 5, there is reason to suppose that the cell triggering mechanism is basically the same in the two cases. Moreover, I have equated mast cells with basophils in considering the contributions of the target cell; although there is evidence of functional as well as morphological differences. For example, rat mast cells have been shown to behave differently to human and rabbit basophils in response to Compound 48/80 (Haye and Schneider 1966). Indeed, there have been suggestions that the rat mast cell might be unique in its behaviour to the wide range of substances which trigger its degranulation.

I have also tended to ignore possible species differences in making direct comparisons of the mode of artificial release of mediators from rat mast cells, for example, with that of γE-mediated reactions in human cell systems. I feel, nevertheless, that the adoption of this general treatment of the subject will prove to be justified; because I strongly suspect that all of the reactions discussed will turn out to be based on a similar general type of mechanism.

Obviously the next step will be to extend investigation to the identification and characterisation of functional sites on and within the target cells. Before such a study can be contemplated, however, it will be necessary to establish a source and method of production of large quantities of highly purified mast cells or basophils. Unfortunately, human mast cells cannot be obtained in sufficient quantity; nor can circulating basophils. There are possiblities of using other sources, however, such as cultured mast cells or dog mastocytoma material. We are also looking into the possibility of using the blood of rats with chemically induced basophilic leukaemia as a convenient source of basophils.

Once this hurdle has been passed it will be necessary to devise suitable methods of sub-cellular fractionation; and of isolating membrane fractions retaining the antibody-binding or activation sites. As far as the latter problem is concerned it might prove possible to adopt similar methods to those being currently used by Allan et al. (1972) in the isolation of lymphoid cell membrane fractions containing, for example, the mitogen-stimulatory site. Another approach which might prove a useful guide is one which has been recently employed in the identification of multiple liver cell membrane enzymes, by use of specific enzyme staining of antigen–antibody precipitin lines formed on immunoelectrophoresis (Blomberg and Perlmann 1971). It will also be important, of course, to attempt to isolate cytoplasmic and membrane enzymes (e.g. adenyl cyclase) in pure form; in an endeavour to throw more light on the nature and location of the initial triggering site.

I suppose it is just possible that if a regulatory enzyme could be isolated, it might show conformational changes when reacted with anaphylactic antibody–antigen complex (or aggregated immunoglobulin) in free solution; an effect which could possibly be exploited in the development of a method for measuring γE antibody activity without the need of a tissue (or cell) sensitisation step. It will also probably prove rewarding to pay further attention to isolated mast granules; in direct tests designed to obtain further evidence of the possibility of a 'second messenger' responsible for conveying the effect of the initial stimulus on the target cell surface to the site of storage of histamine and other mediators of immediate hypersensitivity.

Notes

[1] A relationship between accumulation of cyclic AMP and inhibition of histamine release has now been demonstrated in several laboratories.

[2] Other potential histamine-liberating sequences, now under investigation in our laboratory, are:

288 290		338 340
Lys–Thr–Lys	and	Lys–Ala–Lys

[3] Direct evidence of a greater number of IgE molecules on atopics' basophils has recently been obtained (Ishizaka, T., Montreal Allergy Meeting, 1972).

[4] A more direct role recently attributed to Ca^{2+} (Orr, T.S.C. et al., Nature, 1972, *236*,350) involves their activation of an ATPase which supposedly causes the contraction of microfilaments situated close to the cytoplasmic membrane, resulting in extrusion of the mast granules.

[5] Although the cromone inhibits Synacthen-induced histamine release from rat mast cells in vitro.

CHAPTER 9

The inhibition of immediate hypersensitivity responses

9.1 Introduction

Although there are certain clinical situations, notably parasitic infections (ch. 7), where the outcome of a reagin-mediated reaction could be of benefit to the host it cannot be seriously disputed that immediate hypersensitivity reactions are usually of an adverse nature. A discourse of this type would not be complete, therefore, without some comment on current methods of therapy and prophylaxis, in the light of the recent advances in the experimental investigation of immediate hypersensitivity discussed in preceding chapters.

It should have become apparent that inhibition is possible, theoretically, at every stage of the complex series of events culminating in the release of pharmacological mediators. It seems logical, therefore, to consider these sequentially, starting with the synthesis of anaphylactic antibody.

9.2 Suppression of reaginic antibody synthesis

As was mentioned in earlier chapters, evidence has been recently obtained to suggest that γE antibody formation in certain animal species such as rabbits and rats is – like the production of immunising antibody – under the control of a feed-back regulatory mechanism. This has been indicated by direct studies in which, for example, reagin production in rabbits sensitised with hemocyanin (Strannegård and Belin 1970) and in rats sensitised with dinitrophenylated ascaris extract (Tada and Okumura 1971) was suppressed by homologous γG antibody administered close to the time of sensitisation. There is indirect evidence too to suggest that actively produced γG antibody likewise exerts a suppressive effect on reaginic antibody formation, in rabbits immunised with protein and protein-hapten conjugates (Strannegård and Yurchison 1969). In contrast, a long-lived γM antibody response, such as that which is readily elicited by antigens like hemocyanin, tends to encourage a prolonged reagin response especially after high antigen doses (Strannegård 1971).

The significance of these observations to the control of immediate hypersensitivity reactions in humans is obvious. For instance it raises the question as to whether the well established clinical practice of hyposensitisation by injection of relatively high doses of allergen might not achieve a similar effect, as a result of the production of large amounts of γG antibodies which exert their influence at the reagin synthesis level; besides competing with mast cell-bound reaginic antibody for allergen. This implies that competition for allergen might also be directed towards receptor immunoglobulin on the surface of those immunocompetent cells responsible for γE antibody production, if presently held ideas about the mechanism of susppression of immunising antibody formation by passively administered antibody apply also to reagin synthesis. It is also possible, however, (continuing the analogy) that immunosuppression of reagin formation might involve a direct action of antibody on potential γE antibody forming cells; and it might be relevant in this connection that the treatment of rhesus monkeys with anti-human lymphocyte serum has been found (in coming preliminary studies) to result in an elevation of the serum IgE level (ch. 7). But there is some doubt about the specificity of this effect; and, furthermore, no significant change was observed in the blast transformation response of pollen-sensitive individuals' lymphocytes to specific allergen, in tissue culture, following hyposensitisation (Zeitz et al. 1966). An increase in the P–K activity of allergic individuals' sera following hyposensitisation has been observed by several investigators; but this has usually proved to be only transient in duration. There has, however, been a recent report (Berg and Johansson 1970) of a pronounced increase in the serum γE antibody level of pollen-sensitive children, as measured by the RAST procedure, a few weeks after hyposensitisation by simultaneous injection of different pollen allergens over a 5–7 day period. It is also interesting to note that changes in leucocyte (presumably basophil) reactivity have been claimed to occur (Van Arsdel 1965; Pruzansky et al. 1967) following hyposensitisation. But an extensive study of 40 ragweed-sensitive patients over a 2 year period failed to find any evidence that specific therapy had produced a significant change in the patients' leucocyte activity, as expressed in terms of the amount of allergen needed to effect a 50 per cent release of histamine (Osler et al. 1968). On the other hand, a similar study of the reactivity of the patients' tissue mast cells might have provided a more reliable indication of the clinical effects of hyposensitisation, if this had been feasible.

I suppose that an observed change in mast cell activity following hyposensitisation might be attributable to qualitative changes in the sensitising antibody; but, it will be important to rule out any basic influence on the derivation of the cells themselves, as a variety of reagents are known to induce mast cell proliferation (Benditt and Lagnoff 1964).

Leucocyte testing has also been used to demonstrate that parenteral administration of allergen brings about a reduction in the annual anamnestic response of allergic individuals to airborne pollen allergens (Osler et al. 1968); but a more satisfactory outcome of hyposensitisation therapy would be the complete inhibition of such a response, as was observed in the studies of the suppression of reagin synthesis in rabbits which were mentioned earlier. By analogy, this condition would seem to be most readily achieved in allergic humans by the stimulation of production of large amounts of γG antibody; as opposed to antibody of the γM-type, which would be expected to work against the suppressive effect of the γG blocking antibody. It is suggested (Strannegård and Belin 1969), therefore, that the highest tolerable allergen dose should be used for hyposensitisation; an assumption which is supported by the results of clinical trials in which various dosages of pollen allergen have been tried and which have indicated that doses less than 250 μg of ragweed allergen E (or 2500 PNU whole extract) are essentially ineffective (Norman 1969). In contrast, the administration of low doses of allergen would be expected to favour reagin production, according to studies of the artificial induction of reaginic antibodies in mice (ch. 6); an effect which is possibly attributable indirectly to the ready production of γM antibodies under such circumstances.

It is also apparent from recent work on the experimental production of immediate hypersensitivity in animals that the nature of the adjuvant used is of some influence; aluminium salts, for example, seem to favour reaginic antibody production whereas complete Freund's adjuvant is particularly effective in producing γG-type antibody responses. It could be, therefore that the British practice of using alum-precipitated allergenic extracts in hyposensitisation, in contrast to the American use of mineral oil, would tend to favour reagin production (other factors being equally balanced). Any possible disadvantage of the former procedure on this count has to be weighed, however, against other risks peculiar to the latter practice. As far as I am aware, no clinical trial has been undertaken to compare directly the relative efficacies of the 2 types of adjuvant.

There are potential disadvantages, too, in the use of high doses of allergen in hyposensitisation therapy; as this increases the chances of combination with mast cell-bound reagin and the incidental triggering of histamine release. A suggestion for overcoming this problem, as an alternative to the practice of using anti-histamines, involves the administration of allergen mixed with anti-allergen antibody (of the γG-type); a procedure which has proved effective in suppressing reagin formation in rabbits (Strannegård 1971). This offers, ingeniously, a means of preventing the appearance of large quantities of free allergen in the circulation whilst, at the same time, providing potentially reagin-suppressive γG antibody.

Another approach, which (as De Weck and Schneider 1969, have pointed out in relation to desensitation to drugs) should be theoretically ideal, would be to use a monovalent hapten for hyposensitisation purposes; as this should be capable of neutralising cell-bound reagin without initiating histamine release, because of its inability to meet the antibody-bridging requirements (ch. 3 and fig. 3–10). But before such a procedure could be applied to the treatment of inhalant-sensitive individuals it would be necessary to accomplish the technically difficult task of isolating 'monovalent' fragments by dissociation of purified allergens.

An alternative possibility, involves the chemical modification of the allergen to a form which, by analogy with the development of bacterial toxoids for immunisation purposes, retains the capacity to evoke blocking antibody formation whilst losing the ability to initiate deleterious anaphylactic response. Such a derivative (termed an 'allergoid') has been prepared from rye pollen allergen by formalinization (Marsh et al. 1970), and shown to lack the ability to inhibit allergen-induced histamine release from sensitive individuals' leucocytes. It is hoped, therefore, that it will be possible to use much higher doses of this derivative than would be possible with unmodified allergen, for the immunisation of allergic individuals.

The ultimate ideal is, of course, the achievement of a state of permanent tolerance to the offending allergen; a situation which will not be readily realised in individuals who are already sensitised.

Perhaps it will eventually prove possible to screen the population, by some form of simple genetic test to identify those individuals showing a predisposition to immediate hypersensitivity; and to render them refractory to reaginic antibody formation on subsequent exposure to common sensitogens, by means of an appropriate tolerizing treatment. The suggestion, referred to earlier, that those immunocompetent cells involved in γE antibody formation might be more susceptible to immunosuppression than cells responsible for the production of other classes of immunoglobulin offers hope that the induction of a 'blanket' state of tolerance to all types of sensitogen might be feasible. The alternative task, of dealing with every potential allergen-reagin system separately, would prove a far more complex and formidable proposition.

In the meantime, it is worth mentioning some encouraging findings from a recent study (Norman et al. 1971) of maintenance immunotherapy in ragweed-sensitive hay fever sufferers, in which the level of blocking antibody in the serum was measured by the capacity to inhibit the allergen-induced release of histamine from standard sensitised leucocytes. It was found over a 2 year period, that 8 gradually increasing doses of an aqueous solution of ragweed antigen E (omitting an injection during the season) were sufficient to maintain both clinical improvement and blocking antibody levels without apparently causing any untoward reactions.

9.3 Inhibition of tissue sensitisation

An alternative to blocking reagin synthesis is to inhibit the uptake of sensitising antibody on to the allergic individual's tissues. This presupposes, of course, that the sensitisation of mast cells and basophils occurs at a stage which is distinct from and subsequent to the process of reagin biosynthesis; the free γE antibody in the circulation representing an 'overflow' following such uptake.

As already indicated (chs. 4 and 5) it is possible to inhibit the local passive sensitisation of normal human skin sites, when excess (10–100-fold) human myeloma IgE or its Fc fragment is administered simultaneously or 24 hr prior to the sensitising reaginic antibody. Furthermore, these observations have been repeated in similar studies performed in baboons; but it was found, not unexpectedly, that pre-administered myeloma IgE did not persist for as long in the heterologous primate skin as in isologous human tissue. For example, when the myeloma protein was injected into baboon skin sites 24 hr prior to passive sensitisation with allergic serum a 10-fold higher dose was needed to achieve complete inhibition of cutaneous anaphylactic response (on subsequent allergen challenge) than the effective dose of myeloma IgE administered simultaneously with the sensitising serum (Stanworth 1971B).

The significance of the latter findings to the present discussion is that they indicated that it was feasible to perform inhibition studies in sub-human primates, thereby permitting a much more thorough investigation of the whole question of the blockage of uptake of administered reaginic antibody on to primate tissue. For instance, this has enabled us to extend our earlier studies with myeloma IgE to the attempted inhibition at the systemic level.

It has been shown (Patterson et al. 1965; 1967) that monkeys (*Macaca mulatta*) can be systemically sensitised with relatively large volumes (e.g. 25–40 ml/kg body weight) of serum from ragweed-sensitive individuals, as indicated by their subsequent response to local and systemic allergen challenge. It seemed possible, therefore, that intravenously injected myeloma IgE would behave similarly (if sufficient were administered), by 'homing' on the reagin-binding tissue sites of the monkeys. Our preliminary studies of the turnover of radio-labelled IgE in baboons (McLauglan and Stanworth 1972) mentioned in ch. 7, supported this supposition; for no evidence was obtained for anywhere near the complete excretion of the labelled protein, despite its rapid disappearance from the circulation. It seemed, therefore, that an animal injected systematically with non-antibody (i.e. myeloma) IgE might be rendered refractory to subsequent attempts to sensitise it by the local transfer of allergic serum; or, indeed, to an intravenously injected dose of specific allergen which would otherwise have evoked a state of generalised anaphylactic shock.

Experiments to test this possibility were conducted in pairs of baboons, one of which received an intravenous dose of myeloma IgE in the range of 1–40 mg and the other (control) a comparable amount of human myeloma IgG1 protein. The state of refractoriness of each animal was subsequently assessed regularly, both by PCA testing with a control human allergic serum and by the immediate response to the intradermal injection of polymerised myeloma IgE. But, as there were technical obstacles to the repeated PCA testing in the same animal, the results of the tests with aggregated IgE were considered more reliable. These indicated that a state of refractoriness extending over a period of 6–7 days could be induced by a single intravenous injection of about 8 mg myeloma IgE per kg body weight (Stanworth 1971B); as will be seen from table 9.1.

TABLE 9.1

Results of skin testing a pair of baboons with aggregated IgE before and after systemic administration of myeloma IgG1 or myeloma IgE. (Stanworth, D.R; Housley, J; Bennich, H. and Johansson, S.G.-O; unpublished data.)

Day of test	Reactivity to aggregated IgE (25 μg)	
	Recipient 1	Recipient 2
−7	+++	+++
0	36 mg IgG1 (i.v.)	36 mg IgE (i.v.)
2	+++	−
3	+++	−
6	+++	±
8	+++	+++

These observations raise the question of exploiting a similar type of inhibitory procedure as a form of prophylaxis in the control of immediate hypersensitivity responses in atopic individuals; if a sufficient amount of 'inert' IgE were to become available for this purpose. It is conceivable that the refractory state induced was due to the production of anti-human IgE antibody, however; an effect which was supposedly responsible for a state of refractoriness observed on PCA testing monkeys 2 weeks after being systemically sensitised by transfusion of allergic serum (Patterson et al. 1967). Furthermore, a similar effect induced in monkeys by the intravenous injection of rabbit serum (40 ml) was attributed to the production of monkey anti-rabbit IgE which possessed cross-reactivity for human IgE. We failed, however, to find any evidence (by the RIST method) of the production of anti-human IgE antibodies in baboons which had received high systemic doses of myeloma IgE; and the chance of evoking a similar response in a human recipient of human myeloma IgE would be even less. Nevertheless, it is interesting to note that the deliberate rigorous immunisation of monkeys (*Macacca mulatta* and *speciosa*) with human myeloma IgE in complete Freund's adjuvant resulted in a loss of receptivity to passive sensitisation by human reaginic antibody, which was attributed to the production of monkey anti-human IgE antibody (Feinberg et al. 1971).

A small polypeptide fragment of human IgE, which retained the tissue-binding activity of the whole molecule, but which had lost potential iso-antigenic groupings, would be an ideal inhibitor of systemic sensitisation. Moreover, such a substance would be relatively easy to produce in large quantities by means of modern solid state methods of polypeptide synthesis; thus providing a solution to the problem of acquiring sufficient inhibitor for a large-scale programme of treatment of allergic individuals. Unfortunately (as mentioned in ch. 5) of the wide range of fragments of myeloma IgE so far tested in PCA-inhibition systems, none smaller than the Fc fragment (corresponding to about half of the molecule of 200 000 mol. wt.) has proved inhibitory. It is possible, however, that sub-fragments originating from the N-terminal half of the Fc region of the IgE molecule will prove more effective; for it seems likely that the tissue-binding sites are located in this region of the molecule (ch. 5). There is also the problem of the loss of tertiary structure to be taken into account, however, in the attempted isolation of active immunoglobulin fragments; and, in this connection, the finding that some of the intra-chain disulphide bonds are effective in maintaining the conformational integrity of the IgE molecule could be decisive. Incidentally, if a small tissue-binding polypeptide were to become available it might be possible to encourage its more permanent fixation to the tissues by adopting a similar principle to that on which the 'affinity labelling' of antibody active sites is based.

An alternative method of blocking the reagin-binding sites on the tissues of allergic individuals might be to deliberately promote the elevation of their circulatory IgE level by sensitisation to a clinically unimportant allergen. This idea is prompted by recent observations in the rat (Jarrett et al. 1971); which suggested that the presence of anti-nematode γE antibody on mast cells can impede their sensitisation by γE antibody produced in response to subsequent injection of a protein antigen (ovalbumin). But a problem in exploiting this principle at a therapeutic level would be the difficulty of obtaining a suitable-potentiating allergen, which could be relied upon to remain clinically inert.

A safer approach would be to stimulate the production of γG antibodies against the offending allergen, which would occupy the same tissue receptor sites as γE antibody or perhaps sterically hinder their cell-binding. But although such an effect has been observed in experimental animal systems, for example, in the inhibition by excess γ_2-type antibodies of PCA reactions provoked by guinea pig γ_1-type antibodies, there has been no clear indication to suggest that human γG-type antibodies are capable of binding to reagin-receptor sites on human tissue mast cells. [1]

9.4 Immobilisation of cell-bound reaginic antibody

It has been assumed throughout the previous section that findings from studies involving the inhibition of passive sensitisation of normal recipients' tissues are directly translatable to situations of active sensitisation, where one is dealing with allergic individuals whose tissue sites are presumed to be already occupied by reaginic antibody. Such an assumption, which will need to be verified by systemic inhibition studies in actively sensitised primates, is not necessarily tenable.

It is possible that this problem might be tackled in another way, however; by immobilising tissue-bound reaginic antibody in situ either before or at the time of combination with specific allergen. Considering the former possibility first, the objective would be to dislodge the sensitising antibody in some way from the target cell surface. Neither proteolytic enzymes, nor chemical dissociating agents, would seem to be selective enough for such an application in vivo; despite the observations from animal studies (table 8.1) that certain relatively non-selective agents (such as protein denaturants and thiols) are capable (at certain dosages) of inhibiting histamine release by a process which might involve inactivation of cell-bound sensitising antibody.

In contrast to these relatively crude methods, it might prove possible to develop a reagent capable of specifically neutralising the activation sites which are supposedly formed within the Fc regions of γE antibody molecules following combination with allergen (ch. 5 and 8). For instance, it is conceivable that some bifunctional reagent (similar to those used in the investigation of enzyme–substrate interaction) would be capable of chelating across a 'co-operative dimer' activation site of the type assumed to form between adjacent cell-bound γE molecules following bridging by allergen (ch. 5 and 8); thereby nullifying the triggering action. Or, alternatively chelation might occur across the activation site, formed by adjacent sensitising antibody molecules and substrate (enzyme) on the target cell. Such a reagent would, of course, have to be incapable of causing any structural rearrangement within the cell-bound γE molecules, which could lead to the premature artificial triggering of the amine release mechanism; nor would it have to possess any reactivity for free γE antibody molecules.

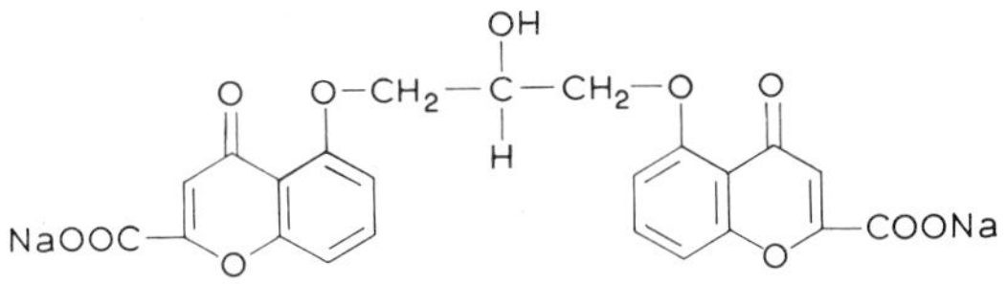

Fig. 9.1. Structure of disodium cromoglycate (Intal).

It is interesting to consider whether the recently developed anti-asthmatic drug Intal (disodium cromoglycate), whose structure is shown in fig. 9.1, might be fortuitously meeting those requirements (Stanworth 1971B). For recent studies in experimentally sensitised rats (Orr et al. 1970) have suggested that if present at the time of antigen challenge this compound permits reagin antibody combination without the release of pharmacologically active substances; and it does not appear to effect the fixation of γE antibodies to normal rat mast cells, nor their subsequent interaction with antigen. Moreover, it appears not to exert its effect at a later stage by acting, for instance, as an inhibitor of those key enzyme steps (ch. 8) which have been incriminated in the release mechanism.

But there are recent indications (reviewed by Cox et al. 1970) which suggest that the mode of action of disodium cromoglycate is not operating at the level just discussed. For instance, it is puzzling why the drug appears to be incapable of inhibiting reagin-mediated histamine release from sensitised human and rabbit leucocytes, or from actively or passively sensitised human skin sites (Assem and Mongar 1970); although, apart from its inhibitory effect on release from reagin-sensitised rat mast cells in vitro and in vivo, it has been shown to inhibit release of histamine and SRS-A from human and monkey lung passively sensitised with reaginic antibody (Sheard and Blair 1970; Assem and Mongar 1970) and of histamine release from guinea pig basophils (Greaves 1969), but only at high doses (2–4 mM). Moreover, as already mentioned in ch. 6, it was also found to suppress histamine release from rat mast cells sensitised with non-reaginic IgG-type antibody (Morse et al. 1969). But perhaps the most interesting observation was the inhibition by disodium cromoglycate of mast cell degranulation and histamine release effected artificially by treatment with phospholipase A (Orr and Cox 1969). It could be that here the cromone is acting as a true enzyme-substrate chelator,[2] in a system which is closely related structurally to the immunological mast cell trigger mechanism (fig. 8.8). But the suggestion that it exerts its effect by stabilisation of the mast cell membrane has yet to be discounted.

It seems reasonable to suppose that further inhibition studies with disodium cromoglycate will contribute to a clearer understanding of the mechanism of immediate hypersensitivity reactions; besides perhaps leading to the development of other anti-allergic drugs which also operate at an immunological rather than a pharmacological level, but which are less tissue specific.

9.5 Pharmacological inhibitors

Even if reagin–allergen combination cannot be averted by the procedures already discussed there is still scope, of course, for inhibition of the effects of the triggering of the target cells. This is possible at 2 stages: 1) at the ensuing enzymic steps leading to disruption of the mast cell granules and the release of the mediators of the allergic responses; 2) at the time of action of these substances on smooth muscle and other target organs; i.e. the 'second' and 'third messenger' stages respectively, by analogy with the supposed mode of action of hormones (ch. 8).

The biochemical processes which are rapidly (i.e. in a matter of seconds) set into train as a result of reagin–allergen interaction at the mast cell surface have yet to be characterised in detail. But, as will have become apparent from ch. 8, there is increasing evidence to suggest that cyclic adenosine 3′-5′-monophosphate (cyclic AMP) is involved in some regulatory capacity; although perhaps not in such a direct manner as its postulated role as a 'second messenger' in the mediation of hormone activity. Nevertheless, it is particularly interesting in this connection that sympathomimetic amines have been recently shown (Assem and Schild 1969) to prevent allergen-induced histamine release from passively sensitised chopped human lung at doses which were less than a thousandth of those of the most active inhibitors (e.g. disodium cromoglycate) previously reported to show this activity. Furthermore, catecholamines such as epinephrine and isoproterenol were shown to inhibit reagin-mediated histamine release from sensitised human leucocytes (Lichenstein and Margolis 1968); and from monkey lung (Ishizaka et al. 1971) as well. These effects, and their antagonism by propranolol, suggest that the inhibitory action is mediated through the stimulation of β-adrenergic receptors; and, because the adenyl cyclase system also appears to be influenced by β-adrenergic agonists and antagonists, it has been concluded that the inhibitory effect of the catecholamines on anaphylactic processes is related to their ability to promote cyclic AMP formation (ch. 8).

Further studies along these lines should lead to the formulation of more selective and effective methods of treating the allergic patient, besides providing explanations of the mode of action of well established drugs. In this latter connection, it is interesting to note that the studies of Assem and Schild (1969) on the inhibition of in vitro histamine release from sensitised human lung have suggested that the clinical effectiveness of isoprenaline and adrenaline in allergic bronchial asthma depends upon their ability to inhibit anaphylactic reactions as well as to relax bronchial smooth muscle.

Finally, if every other treatment fails there is always the possibility of preventing the substances released from the target cells (i.e. vasoactive amines, SRS-A etc.) from reaching their sites of action. But, as has become particularly apparent from the use of experimental animals in the study of mechanisms of anaphylactic reactions (ch. 6), immediate hypersensitivity responses are frequently heterogeneous in as much as they involve several different target cell–antibody–allergen systems responsible for the release of different mediators. Thus, it could be shown for example, that anti-histamines (such as mepyramine maleate and tripolidine hydrochloride) suppress γ_1-type antibody mediated PCA reactions in guinea pigs; but have little effect on PCA reactions in guinea pigs passively sensitised with heterologous (rabbit)γ_2-type antibody, which appear to be mediated primarily by lysosomal products from polymorphonuclear leucocytes (Movat et al. 1967). To take another example, there appear to be 3 different anaphylactic mechanisms operative in experimentally sensitised rats (fig. 6.2). Moreover, it has been observed (Orange et al. 1968) that diethyl carbamazine (hetrazan) inhibits the antigen-induced release of slow reacting substance (SRS-A) from rat peritoneal mast cells, which is thought to be mediated by γE antibody–antigen complex; but it does not inhibit histamine release from the same cells by a mechanism dependent upon a different class of antibody (namely IgGa).

It will obviously be important to establish just how closely selective inhibitory effects observed in model systems of this sort can be expected to be realised in allergic individuals treated with similar drugs.

It is, finally, worth mentioning that there are other clinical situations – involving the non-anaphylactic release of histamine and other vasoactive amines – where the use of antagonists of the type mentioned above is of particular advantage. I am referring to the clinical use of drugs which themselves may, under certain circumstances, cause histamine release; for example, polymyxin B (Ellis et al. 1970) and Synacthen, both basic polypeptides which have the ability to effect histamine release from mast cells in experimental systems by a mechanism which shows many features in common with the anaphylactic release process (ch. 8). This is a situation where the methods of controlling true immediate sensitivity responses discussed in the previous 3 sections are not applicable.

Notes

[1] Our recent evidence (see note 2, p. 126) of the blocking of human IgE-mediated PCA reactions in baboons by pre-injection of human IgE-4 could be of relevance here.

[2] But, apparently, its chemical behaviour in solution offers no reason to suppose such a mode of action.

CHAPTER 10

Future horizons

The rate of progress in the experimental study of immediate hypersensitivity is reflected in the chronological table shown in fig. 10.1, referring to major phases in the investigation of γE antibody.

When I first came into this field in 1949 little was known about the chemical basis of immediate hypersensitivity phenomena; and even after the development of refined methods of isolating and identifying plasma proteins (ch. 4), reaginic antibodies continued to evade characterisation and inhalant allergens proved not to be the easiest of proteins to purify.

As will have become apparent from the previous chapters, how-

1921	CLINICAL OBSERVATIONS (PRAUSNITZ)	
	BIOLOGICAL STUDIES	
1939		
	PHYSICAL-CHEMICAL CHARACTERISATION	
1964		'In vitro' assays
	ISOLATIONAL/IMMUNOLOGICAL CLASSIFICATION	
1967		Myeloma form discovered
	STRUCTURAL ANALYSIS	
		Animal models
	MODE OF FORMATION/FUNCTION (BIOCHEMICAL/PHARMACOLOGICAL STUDIES)	
	CLINICAL APPLICATIONS	

Fig. 10.1. Chronological summary of major phases in the investigation of the nature and function of reagin (γE antibody) (reproduced from Stanworth 1971).

ever, the situation has changed dramatically within the last few years; so that the emphasis is shifting rapidly from the identification and characterisation of the antigens and antibodies involved in anaphylactic responses to a consideration of the manner in which their interaction at the target cell surface triggers the release of the pharmacological mediators of the clinical end-effects. Hence, the initiative is passing into the hands of the biophysicist and biochemist; but there are still many problems to concern the immunochemist, as well as to divert the attentions of the cellular immunologist.

As already mentioned (ch. 5), the definition of the complete primary structure of a γE myeloma protein will undoubtedly provide important new insights into the role of the antibody in the mediation of immediate hypersensitivity reactions. But, if recent experiences in the elucidation of the structural basis of the activity of hemoglobin (Perutz 1970) can be taken as a guide, the task will not be complete until the quaternary (let alone the tertiary) structure of the γE molecule has been fully defined. Even then, it will be important to recognise the pitfalls which can be encountered in extrapolating from the pathological to the normal situation.

This underlines a need for technical improvement in the methods now being used in various laboratories in attempts to recover workable yields of antibody IgE from large volumes of potent allergic sera, and sera from parasite-infected individuals. In this connection it is just possible that the use of columns of appropriate human or sub-human primate tissue would prove a useful alternative to the employment of sorbent-coupled anti-IgE antibody (which separates IgE as antigen), because these would be expected to bind γE antibodies through their Fc regions (rather than through their Fab regions). But it would be necessary to establish first that the conditions needed to retrieve the bound antibody (e.g. low *p*H or high salt concentration) effected release without causing denaturation. Alternatively, it is possible that an ultrasonic procedure now being applied to the recovery of antibody (γG, γM etc.) from actively and passively sensitised erythrocytes (Bird 1971) might be adapted to the retrieval of active γE-type antibody from mast cells or basophils.

It is questionable, however, whether sufficiently high yields of γE antibody for structural studies would be attainable from cell or tissue elution procedures. Furthermore, if an analogy can be drawn from studies of the mode of binding of γG-type antibodies to guinea pig lung tissue (Mongar and Winne 1966), one would run into the problem of an increasing difficulty in reversing passive sensitisation as the time of contact of antibody with tissue increases; owing, it is assumed, to the attachment of antibody by more than the minimum number of 2 sites postulated for sensitisation.

The isolation and characterisation of allergens can also be expected to benefit from the availability of newly developed, highly resolving methods of protein fractionation. For example, techniques such as preparative polyacrylamide electrophoresis would seem to be particularly suited to the separation of these relatively small, highly charged, molecules; and already, as mentioned in ch. 3, isoelectric focusing has proved useful for this purpose. Here too, as in the characterisation of reaginic antibody, it will be essential to elucidate the tertiary and quaternary structures of well-defined natural allergens if a convincing case is to be made in support of the idea that bridging of cell-bound sensitising antibodies by allergen is a general induction process not restricted to artificial hapten-protein 'allergens'. In particular, it will be essential to employ the tools of the physico-chemist if allergens are to be revealed as oligomers comprising at least 2 protomers.

As already mentioned in ch. 3, there is reason to suppose that it will ultimately prove possible to predict that new commercially produced substances showing certain structural characteristics are likely to be sensitogenic. In this event, it would be hoped that the substance concerned would first be subjected to intensive testing in sub-human primates, to establish whether administration by various routes (particularly by inhalation) led to the production of reaginic(γE)-type antibodies and the induction of a state of immediate hypersensitivity. Only by adopting such measures will problems, such as have arisen by the introduction of enzymes into washing powders, be avoided.

These strictures apply particularly to the use of new pharmaceutical agents, some of which themselves have proved to possess an ability to induce the release of histamine and other vasoactive amines non-specifically. The position here is complicated by lack of knowledge yet about the nature and mode of action of the non-γE-types of antibodies which are thought to be implicated in some cases of drug-sensitivity. There is an urgent need, therefore, for further investigation into this aspect of immediate hypersensitivity, which is of considerable clinical importance. It might first be worthwhile looking carefully into the possible involvement of a particular γG sub-class; and, in this connection, it could well be significant that humans immunised with pure polysaccharides such as dextran respond by producing precipitating antibody restricted to the γG2 sub-class. It would also seem to be of possible significance that human hypersensitivity to dextran has not proved transferable in a P–K system. Could it be that γG2-type anaphylactic antibodies are involved here, too; but that their incapacity to sensitise heterologous (guinea pig) tissue extends also to the isologous situation? It should be added, however, that there is no evidence that any of the 3 other human γG sub-classes bind to isologous tissue either.

Another requirement, as far as the investigation of drug-sensitivities is concerned, is the development of a simple and reliable test which can be readily performed by the clinician. Although, the initial promise of the basophil degranulation test has not been substantiated, it might eventually prove possible to adapt one of the several in vitro techniques discussed in ch. 2 for this purpose.

Returning to the area of basic research, the in vitro study of the consequences of reagin(γE antibody)–allergen interaction at the target cell surface is at the moment complicated by the presence of an insoluble (cellular) phase. This demands, therefore, different treatments to those usually employed in (for example) kinetic studies of soluble antibody–antigen interaction systems. Two urgent requirements here are the development of efficient methods of obtaining highly homogeneous and viable target cell (mast cell and basophil) preparations; and the development of new physicochemical and biophysical methods of measuring the nature and outcome of the triggering stimulus effected by reagin–allergen combination.

It is quite possible that the application of zonal-centrifugation and related density-gradient sedimentation procedures will provide a means of obtaining high yields of viable cells. For instance, a newly developed method of centrifugal elutriation, using a specially designed rotor, has already provided promising preliminary results in the isolation of granulocytes (McEwen et al. 1968) and mast cells (Glick et al 1971).

Ultimately, of course, it will be hoped to isolate cytoplasmic and granular membranes, as well as sub-cellular fractions, by the methods now being widely applied to the characterisation of other (more readily handled) cell types. Before this goal is realised, however, it will be necessary to find sufficiently rich sources of mast cells and basophils. One promising approach, now under active investigation in some laboratories, is the culture of mast cells in liquid suspensions, or by an agar colony technique, similar to that which has been successfully employed in the culturing and cloning of granulocytes and macrophages from human bone marrow (Pike and Robinson 1970). It is conceivable, too, that the capacity of granulocytes to bind to glass surfaces could be exploited in the selective separation of basophils; provided that a suitable means of recovery could be devised which did not lead to cell destruction. As already mentioned in ch. 8, other useful sources of target cells could be mastocytomas grown in dogs (and mice); and basophils from rats in which a basophilic leukemia has been induced by chemical means.

Furthermore, there is growing evidence to suggest that release processes initiated in such cells by certain artificial liberators (such as Compound 48/80, and some basic polypeptides) simulate fairly closely the reagin–allergen trigger mechanism; thus offering a useful alternative approach to studies requiring the isolation of adequate amounts of reaginic-type antibodies from experimentally-sensitised animals' sera. But, ultimately it will be necessary to confirm observations on such systems by resort to the study of human cell reactions.

Turning to the crucial question of the elucidation of the nature of the trigger reaction, there is now an urgent need for the development of new approaches. One possibility, which we have been investigating in my own laboratory, is the use of a highly sensitive batch microcalorimeter to measure the small heat changes occurring when allergen reacts with bound reaginic antibody at the basophil (or mast cell) surface. A thorough preliminary series of trial experiments (Stanworth et al. 1972) have demonstrated the potential of this method, which permits the use of target cells under strict physiological conditions (i.e. enshrouded within a thermostated air-bath at 37°). But, although we were able to balance out non-specific effects by adopting a differential approach, it has become apparent that certain technical improvements in the design and performance of the instrument will be needed before we can expect to obtain reliable and meaningful results.

Another technique, which might eventually find application in this field, is the measurement of changes in electrical impedance across the cell membrane; because the transverse impedance of thin lipid films separating 2 aqueous saline solutions containing a small concentration of antibody or enzyme has been shown to decrease markedly following reaction with antigen or substrate respectively (Castillo et al. 1966).

Obviously there is much development work to be done before this, and other types of refined physico-chemical procedure (such as depolarisation of fluorescence, to take another example), can be applied directly to the measurement of changes occurring at the surface of viable mast cells or basophils following reagin–allergen interaction. In the meantime, there should be much valuable 'spin off' from the wealth of biophysical and biochemical investigations now being directed with increasing vigour in many laboratories towards the characterisation of the membranes of erythrocytes and other cell types. Promising approaches in this area, which might well soon begin to find application to the study of mast cell membranes, include the use of specific antibodies directed against cell surface antigens; in order to label specific protein regions of the membrane prior to subsequent electron microscopic examination by use of a freeze-etching technique (e.g. Da Silva et al. 1971; Nicholson et al. 1971). Alternatively, a method (Bretscher et al. 1971) of attaching radioactive label to proteins exposed on the surface of cell membranes has been devised, with a similar aim in mind. Interesting conclusions to be tentatively drawn from these types of approach are that erythrocyte membranes possess quite different outside and inside faces, and are comprised mainly of a lipid bilayer with different types of protein distributed about both faces. Moreover, there is evidence now that certain major protein constituents, some of which contain large amounts of conjugated carbohydrate, are exposed on the outer surface and stretch right across the membrane.

Assuming that mast cells and basophil membranes show similar types of architectural feature, it is possible that similarly scattered – but structurally distinguishable – protein constituents comprise the separate sites which are supposedly concerned with reagin-binding and the cell triggering process (ch. 8). On the other hand, one can expect that the particular array[1] of such sites, as well as their chemical characteristics, will prove to be factors responsible for the finding that only cells of this type appear to be capable of acting as targets for reagin–allergen mediated anaphylactic reactions.

In order to obtain more definitive experimental evidence in support of these suggestions it will be necessary first to recover mast cell membrane fragments in which the particular activities are retained; possibly by application of procedures similar to those now being employed in the isolation of active lymphoid cell membrane constituents (ch. 8), where (for example) deoxy-cholate has proved a valuable disrupting agent. This sort of direct approach could lead ultimately to the characterisation of the reagin-receptor groups; as well as the sites triggered by antibody–allergen interaction, which might perhaps be most easily identified by the use of radio-labelled artificial releasing agents. It might also result in the identification of key regulatory membrane enzymes, fulfilling similar roles to those suspected of being implicated in the sites of hormone triggering action on different types of target cells.

It is to be hoped, too, that further studies with purified mast cell preparations and sub-cellular constituents will facilitate the definition of those secondary events which culminate in the release of the pharmacological mediators. In this sphere there is still much to be learnt about the role of cyclic AMP and other 'secondary messengers' involved in conveying the effects of the initial stimulus at the mast cell surface to the granules containing the vasoactive amines. The use of radio-labelled tracers should prove particularly rewarding, in this connection; and the application of improvements in electron microscopic technique can be expected to throw further light on the train of morphological changes involved.

It is becoming increasingly recognised that cell triggering processes in general, whether they involve stimulation of lymphocytes by specific antigen (on non-specifically by phytomitogens), activation of phagocytosing cells by antigen–antibody complexes or induction of amine release from mast cells by reagin–allergen interaction, possess certain basic features in common. Hence, it can be confidently expected that new knowledge gleaned about the mechanism of reagin-mediated histamine release at the cellular level will prove to be more than a little relevant to the understanding of other, basic, immunological processes. Furthermore, it is worth noting in this connection, that in the study of the histamine-release mechanism it is possible to investigate the mode of uptake of the mediatory antibody on to the target cell; a process which has not proved possible yet as far as the study of lymphocyte receptor immunoglobulin is concerned.

As already mentioned in ch. 7, there could be other pathological situations where γE antibody-mediated reactions are involved. For instance, the localisation of IgE in the glomeruli of patients with nephrotic syndrome has prompted the suggestion that this immunoglobulin plays some form of pathogenic role in this condition (Gerber and Paronetto 1971). It might also be of some significance, in this context, that mast cells were observed to appear early and in excess in the peri-articular tissues of rats during the phase of onset of experimental adjuvant arthritis (Gryfe et al. 1971).

But it is, of course, towards the understanding of the aetiology of human hypersensitivity conditions of the asthma-hayfever-urticaria type that future studies are expected to make the greatest contribution. It can be confidently predicted that the next decade will see the detailed elucidation of the mechanism of immediate-type hypersensitivity reactions; which could well lead to the development of more effective methods of control and even prevention.

In the meantime, plenty of problems remain to test the resources and ingenuity of the immunochemist. For instance, what is the chemical basis of the hypersensitivity response; which reveals such fine differences in specificity between one atopic individual and another although both are exposed to the same range of inhalants? I suspect that only the approach of a Landsteiner will finally resolve fascinating questions of this type; which will demand a consideration of the fine structure of the host's own tissue antigens as well as that of the offending sensitogens. In similar vein, I suppose that passive tissue sensitisation by reaginic (γE)-type antibody could be likened to a graft-host reaction at the molecular level.

Finally, there is the question of the somewhat unusual structure of γE antibodies to consider. On teleological grounds it could perhaps be argued that the extra structural domain within the heavy chain has evolved to cope with an additional role, namely the mounting of a hypersensitising (as opposed to immunising) response; which presupposes that anaphylactic reactions are of some benefit to the host. But, on the other hand, the presence of this structural characteristic, which is also seen in the μ chains of γM-globulins (and in the heavy chains of γD-globulins), might have arisen from a 'cross-over' (to use the language of the immunogeneticist). Nevertheless, it is perhaps not altogether fortuitous that those polypeptide chains which are involved directly in cell surface triggering mechanisms (i.e. the μ chains in lymphocyte receptors and ϵ chains of reagin on sensitised mast cells and basophils) both possess 3 structural domains (demarcated by intra-chain S-S bridges) within their Fc regions.

Note

[1] It seems particularly significant that recent EM Studies (Sullivan, A.L. et al., J. Exp. Med.; 1971, *134*, 1403) have provided evidence of a temperature dependence of the distribution of endogenous IgE on human basophils not unlike that of the surface immunoglobulins revealed on mouse lymphocytes by immunofluorescence.

References

Aas, K. (1967). Studies of hypersensitivity to fish. Studies of different fractions of extracts from cod muscle tissue. Int. Arch. Allergy *31*, 239.

Aas, K. (1968). Studies of hypersensitivity to fish. Universitets-Forlagets Trykningssentral.

Aas, K. and Jebsen, J.W. (1967). Studies of hypersensitivity to fish. Partial purification and crystallisation of a major allergenic component of cod. Int. Arch. Allergy *32*, 1.

Aas, K. and Elsayed, S.M. (1969). Characterisation of a major allergen (cod). Effect of enzymic hydrolysis on the allergenic activity. J. Allergy *44*, 333.

Ackroyd, J.F. (1954). The role of sedormid in the immunological reaction that results in platelet lysis in sedormid purpura. Clin. Sci. *13*, 409.

Allan, D., Auger, J. and Crumpton, M.J. (1972). Glycoprotein receptors for Concanavalin A isolated from guinea pig lymphocyte plasma membranes by affinity chromatography in sodium deoxycholate. Nature New Biol. *236*, 23.

Ammann, A.J., Cain, W.P., Ishizaka, K., Hong, R. and Good, R.A. (1969). Immunoglobulin E deficiency in ataxia-telangiectasia. New Eng. J. Med. *281*, 469.

Amundsen, E., Ofstad, E. and Hagen, P.O. (1969). Histamine release induced by synergistic action of kallikrein and phospholipase A. Arch. Intern. Pharmacodyn. *178*, 104.

Andersen, B.R. and Vannier, W.E. (1964). The sedimentation properties of the skin-sensitising antibodies of ragweed-sensitive patients. J. Exp. Med. *120*, 3I.

Andersen, B.R., Abele, D.C. and Vannier, W.E. (1966). Effect of mild periodate oxidation on antibodies. J. Immunol. *97*, 913.

Arbesman, C.E., Girard, J.P. and Rose, N.R. (1964). Demonstration of human reagin in the monkey. I. In vitro passive sensitization of monkey ileum with sera of untreated atopic patients. J. Allergy *35*, 535.

Arbesman, C.E., Dolovich, J., Wicher K., Dushenski, C.A., Reisman, R.E. and Tomasi, T.B. (1968). Proc. 6th Int. Congr. Allergology (Montreal).

Arbesman, C.E., Ito, K., Wypch, J.I. and Wicher, K. (1972). Measurement of serum IgE by a one-step single radial radiodiffusion method. J. Allergy *49*, 72.

Archer, G.T. (1959). The release of histamine from mast cells of the rat. Aust. J. Exp. Biol. Med. Sci. *37*, 383.

Askonas, B.A., White, R.G. and Wilkinson, P.C. (1965). Production of γ_1 and γ_2-anti-ovalbumin by various lymphoid tissues of the guinea pig. Immunochem. *2*, 329.

Assem, E.S.K. and Schild, H.O. (1968). Detection of allergy to penicillin and other antigens by in vitro passive sensitisation and histamine release from human and monkey lung. B.M.J. *3*, 272.

Assem, E.S.K. and Schild, H.O. (1969). Inhibition by sympathomimetic amines of histamine release induced by antigen in passively sensitised human lung. Nature *224*, 1028.

Assem, E.S.K. and Mongar, J.L. (1970). Inhibition of allergic reactions in man and other species by cromoglycate. Int. Arch. Allergy *38*, 68.

Augustin, R. (1955). Chemical, biochemical and immunological advances in allergy with special reference to pollens and their standardization. Quart. Rev. Allergy Appl. Immunol. *9*, 504–560.

Augustin, R. (1967). Demonstration of reagins in the sera of allergic subjects. In: *Handbook of Experimental Immunology,* ed. D.M. Weir (Blackwell).

Augustin, R, Connolly, R.C. and Lloyd, G.M. (1964). Atopic reagins as a prototype of cytophilic antibodies. In: Protides of the biological fluids, 11th Colloq. Bruges, 1963, ed. H. Peeters, (Elsevier Publishing Co., Amsterdam) p. 56.

Austen, K.F. (1968). Discussion in: C.I.O.M.S. Symp., Biochemistry of the acute allergic reactions, eds. Austen, K.F. and Becker, E.L. (Blackwell) p. 114.

Austen, K.F. and Brocklehurst, W.E. (1961). Anaphylaxis in chopped guinea pig lung. II. Enhancement of the anaphylactic release of histamine and slow reacting substance by certain dibasic aliphatic acids and inhibition by monobasic fatty acids. J. Exp. Med. *113*, 541.

Austen, K.F. and Valentine, M.D. (1968). Complement-dependent histamine release from rat peritoneal mast cells by rabbit anti-rat gamma globulin (Ra anti-RGG) and rabbit anti-rat mast cell (Ra anti-RMC) antibodies. In: Biochemistry of the acute allergic reactions, C.I.O.M.S. Symp., eds. K.F. Austen and E.L. Becker, (Blackwell) p. 231.

Barbaro, J.F. and Zvaifler, N.J. (1966). Antigen induced histamine release from platelets of rabbits producing homologous *PCA* antibody. Proc. Soc. Exp. Biol. Med. *122*, 1245.

Barker, S.A., Cruickshank, C.N.D. and Morris, J.H. (1963). Structure of a galactomannan-peptide allergen from *Trichophyton mentagrophytes.* Biochim. Biophys. Acta *74*, 239.

Barth, E.E.E., Jarrett, W.F.H. and Urquhart, G.M. (1966). Studies on the mechanism of the self-cure reaction in rats infected with *Nippostrongylus brasiliensis.* Immunol. *10*, 459.

Batchelor, F.R., Dewdney, J.M. and Gazzard, D. (1965). Penicillin allergy: the formation of the penicilloyl determinant. Nature (Lond.) *206*, 362.

Batchelor, F.R. and Dewdney, J.M. (1968). Some aspects of penicillin allergy. Proc. Roy. Soc. Med. *61*, 897.

Becker, E.L. (1968). Nature and significance of antigen-antibody activated esterases. In: C.I.O.M.S. Symp., Biochemistry of the acute allergic reactions, eds. K.F. Austen and E.L. Becker, (Blackwell) p. 199.

Becker, E.L. and Rappaport, B.Z. (1948). Quantitative studies in skin testing. II. The form of the dose-response curve utilising a quantitative response. J. Allergy *19*, 317.

Beede, R.B., Rose, N.R. and Arbesman, C.E. (1958). Sensitivity to animals: a case report with immunologic studies. II. Serologic aspects. J. Allergy *29*, 139.

Belin, L., Falsen, E., Hoborn, J. and André, J. (1970). Enzyme sensitization in consumers of enzyme-containing washing powder. Lancet ii, 1153.

Benacerraf, B. (1967). The anaphylactic antibodies of mammals including man. Personal communication (cited in Bloch. Prog. Allergy *10*, 84).

Benacerraf, B., Ovary, Z., Bloch, K.K. and Franklin, E.C. (1963). Properties of guinea pig 7*S* antibodies. I. Electrophoretic separation of two types of guinea pig 7*S* antibodies. J. Exp. Med. *117*, 937.

Benacerraf, B., Nussenzweig, V., Maurer, P.H. and Stylos, W. (1969). Relationship between the net electrical charge of antigens and specific antibodies. An example of selection by antigen of cells producing highest affinity antibody. In: *Topics in Immunology*, eds. M. Sela and M. Prywes (Academic Press).

Benditt, E.P. and Lagnoff, D. (1964). Proliferation of mast cells induced by a variety of reagents. Prog. Allergy *8*, 195.

Bennich, H. (1968). Immunoglobulin ND(IgE). Chemical and physical studies. Acta Universitatis Upsaliensis No. 53.

Bennich, H. and Johansson, S.G.O. (1968). Studies on a new class of human immunoglobulins. II. Chemical and physical properties. Nobel Symp. 3, 199, ed. J. Killander (Almqvist and Wiksell, Stockholm).

Bennich, H., Ishizaka, K., Johansson, S.G.O., Rowe, D.S., Stanworth, D.R. and Terry, W.D. (1968). Immunoglobulin E, a new class of human immunoglobulin. Bull. World Health Org. *38*, 151.

Bennich, H., Ishizaka, K., Ishizaka, T. and Johansson, S.G.O. (1969). A comparative antigenic study of γE-globulin and myeloma IgND. J. Immunol. *102*, 826.

Bennich, H. and Johansson, S.G.O. (1970). Immunoglobulin E and immediate hypersensitivity. Vox. Sang. *19*, 1.

Bennich, H. and Johansson, S.G.O. (1971). The structure and function of human immunoglobulin E. Adv. Immunol. *13*, 1.

Berdal, P. (1952). Serologic investigation of the edema fluid from nasal polyps. J. Allergy *23*, 11.

Berg, T. and Johansson, S.G.O. (1969A). IgE concentrations in children with atopic diseases. Int. Arch., Allergy. *36*, 219.

Berg, T. and Johansson, S.G.O. (1969B). Immunoglobulin levels during childhood, with special regard to IgE. Acta Paediat. Scand. *58*, 513.

Berg, T. and Johansson, S.G.O. (1970). IgE specific reagins during hyposensitization. Acta. Paediat. Scand. *59*, Suppl. 206, p. 85.

Berg, T., Bennich, H. and Johansson, S.G.O. (1971). In vitro diagnosis of atopic allergy. I. A comparison between provocation tests and the radioallergosorbent test. Int. Arch. Allergy *40*, 770.

Berken, A. and Benaceraff, B. (1966). Properties of antibodies cytophilic for macrophages. J. Exp. Med. *123*, 119.

Berrens, L. (1971). The chemistry of atopic allergens. Monographs in Allergy, Vol. *7*, (Karger).

Berrens, L. and Bleumink, E. (1965). Spectroscopic evidence for N-glycosidic linkages in atopic allergens. Int. Arch. Allergy *28*, 150.

Berrens, L., Morris, J.H. and Versie, R. (1965). 'The complexity of house dust, with special reference to the presence of human dandruff allergent. Int. Arch. Allergy. *27*, 129.

Berrens, L. and Versie, R. (1967). Antigenic relationships in atopy. II. Cross-reactions of anti-house dust sera with inhalant glycoprotein allergens from different sources. Acta Allergolica *22*, 347.

Berson, S.A., Yalow, R.S., Bauman, A., Rothschild, M.A. and Newerly, K. (1956). Insulin-I^{131} metabolism in human subjects: Demonstration of insulin binding globulin in the circulation of insulin treated subjects. J. Clin. Invest. *35*, 170.

Berson, S.A. and Yalow, R.S. (1962). Immunoassay of plasma insulin In: Ciba Colloq. of Endocrinology *14*, 182.

Billingham, R.E. and Medawar, P.B. (1952). The freezing, drying and storage of mammalian skin. J. Exp. Biol. *29*, 454.

Binaghi, R., Liacopoulos-Briot, M., Halpern, B.N. and Liacopoulos, P. (1960). Influence of the ionic strength of the medium on the anaphylactic sensitisation of isolated tissues in vitro. Nature *187*, 697.

Binaghi, R., Liacopoulos, P., Halpern, B.N. Liacopoulos-Briot, M. (1962). Interference of non-specific gamma-globulins with passive anaphylactic sensitisation of isolated guinea pig intestine. Immunol. *5*, 205.

Binaghi, R.A. and Benacerraf, B. (1964). The production of anaphylactic antibodies in the rat. J. Immunol. *92*, 920.

Binaghi, R.A., Benacerraf, B., Bloch, K.J. and Kourilsky, F.M. (1964). Properties of rat anaphylactic antibody. J. Immunol. *92*, 927.

Bird, G. (1971). Personal communication.

Blackley, C.H. (1873) (Reprinted 1959). Experimental researches on the causes and nature of catarrhus aestivus (Hay fever or Hay asthma). Dawson's of Pall Mall, London.

Blandford, G. (1970). Arthus reaction and pneumonia. B.M.J. 1, 758.

Bleumink, E. and Berrens, L. (1966). Synthetic approaches to the biological activity of β-lactoglobulin in human allergy to cow's milk. Nature (Lond.) *212*, 541.

Bleumink, E. and Young, E. (1968). Identification of the atopic allergen in cow's milk. Int. Arch. Allergy *34*, 521.

Bleumink, E. and Young, E. (1969). Studies on the atopic allergen in hen's egg. I. Identification of the skin-reactive fraction in egg white. Int. Arch. Allergy *35*, 1

Bloch, K.J. (1967). The anaphylactic antibodies of mammals including man. Prog. Allergy *10*, 84.

Blomberg, F. and Perlmann, P. (1971). Immunochemical characterisation of enzyme activities in liver plasma membranes of the rat. Exp. Cell Res. *66*, 104.

Bloom, G.D. and Haegermak, D. (1967). Studies on morphological changes and histamine release induced by bee venom, n-decylamine and hypotonic solutions in rat peritoneal mast cells. Acta Physiol. Scand. *71*, 257.

Bolton, F.G. (1956). Thrombocytopenic purpura due to quinidine. II. Serologic mechanisms. Blood *11*, 547.

Borsos, T., Dourmashkin, R.R. and Humphrey, J.H. (1964). Lesions in erythrocyte membranes caused by immune hemolysis. Nature *202*, 251.

Borsos, T. and Rapp, H.J. (1965). Complement fixation on cell surfaces by 19*S* and 7*S* antibodies. Science *150*, 505.

Boura, A., Mongar, J.L. and Schild, H.O. (1954). Improved automatic apparatus for pharmacological assays on isolated antigens. Brit. J. Pharmacol. *9*, 24.

Bowman, K.L. and Walzer, M. (1953). Studies in reaginic and histamine wheals. I. The effects of reaginic and histaminic wheals upon the subsequent responsiveness of passively sensitised cutaneous sites. J. Allergy *24*, 126.

Boyden, S.V. (1951). Adsorption of proteins on erythrocytes treated with tannic acid and subsequent hemagglutination by anti-protein sera. J. Exp. Med. *93*, 107.

Brandtzaeg, P., Fjellanger, I. and Gjeruldsen, S.-T. (1967). Localization of immunoglobulins in human nasal mucosa. Immunochem. *4*, 57.

Brattsten, I., Colldahl, H. and Laurell, A.H.F. (1955). The distribution of reagins in the serum protein fractions-obtained by continuous zone electrophoresis. Acta Allergol. *8*, 339.

Bretscher, M. (1971). A major protein which spans the human erythrocyte membrane. J. Mol. Biol. *59*, 351.

Bretscher, M.S. (1971). The proteins of erythrocyte membranes: where are they? In: Proc. Biochem. Soc. Colloq: The proteins of membranes, p. 4.

Britton, C.J.C. and Coombs, R.R.A. (1955). The serological examination of sera from normal persons and from hayfever patients both before and after specific hyposensitization for heat stable antibodies to the proteins of timothy grass pollen. Acta Allergol. *8*, 31.

Brocklehurst, W.E., Humphrey, J.H. and Perry, W.L.M. (1961). The in vitro uptake of rabbit antibody by chopped guinea pig lung and its relationship to anaphylactic sensitization. Immunol. *4*, 67.

Brocteur, J. and Versie, R. (1967). Mise en évidence de divers facteurs de groupes sanguins dans des extracts allergeniques de poussières de maison. Acta Allergol. *22*, 118.

Brostoff, J., Greaves, M.F. and Roitt, I.M. (1969). IgE in lymphoid cells from pollen-stimulated cultures. Lancet i, 803.

Buckley, R.H. and Metzgar, R.S. (1965). The use of non-human primates for studies of reagins. J. Allergy *36*, 382.

Budd, G.C., Daržynkiewicz, Z. and Barnard, E.A. (1967). Intracellular localization of specific proteases in rat mast cells. Nature *213*, 1202.

Bukhari, A.Q.S. (1967). Studies on the passive sensitization of human lung. Ph.D. Thesis, Univ. of Edinburgh.

Butcher, R.W., Robison, G.A., Hardman, J.G. and Sutherland, E.W. (1968). The role of cyclic *AMP* in hormone action. Adv. Enzyme Regulation *6*, 357.

Callerame, M.L., Condemi, J.J., Ishizaka, K., Johansson, S.G.O. and Vaughan, J.H. (1971). Immunoglobulins in bronchial tissues from patients with asthma, with special reference to immunoglobulin E. J. Allergy *47*, 187.

Caspary, E.A. and Comaish, S. (1967). Release of serotonin from human platelets in hypersensitivity states. Nature *214*, 286.

Cass, R.M. and Anderson, B.R. (1968). The disappearance rate of skin-sensitising antibody activity after intradermal injection. J. Allergy *42*, 29.

Castillo, J. Del, Rodriguez, A., Romero, A. and Sanchez, V. (1966). Lipid films as tranducers for detection of antigen-antibody and enzyme-substrate reactions. Science *153*, 185.

Catt, K.J. (1970). ABC of endocrinology. I. Hormones in general. Lancet i, 763.

Catt, K.J., Niall, H.D. and Tregear, G.W. (1966). Solid-phase radioimmunoassay of human growth hormone. Biochem. J. *100*, 31C.

Catt, K.J., Niall, H.D. and Tregear, G.W. (1967). Solid-phase radio-immunoassay. Nature *213*, 825.

Catt, K.J., Niall, H.D. and Tregear, G.W. (1967). Solid-phase disc radio-immunoassay for human growth hormone. J. Lab. Clin. Med. *70*, 820.

Catt, K.J., and Tregear, G.W. (1967). Solid-phase radio-immunoassay in antibody coated tubes. Science *158*, 1570.

Catty, D. (1969). The immunology of nematode infections; trichinosis in guinea-pigs as a model. Monographs in Allergy *5*.

Caulfield, A.H.W., Brown, M.H. and Waters, E.T. (1936). Suitability of the monkey (*Macacus rhesus*) as a recipient for the Prausnitz-Küstner reaction. Proc. Soc. Exp. Biol. Med. *35*, 109.

Chakravarty, N. (1960). The mechanism of histamine release in anaphylactic reaction in guinea pig and lung. Acta Physiol. Scand. *48*, 146.

Chan, P.C.Y. and Porter, R.R. (1967). In vitro assay of reaginic antibodies to horse serum albumin. Immunol. *13*, 633.

Chopra, S.L., Kovacs, B.A., Goodfriend, L. and Rose, B. (1965). In vitro detection of reagins to ragweed. Federation Proc. *24*, 633.

Chopra, S.L., Kovacs, B.A., Rose, B. and Goodfriend, L. (1966). Detection of human reagins by Schultz-Dale technique using human appendix. Int. Arch. Allergy *29*, 393.

Chu, C.H.U. (1963). On the formation and function of mast cell granules. Anat. Rec. *145*, 217 (Abstract).

Clark, J.M. and Higginbotham, R.D. (1968). Significance of the mast cell response to a lysosomal protein. J. Immunol. *101*, 488.

Coca, A.F. and Cooke, R.A. (1923). On the classification of the phenomena of hypersensitiveness. J. Immunol. *8*, 163.

Coca, A.F. and Grove, E.F. (1925). Studies in hypersensitiveness. A study of the atopic reagins. J. Immunol. *10*, 445.

Coe, J. (1966). 7S γ_1 and 7S γ_2 antibody response in the mouse. I. Influence of strain, antigen and adjuvant. J. Immunol. *96*, 744.

Cohen, S. (1968). The requirements for the association of two adjacent rabbit γG-antibody molecules in the fixation of complement by immune complexes. J. Immunol. *100*, 407.

Coloquhoun, D. (1968). The rate of equlibration in a competitive n drug system and the auto-inhibitory equations of enzyme kinetics: some properties of simple models for passive sensitization. Proc. Roy. Soc. (London), B, *170*, 135.

Connell, G.E. and Porter, R.R. (1971). A new enzymic fragment (Facb) of rabbit immunoglobulin G. Biochem. J. *124*, 53P.

Connell, J.T. and Sherman, W.B. (1965). Relationship of passive cutaneous anaphylaxis to antibodies in the serum of ragweed hayfever patients after injection treatment. J. Immunol. *94*, 498.

Connell, J.T. and Sherman, W.B. (1969) Changes in skin-sensitising antibody after injections of aqueous pollen extract. J. Allergy *43*, 22.

Cooke, R.A., Barnard, J.H., Hebald, S. and Stull, A. (1935). Serologic evidence of immunity with coexisting sensitization in a type of human allergy (hay fever). J. Exp. Med. *62*, 733.

Cooke, R.A., Loveless, M. and Stull, A. (1937). Studies on immunity in a type of human allergy (hay fever): serologic response of non-sensitive individuals to pollen injections. J. Exp. Med. *66*, 689.

Coombs, R.R.A. (1955). Serological problems in allergy. Int. Arch. Allergy *6*, 252.

Coombs, R.R.A., Jonas, W.E., Lachmann, P.J. and Feinstein, A. (1965). Detection of IgA antibodies by the red cell linked antigen-antiglobulin reaction: antibodies in the sera of infants to milk proteins. Int. Arch. Allergy *27*, 321.

Coombs, R.R.A., Hunter, A., Jonas, W.E., Bennich, H., Johansson, S.G.O. and Panzani, R. (1968). Detection of IgE (IgND) specific antibody (probably reagin) to castor-bean allergen by the red-cell-linked antigen-antiglobulin reaction. Lancet i, 1115.

Cooper, J.R. and Cruickshank, C.N.D. (1966). Improved method for direct counting of basophil leucocytes. J. Clin. Path. *19*, 402.

Cox, J.S.G., Beach, J.E., Blair, A.M.J.N., Clarke, A.J., King, J., Lee, T.B., Loveday, D.E.E., Moss, G.F., Orr, T.S.C., Ritchie, J.T. and Sheard, P. (1970). Disodium cromoglycate (Intal). Adv. Drug Res. *5*, 115.

Crunkhorn, P. and Meacock, S.C.R. (1971). The effect of adrenalectomy on the production of homocytotropic antibody in rats. Immunol. *20*, 91.

Dale, H.H. (1913). The anaphylactic reaction of plain muscle in the guinea pig. J. Pharmacol. *4*, 167.

Dale, M.M. and Ziletti, L. (1970). The Schultz-Dale response of the longitudinal muscle strip preparation of the guinea-pig ileum. Brit. J. Pharmacol. *39*, 542.

Daržynkiewicz, Z. and Barnard, E.A. (1967). Specific proteases of the rat mast cell. Nature *213*, 1198.

Da Silva, P.P. and Branton, D. (1970). Membrane splitting in freeze-etching; covalently bound ferritin as a membrane marker. J. Cell. Biol. *45*, 598.

Da Silva, P.P., Douglas, S.D. and Branton, D. (1971). Localization of A antigen sites on human erythrocytes ghosts. Nature *232*, 194.

Davey, M.J. and Asherson, G.L. (1967). Cytophilic antibody. I. Nature of the macrophage receptor. Immunology *12*, 13.

Davies, G.E. (1971). Personal communication.

De Besche, A. (1923). Studies on the reactions of asthmatics and on passive transference of hypersusceptibility. Am. J. Med. Sci. *166*, 265.

De Weck, A.L. (1968). The formation of penicillin antigens. Proc. Roy. Soc. Med. *61*, 894.

De Weck, A.L. and Schneider, C.H. (1968). Immune and non-immune responses to monovalent low molecular weight penicilloyl-polylysines and penicilloyl-bacitracin in rabbits and guinea pigs. Immunol. *14*, 457.

De Weck, A.L. and Schneider, C.H. (1969). Molecular and stereochemical properties required of antigens for the elicitation of allergic reactions. In: Bayer Symp., Vol. 1, *Problems in Immunology* (Springer Verlag).

Diamant, B. and Uvnäs, B. (1961). Evidence for energy-requiring processes in histamine release and mast cell degranulation in rat tissues induced by compound 48/80. Acta Physiol. Scand. *53*, 315.

Dobson, C., Morseth, D.J. and Soulsby, E.J.L. (1971). Immunoglobulin E-type antibodies induced by *Ascaris suum* infections in guinea pigs. J. Immunol. *106*, 128.

Donovan, R., Johansson, S.G.O., Bennich, H. and Soothill, J.F. (1970). Immunoglobulins in nasal polyp fluids. Int. Arch. Allergy *37*, 154.

Dowben, R.M. (1969). Composition and structure of membranes. In: *Biological Membranes*, ed. R.M. Dowben (Churchill, London) p. 1.

Dubos, R. (1971). Toxic factors in enzymes used in laundry products. Science *173*, 259.

Edman, K.A.P., Mongar, J.L. and Schild, H.O. (1964). The role of SH and SS groups in the anaphylactic reaction. J. Physiol. (London) *170*, 124.

Eisen, H.N., Little, J.R., Osterland, C.K. and Simms, E.S. (1967). A myeloma protein with antibody activity. Cold Spring Harbour Symposium Quant. Biol. *32*, 75.

Ellis, H.V., Johnson, A.R., and Moran, N.C. (1970). Selective release of histamine from rat mast cells by several drugs. J. Pharmacol. Exp. Therap. *175*, 627.

Elsayed, S.M. and Aas, K. (1970). Characterisation of a major allergen (cod). Chemical composition and immunological properties. Int. Arch. Allergy *38*, 536.

Elsayed, S., Aas, K. and Christensten, T. (1971). Partial characterisation of homogeneous allergens (cod). Int. Arch. Allergy *40*, 439.

Elsayed, S. and Aas, K. (1971A). Isolation of purified allergens (cod) by iso-electric focusing. Int. Arch. Allergy *40*, 428.

Elsayed, S. and Aas, K. (1971B). Characterisation of a major allergen (cod). Observations on effect of denaturation of the allergenic activity. J. Allergy *47*, 283.

Engelman, D.M. (1971). Lipid bilayer structure in the membrane of *Mycoplasma laidlawii*. J. Mol. Biol. *58*, 153.

Epstein, F.H. and Whittam, R. (1966). The mode of inhibition by calcium of cell-membrane adenosine triphosphatase activity. Biochem. J. *99*, 232.

Fairbanks, G., Steck, T.L. and Wallach, D.F.H. (1971), Electrophoretic analysis of the major polypeptides of the human erythrocyte membranes. Biochem. *10*, 2606.

Farr, R.S. (1958). A quantitative immuno-chemical measure of the primary interaction between I*BSA and antibody. J. Infect. Dis. *103*, 239.

Faulk, W.P., Pondman, K.W. and Fudenberg, H.H. (1969). Homocytotropic antibodies in the primary and secondary immune response. Israel. J. Med. Sci. *5*, 245.

Feinberg, R. (1954). Detection of non-precipitating antibodies coexisting with precipitating antibodies using I^{131}-labelled antigen. Federation Proc. *13*, 493.

Feinberg, S.M., Becker, R.J., Slavin, R.G., Feinberg, A.R. and Sparks, D.B. (1962). The sensitizing effects of emulsified pollen antigens in atopic subjects naturally sensitive to an unrelated antigen. J. Allergy *33*, 285.

Feinberg, S.M., Feinberg, A.R. and Lee, F. (1969). Hypersensitivity responses in monkeys. III. The influence of various tranquilizers and other drugs on immediate skin reactions. J. Allergy *43*, 81–88.

Feinberg, S.M., Feinberg, A.R. and Lee, F. (1971). Hypersensitivity responses in monkeys. IV. Sensitization to human sera and non-acceptance of reagin. J. Allergy *46*, 231.

Feinstein, A. and Rowe, A.J. (1965). Molecular mechanisms of formation of an antigen-antibody complex. Nature (Lond.) *205*, 147.

Feldberg, W. and Miles, A.A. (1953). Regional variations of increased permeability of skin capillaries induced by a histamine liberator and their relation to the histamine content of the skin. J. Physiol. *120*, 205.

Finke, S.R., Phillips, G.B. and Middleton, E. (1966). Histamine release from human leucocytes by lysolecithin and the effect of in vitro anaphylaxis on leucocyte lipids. J. Lab. Clin. Med. *67*, 601.

Fireman, P., Vannier, W.E. and Goodman, H.C. (1963). The association of skin-sensitising antibody with the β_2A-globulins in sera of ragweed-sensitive patients. J. Exp. Med. *117*, 603.

Fireman, P., Boesman, M. and Gitlin, D. (1967). Heterogeneity of skin-sensitising antibodies. J. Allergy *40*, 259.

Fischer, H. (1964). Lysolecithin and the action of complement. Annal. N.Y. Acad. Sci. *116*, 1063.

Fisher, J.P. and Connell, J.T. (1962). Passive cutaneous anaphylaxis in the guinea pig with serum of allergic patients treated with ragweed extract emulsions. J. Allergy *33*, 59.

Fisherman, E.W. (1962). Induction of immediate cutaneous reactivity to an antigen (Ascaris) in cancerous and non-cancerous individuals. J. Allergy *33*, 12.

Fitzpatrick, M.E., Connolly, R.C., Lea, D.J., O'Sullivan, S.A., Augustin, R. and Macaulay, M.B. (1967). In vitro detection of human reagins by double layer leucocyte agglutination method and controlled blind study. Immunol. *12*, 1.

Forsgren, A. and Sjöquist, J. (1966). Protein A from *S. aureus*. I. Pseudo-immune reaction with human γ-globulin. J. Immunol. *97*, 822.

Frangione, B., Milstein, C. and Pink, J.R. (1969). Structural studies of immunoglobulin G. Nature *221*, 145.

Frankland, A.W. (1955). High and low dosage pollen extract treatment in Summer hay fever and asthma. Acta Allergol. *9*, 183.

Franklin, E.C. and Stanworth, D.R. (1961). Antigenic relationships between immunoglobulins and certain related paraproteins in man. J. Exp. Med. *114*, 521.

Franklin, W. and Lowell, F.C. (1967). A comparison of two dosages of ragweed extract in the treatment of pollenosis. J. Amer. Med. Assoc. *201*, 95.

Freeman, J. (1924). Discussion on paroxysmal rhinorrhoea. Proc. Roy. Soc. Med., Sect. Laryngol. *18*, 29.

Freeman, M.J., Braleey, H.C., Kaplan, R.M. and McArthur, W.P. (1969). Occurrence and properties of rabbit homocytotropic antibody. Int. Arch. Allergy *36*, 530.

Fudenburg, H.H., Drews, G. and Nisonoff, A. (1964). Serologic demonstration of dual specificity of bivalent hybrid antibody. J. Exp. Med. *119*, 151.

Furness, G. and Maitland, H.B. (1952). Studies on cotton dust in relation to byssinosis. I. Bacteria and fungi in cotton dust. Brit. J. Industr. Med. *9*, 138.

Gerber, M.A. and Paronetto, F. (1971). IgE in glomeruli of patients with nephrotic syndrome. Lancet i, 1097.

Gill, T.J., Kunz., H.W. and Papermaster, D.S. (1967). Studies on synthetic polypeptide antigens. XVII. The role of composition, charge, and optical isomerism in the immunogenicity of synthetic polypeptides. J. Biol. Chem. *242*, 3308.

Gillepsie, E., Levine, R.J. and Malawista, S.E. (1968). Histamine release from rat peritoneal mast cells: inhibition by colchicine and potentiation by deuterium oxide. J. Pharmacol. Exp. Therap. *164*, 158.

Ginsburg, H. and Lagunoff, D. (1967). The in vitro differentiation of mast cells. Culture of cells from immunised mouse lymph nodes and thoracic duct lymph on fibroblast monolayers. J. Cell Biol. *35*, 685.

Girard, J.P., Rose, N.R., Kunz, M.L., Kobayashi, S. and Arbesman, C.E. (1967). In vitro lymphocyte transformation in atopic patients induced by antigens. J. Allergy *39*, 65.

Glock, D., Redlich, D. Von, Juhos, E.Th. and McEwen, C.R. (1971). Separation of mast cells by centrifugal elutriation. Exp. Cell Res. *65*, 23.

Gocke, D.J. and Osler, A.G. (1965). In vitro damage of rabbit platelets by an unrelated antigen-antibody reaction. J. Immunol. *94*, 236.

Goldfarb, A.R. (1968). Separation of new skin-reactive antigens from dwarf ragweed pollen, J. Immunol. *100*, 902.

Goldfarb, A.R. and Kaplan, M. (1967). Qualitative and quantitative variations in dwarf ragweed pollens. J. Allergy *40*, 237.

Goldman, A.S., Anderson, D.W., Sellars, W.A., Saperstein, S., Kniker, W.T. and Halpern, S.R. (1963A). I. Oral challenge with milk and isolated milk proteins in allergic children. Pediatrics *32*, 425.

Goldman, A.S., Sellars, W.A., Halpern, S.R., Anderson, D.W., Furlow, T.E. and Johnson, C.H. (1963B). II. Skin testing of allergic and normal children with purified milk proteins. Pediatrics *32*, 572.

Goodfriend, L., Kovacs, B.A. and Rose, B. (1966A). Use of monkey lung tissue for in vitro detection of reagins in human atopic sera. J. Allergy, *37*, 122.

Goodfriend, L., Kovacs, B.A. and Rose, B. (1966B). In vitro sensitisation of monkey lung fragments with human ragweed atopic serum. Int. Arch. Allergy *30*, 511.

Goodfriend, L., Perelmutter, L. and Rose, B. (1966). Relationship between ragweed reagins and serum immunoglobulins. Int. Arch. Allergy *30*, 542.

Goodfriend, L. and Luhovyj, I. (1968). In vitro detection of reagins in human atopic sera by monkey skin suspension technique. Int. Arch. Allergy *33*, 171.

Goodfriend, L. and Perelmutter, L. (1968). Properties of two chromatographically distinct reagins in the sera of ragweed atopic individuals. Int. Arch. Allergy *33*, 89.

Goodfriend, L., Hubscher, T. and Radermecker, M. (1969). The monocytotopic nature of reaginic antibodies. In: *Cellular and humoral mechanisms in anaphylaxis and allergy*, ed. H.L. Movat, (S. Karger) p.90.

Goodman, J.W. (1964). Immunologically active fragments of rabbit gamma globulin. Biochem. *3*, 857.

Goodman, J.W. (1965). Heterogeneity of rabbit γ-globulin with respect to cleavage by papain. Biochem. *4*, 2350.

Graham, H.T., Lowry, O.H., Wheelwright, F., Lenz, M.A. and Parish, H.H. (1955). Distribution of histamine among leucocytes and platelets. Blood *10*, 467.

Greaves, M.F. (1973). Antigenic recognition mechanisms. Haematologia. In press.

Greaves, M.W. (1968A). The mechanism of anaphylactic histamine release from rabbit leucocytes. Immunol. *15*, 743.

Greaves, M.W. (1968B). The role of the basophil leucocyte in anaphylaxis. PhD Thesis, Univ. of London.

Greaves, M.W. (1969). The effect of disodium cromoglycate and other inhibitors on in vitro anaphylactic histamine release from guinea pig basophil leucocytes. Int. Arch. Allergy *36*, 497.

Greaves, M.W. and Mongar, J.L. (1968). The histamine content of rabbit leucocytes and its release during in vitro anaphylaxis. Immunol. *15*, 733.

Green, M. and Lim, K.H. (1971). Bronchial asthma with Addison's disease. Lancet i, 1159.

Green, N.M. (1971). Possible modes of organisation of protein molecules in membranes. In: Proc. Biochem. Soc. Colloq, The proteins of membranes, p. 1.

Griffin, D., Tachibana, D.K., Nelson, B and Rosenberg, L.T. (1967). Contribution of tryptophan to the biologic properties of anti-dinitrophenyl antibodies. Immunochem. *4*, 23.

Grove, E.F. (1928). Studies in specific hypersensitiveness. XXXI. On passive transfer to atopic hypersensitiveness to monkeys. J. Immunol. *15*, 3.

Gryfe, A., Sanders, P.M. and Gardner, D.L. (1971). The mast cell in early rat adjuvant arthritis. Ann. Rheum. Dis. *30*, 24.

Gustafson, G.T., Stålenheim, G., Forsgren, A. and Sjöquist, J. (1968). Protein A from *Staphylococcus aureus*. IV. Production of anaphylaxis-like cutaneous and systemic reactions in non-immunized guinea pigs. J. Immunol. *100*, 530.

Haddad, J.H., Marsh, D.G. and Campbell, D.H. (1972). Studies on 'allergoids' prepared from naturally occurring allergens. II. Evaluation of allergenicity and assay of formalinized mixed grass pollen extracts. J. Allergy *49*, 197.

Haimovich, J., Sela, M., Dewdney, J.M. and Batchelor, F.R. (1967). Anti-penicilloyl antibodies detection with penicilloylated bacteriophage and isolation with a specific immunoadsorbent. Nature *214*, 1369.

Haimovich, J. and Sela, M. (1969). Protein-bacteriophage conjugates: application in detection of antibodies and antigens. Science *164*, 1279.

Hale, R., Cawley, L.P., Holman, J.G. and Minerd, B. (1967). Radio immunoelectrophoretic studies of antigen-binding capacity of atopic sera. Ann. Allergy *25*, 88.

Halpern, B.N. (1967). Personal Communication.

Halpern, B.N., Liacopoulos, P., Liacopoulos-Briot, M., Binaghi, R. and Van Neer, F. (1959). Patterns of in vitro sensitization of isolated smooth muscle tissues with precipitating antibody. Immunol. *2*, 351.

Halpern, B.N., Ky, T. and Robert, B. (1967). Clinical and immunological study of an exceptional case of reaginic type sensitisation to human seminal fluid. Immunol. *12*, 247.

Hanson, L.A. and Johansson, B. (1961). Immune electrophoretic studies of bovine milk and milk products. Acta Paediat. (Uppsala) *50*, 484.

Hastie, R. (1971). The antigen-induced degranulation of basophil leucocytes from atopic subjects, studied by phase-contrast microscopy. Clin. Exp. Immunol. *8*, 45.

Hawker, R., McLaughlan, P. and Stanworth, D.R. (1971). Unpublished observations.

Haye, K.R. (1965). Studies on the degranulation of basophil leucocytes in vitro in relation to allergic reactions. M.D. Thesis, Birmingham University.

Haye, K.R. and Schneider, R. (1966). The difference in behaviour of basophil leucocytes and mast cells towards compound 48/80. Brit. J. Pharmacol. *28*, 282.

Henney, C.S. (1965). Biological characteristics of structurally altered γG-globulin. PhD Thesis, Birmingham University.

Henney, C.S., Stanworth, D.R. and Gell, P.G.H. (1965). Demonstration of the exposure of new antigenic determinants following antigen-antibody combination. Nature *205*, 1079.

Henney, C.S. and Stanworth, D.R. (1966). Effect of antigen on the structural configuration of homologous antibody following antigen-antibody combination. Nature *210*, 1071.

Henney, C.S. and Ishizaka, K. (1968). Antigenic determinants specific for aggregated γG-globulins. J. Immunol. *100*, 718.

Henson, P.M. and Cochrane, C.G. (1969). A rabbit passive cutaneous anaphylactic reaction requiring complement, platelets and neutrophils. J. Exp. Med. *129*, 153.

Heremans, J. (1960). Les globulines sériques du système gamma. Leur nature et leur pathologie (Masson, Paris).

Heremans, J.F. and Vaerman, J.P. (1962). β_2A-globulin as a possible carrier of allergic reaginic activity. Nature *193*, 1091.

Higginbotham, R.D. and Karnella, S. (1971). The significance of the mast cell response to bee venom. J. Immunol. *106*, 233.

Hogarth-Scott, R.S., Howlett, B.J., McNicol, K.N., Simons, M.J. and Williams, H.E. (1971). IgE levels in the sera of asthmatic children. Clin. Exp. Immunol. *9*, 571.

Högberg, B. and Uvnäs, B. (1957). The mechanism of disruption of mast cells produced by compound 48/80. Acta Physiol. Scand. *41*, 345.

Högberg, B. and Uvnäs, B. (1960). Further observations on the disruption of rat mesentery mast cells caused by compound 48/80, antigen-antibody reaction, lecithinase A and decylamine. Acta Physiol. Scand. *48*, 133.

Horsfield, D.G.I. (1965). The effect of compound 48/80 on the rat mast cell. J. Path. Bact. *90*, 599.

Howard, A. and Virella, G. (1970). The separation of pooled human IgG into fractions by isoelectric focusing, and their electrophoretic and immunological properties. In: 17th Bruges Symp., Protides of the Biol. Fluids (1969), ed. H. Peeters, p. 449.

Hubscher, T., Watson, J.I. and Goodfriend, L. (1970A). Target cells of human ragweed-binding antibodies in monkey skin. I. Immunofluorescent localisation of cellular binding. J. Immunol. *104*, 1187.

Hubscher, T., Watson, J.I. and Goodfriend, L. (1970B). Target cells of human ragweed-binding antibodies in monkey skin. II. Immunoglobulin nature of ragweed binding antibodies with affinity for monkey skin mast cells. J. Immunol. *104*, 1196.

Humphrey, J.H. (1973). The nature of complement-induced lesions in membranes. Haematologia. In press.

Humphrey, J.H. and Porter, R.R. (1957). Reagin content of chromatographic fractions of human gamma-globulin. Lancet ii, 196.

Humphrey, J.H. and Dourmashkin, R.R. (1965). Electron microscope studies of immune cell lysis. In: Complement, eds. G.E.W. Wolstenholme and J. Knight (Churchill, London) p. 175.

Hunter, A., Feinstein, A. and Coombs, R.R.A. (1968). Immunoglobulin class of antibodies to cow's milk casein in infant sera and evidence for low molecular weight IgM antibodies. Immunol. *15*, 381.

Hunter, W.M. and Greenwood, F.C. (1962). Preparation of Iodine-131 labelled human growth hormone of high activity. Nature *194*, 495.

Hurlimann, J. and Ovary, Z. (1965). Relationship between affinity of anti-dinitrophenyl antibodies and their biologic activities. J. Immunol. *95*, 768.

Ingelman, B., Gröwall, A., Gelin, L. and Eliasson, R. (1969). Properties and applications of dextrans (Almqvist and Wiksell, Stockholm).

Ishizaka, K. (1963). Gamma globulin and molecular mechanisms in hypersensitivity reactions. Prog. in Allergy *7*, 32.

Ishizaka, K. (1970). The significance of immunoglobulin E in reaginic hypersensitivity. Annals Allergy *28*, 189.

Ishizaka, K. and Campbell, D.H. (1959). Biological activity of soluble antigen-antibody complex. V. Change of optical rotation by the formation of skin reactive complexes. J. Immunol. *83*, 318.

Ishizaka, K., Ishizaka, T. and Hornbook, M.M. (1963). Blocking of Prausnitz-Küstner sensitization with reagin by normal human β_2A-globulin. J. Allergy *34*, 395.

Ishizaka, K., Ishizaka, T. and Hornbrook, M.M. (1964). Immunochemical aspects of P-K reaction. Federation Proc. *23*, 402 (Abstr.).

Ishizaka, K., Ishizaka, T. and Hornbrook, M.M. (1966A). Physico-chemical properties of human reaginic antibody. IV. Presence of a unique immunoglobulin as carrier of reaginic activity. J. Immunol. *97*, 75.

Ishizaka, K., Ishizaka, T. and Hornbrook, M.M. (1966B). Physico-chemical properties of reaginic antibody. V. Correlation of reaginic activity with γE-globulin antibody. J. Immunol. *97*, 840.

Ishizaka, K., Ishizaka, T. and Lee, E.H. (1966C). Physico-chemical properties of reaginic antibody. II. Characteristic properties of reaginic antibody from γA isohemagglutinin and γD-globulin. J. Allergy *37*, 336.

Ishizaka, K. and Ishizaka, T. (1966). Physico-chemical properties of reaginic antibodies. I. Association of reaginic activity with an immunoglobulin other than γA or γG-globulin. J. Allergy *37*, 169.

Ishizaka, K. and Ishizaka, T. (1967). Identification of E-antibodies as carrier of reaginic activity. J. Immunol. *99*, 1187.

Ishizaka, K., Ishizaka, T. and Arbesman, C.E. (1967). Induction of passive cutaneous anaphylaxis in monkeys by human γE antibody. J. Allergy *39*, 254.

Ishizaka, K., Ishizaka, T. and Hornbrook, M.M. (1967). Allergen-binding activity of γE, γG and γA antibodies in sera from atopic patients. J. Immunol. *98*, 490.

Ishizaka, K., Ishizaka, T. and Menzel, A.E.O. (1967). Physico-chemical properties of reaginic antibody. VI. Effect of heat on γE, γG and γA antibodies in the sera of ragweed sensitive patients. J. Immunol. *99*, 610.

Ishizaka, K., Ishizaka, T. and Terry, W.D. (1967). Antigenic structure of γE-globulin and reaginic antibody. J. Immunol. *99*, 849.

Ishizaka, K. and Ishizaka, T. (1968A). Human reaginic antibodies and immunoglobulin E. J. Allergy *42*, 330.

Ishizaka, K. and Ishizaka, T. (1968B). Reversed type allergic skin reactions by anti-γE-globulin antibodies in humans and monkeys. J. Immunol. *100*, 554.

Ishizaka, K. and Ishizaka, T. (1968). Induction of erythema wheal reactions by soluble antigen-γE antibody complexes in humans. J. Immunol. *101*, 68.

Ishizaka, K. and Ishizaka, T. (1968). Physicochemical properties of human reaginic antibodies. VIII. Effect of reduction and alkylation on γE antibodies. J. Immunol. *102*, 69.

Ishizaka, K., Ishizaka, T. and Tada, T. (1969). Immunoglobulin E in the monkey. J. Immunol. *103*, 445.

Ishizaka, K. and Ishizaka, T. (1970). Biological function of γE antibodies and mechanisms of reaginic hypersensitivity. Clin. Exp. Immunol. *6*, 25.

Ishizaka, K., Tomioka, H. and Ishizaka, T. (1970). Mechanism of passive sensitization. I. Presence of IgE and IgG molecules on human leucocytes. J. Immunol. *105*, 1459.

Ishizaka, K. and Ishizaka, T. (1971). Mechanisms of reaginic hypersensitivity: a review. Clin. Allergy *1*, 9.

Ishizaka, T., Ishizaka, K., Salmon, S. and Fudenburg, H. (1967). Biologic activities of aggregated γ-globulins. VIII. Aggregated immunoglobulins of different classes. J. Immunol. *99*, 82.

Ishizaka, T., Ishizaka, K., Orange, R.P. and Austen, K.F. (1971). Pharmacologic inhibition of antigen-induced release of histamine and slow reacting substance of anaphylaxis (SRS-A) mediated by human γE antibody. J. Immunol. *106*, 1267.

Ishizaka, T., Taa, T. and Ishizaka, K. (1968). Fixation of C and C1a by rabbit γG and γM antibodies with particulate and soluble antigens. J. Immunol. *100*, 1145.

James, K. (1965). A study of the α2-macroglobulin homologues of various species. Immunol. *8*, 55.

James, K. and Stanworth, D.R. (1965). Studies on the chromatography of purified proteins on DEAE cellulose. II. The chromatographic characteristics of purified serum proteins. J. Chromat. *15*, 336.

Jaques, R. (1965). Non-specific effects of synthetic corticotrophin polypeptides. Int. Arch. Allergy *28*, 221.

Jaques, R. and Brugger, M. (1969). Synthetic polypeptides related to corticotrophin acting as histamine liberators. Pharmacol. *2*, 361.

Jarrett, E.E.E., Orr, T.S.C. and Riley, P. (1971). Inhibition of allergic reaction due to competition for mast cell sensitization sites by two reagins. Clin. Exp. Immunol. *9*, 585.

Jarrett, W.F.H., Miller, H.R.P. and Murray, M. (1969). Immunological mechanisms in mucous membranes. In: Symposium on Resistance to infectious diseases (Univ. of Saskatchewan).

Jasani, B. (1971). Personal communication.

Jasani, B. and Stanworth, D.R. (1971). To be published.

Jefferis, R., Weston, P.D., Stanworth, D.R. and Clamp, J.R. (1968). Relationship between the papain sensitivity of human γG immunoglobulins and their heavy chain subclass. Nature, *219*, 646.

Johansson, S.G.O. (1967). Raised levels of a new immunoglobulin class (IgND) in asthma. Lancet ii, 1.

Johansson, S.G.O. (1968). Serum IgND levels in healthy children and adults. Int. Arch. Allergy *34*, 1.

Johansson, S.G.O. (1968). Immunoglobulin ND(IgE). Clinical and immunological studies. Acta Universitatis Upsaliensis No. 52.

Johansson, S.G.O. and Bennich, H. (1967). Immunological studies of an atypical (myeloma) immunoglobulin. Immunol. *13*, 381–394.

Johansson, S.G.O., Bennich, H. and Wide, L. (1968). A new class of immunoglobulin in human serum. Immunol. *14*, 265.

Johansson, S.G.O., Bennich, H., Berg, T. and Högman, C. (1970). Some factors influencing serum IgE levels in atopic diseases. Clin. Exp. Immunol. *6*, 43.

Johnson, A.R. and Moran, N.C. (1970). Inhibition of the release of histamine from rat mast cells: the effect of cold and adrenergic drugs on release of histamine by compound 48/80 and antigen. J. Pharmacol. Exp. Therap. *175*, 632.

Johnson, P. and Thorne, H.V. (1958). Grass pollen extracts. I. The general properties of aqueous extracts of rye grass pollen. Int. Arch. Allergy *13*, 257.

Johnson, P. and Marsh, D.G. (1965). Isoallergens from rye grass pollen. Nature (Lond.) *206*, 935.

Johnson, P. and Marsh, D.G. (1966A). Allergens from common rye grass pollen (*Lolium perenne*). I. Chemical composition and structure. Immunochem. *3*, 91.

Johnson, P. and Marsh, D.G. (1966B). Allergens from common rye grass pollen (*Lolium perenne*). II. The allergenic determinants and carbohydrate moiety. Immunochem. *3*, 101.

Johnston, D.E. and Dutton, A. (1968). The value of hyposensitisation therapy for bronchial asthma in children. A 14 year study. Pediatrics *42*, 793.

Jones, V.E. and Ogilvie, B.M. (1971). Protective immunity to *Nippostongylus brasiliensis*: the sequence of events which expels worms from rat intestine. Immunol. *20*, 549.

Juhlin, L., Johansson, S.G.O., Bennich, H., Högman, C. and Thyresson, N. (1969). Immunoglobulin E in dermatoses. Levels in atopic dermatisis and urticaria. Arch. Dermatol. *100*, 12.

Kabat, E.A., Turino, G.M., Tarrow, A.B. and Maurer, P.H. (1957). Studies on the immunochemical basis of allergic reactions to dextran in man. J. Clin. Invest. *36*, 1160.

Kabat, E.A. and Bezer, A.E. (1958). The effect of variation in molecular weight on the antigenicity of dextran in man. Arch. Biochem. Biophys. *78*, 306.

Kabat, E.A. and Mayer, M.M. (1961). Experimental Immunochemistry, 2nd edition (Charles. C. Thomas, Springfield, Illinois, U.S.A.).

Kalter, S.S. (1969). Baboons. In: *Primates in medicine,* Vol. 2, ed. W.I.B. Beveridge (Karger) p. 45.

Kanyerezi, B., Jaton, J.C. and Bloch, K.T. (1971). Human rat γE: serologic evidence of homology. J. Immunol. *106*, 1411.

Katz, G. and Cohen, S. (1941). Experimental evidence for histamine release in allergy. J. Am. Med. Assoc. *117*, 1782.

Kay, A.B. (1970). Studies on eosinophil leucocyte migration. II. Factors specifically chemotactic for eosinophils and neutrophils generated from guinea pig serum by antigen-antibody complexes. Clin. Exp. Immunol. *7*, 723.

Kay, A.B., Stechschulte, D.J. and Austen, K.F. (1971). An eosinophil leukocyte chemotactic factor of anaphylaxis. J. Exp. Med. *133*, 602.

Keller, R. (1961). Zum Mechanismus der Mastzell-disruption. Path. Microbiol. *24*, 932.

Keller, R. (1964). Zytolytische Aktivität von Lysolecithin. Helv. Physiol. Pharmocal. Acta *22*, C24.

Keller, R. (1966). Tissue mast cells in immune responses. Monographs in Allergy, Vol. 2 (American Elsevier Publ. Inc.).

Keller, R. (1971). Cited in V.E. Jones and B.M. Ogilvie. Immunol. *20*, 549.

Keogh, R. (1970). A study of the immunochemical heterogeneity of rabbit immunoglobulin-G. PhD. Thesis, Birmingham University.

Keogh, R. and Stanworth, D.R. (1972). The heterogeneity of rabbit immunoglobulin G. In preparation.

King, C.A. and Francis, G.E. (1967). Absorption of heterologous γ-globulins by chopped guinea pig lung. Immunol. *13*, 1.

King, T.P. and Norman, P.S. (1962). Isolation studies of allergens from ragweed pollen. Biochem. *1*, 709.

King, T.P., Norman, P.S. and Connell, J.T. (1964). Isolation and characterisation of allergens from ragweed pollen. II. Biochem. *3*, 458.

King, T.P., Norman, P.S. and Lichtenstein, L.M. (1967A). Isolation and characterisation of allergens from ragweed pollen. IV. Biochem. *6*, 1992.

King, T.P., Norman, P.S., and Lichenstein, L.M. (1967B) Studies of ragweed pollen allergens. V. Annals Allergy *25*, 541.

Kleine, N., Matthes, M. and Müller (1957). Untersuchungen über die Trübungsreaktion nach Hoigne zum Nachweis einer Allergensensibilisierung. Klin. Wochschr. *35*, 132.

Kletter, B., Gery, I., Frier, S., Noah, Z. and Davies, M.A. (1971). Immunoglobulin E antibodies to milk proteins. Clin. Allergy *1*, 249.

Klibansky, C., London, Y., Frenkel, A. and De Vries, A. (1968). Enhancing action of synthetic and natural basic polypeptides on erythrocyte-ghost phospholipid hydrolysis by phospholipase A. Biochim. Biophys. Acta *150*, 15.

Knox, R.B. and Heslop-Harrison, J. (1969). Cytochemical localization of enzymes in the wall of the pollen grain. Nature (Lond.) *223*, 92.

Knox, R.B. and Heslop-Harrison, J. (1970). Scanning electron microscopy of fresh leaves of pinguicula. Science *167*, 172.

Knox, R.B., Heslop-Harrison, J. and Reed, C. (1970). Localization of antigens associated with the pollen grain wall by immunofluorescence. Nature (Lond.) *225*, 1066.

Kobayashi, S., Girard, J.P. and Arbesman, C.E. (1967). Demonstration of human reagin in monkey tissues. III. In vitro passive sensitisation of monkey ileum with sera of atopic patients. Physiologic and enhancing experiments. J. Allergy *40*, 26.

Korotzer, J.L., Haddad, Z.H. and Lopapa, A.F. (1971). Detection of human IgE by a modified rat mast cell degranulation technique. Immunol. *20*, 245.

Kravis, L.P., Lecks, H.I. and Whitney, T. (1965). Basophil degranulation tests in atopic allergic states: a pilot study of ragweed pollen sensitive patients. J. Allergy *36*, 23.

Kremzner, L.T. and Wilson, I.B. (1961). A procedure for the determination of histamine. Biochim. Biophys. Acta *50*, 364.

Kruger, P.G., Diamant, B. and Scholander, L. (1970). Non-degranulating structural changes of rat mast cells induced by antigen and Toluidine Blue. Exp. Cell Res. *63*, 101.

Kuhns, W.J. (1961). Disappearance of diphtheria antitoxin from skin. Proc. Soc. Exp. Biol. Med. *108*, 63.

Kunz, M.L., Reisman, R.E. and Arbesman, C.E. (1967). Evaluation of penicillin hypersensitivity by newer immunological procedures. J. Allergy *40*, 135.

Lachmann, P.J., Munn, E.A. and Weissmann, G. (1970). Complement-mediated lysis of liposomes produced by the reactive lysis procedure. Immunol. *19*, 983.

Layton, L.L. (1965). Passive transfer of human atopic allergies into primates. J. Allergy *36*, 523.

Layton, L.L., Lee, S. and De Eds, F. (1961). Diagnosis of human allergy utilising passive skin-sensitisation in the monkey (*Macaca irus*). Proc. Soc. Exp. Biol. Med. *108*, 623.

Layton, L.L., Lee, S. and Yamanka, E. (1962). Allergen testing in monkeys passively sensitised by hayfever and asthma reagins of human sera. Nature *193*, 988.

Layton, L.L., Greer, W.E., Green, F.C. and Yamanaka, E. (1963). Passive transfer of human atopic allergies to catarrhine and platyrrhine primates of suborder anthropoidea. Int. Arch. Allergy *23*, 176.

Leddy, J.P., Freeman, G.L., Luz, A. and Todd, R.H. (1962). Inactivation of the skin-sensitizing antibodies of human allergy by thiols. Proc., Soc. Exp. Biol. Med. *111*, 7. 7.

Leemann, W., De Weck, A.L. and Schneider, C.H. (1969). Hypersensitivity to carboxymethyl cellulose as a cause of anaphylactic reactions to drugs in cattle. Nature (Lond.) *223*, 621.

Leonard, B.J., Eccleston, E., Jones, D., Lowe, J. and Turner, E. (1971). Basophilic leukaemia in the rat induced by a β-chlorethylamine-ICI 42464. Paper presented to the British Pathology Society.

Levin, R.A. (1967). An indirect basophil degranulation slide test for detection of immediate type hypersensitivity reactions. J. Immunol. *48*, 150.

Levine, B.B. (1965A). The nature of the antigen-antibody complexes which initiate anaphylactic reactions. I. A quantitative comparison of the abilities of non-toxic univalent, toxic univalent and multivalent benzyl penicilloyl haptens to evoke passive cutaneous anaphylaxis in the guinea pig. J. Immunol. *94*, 111.

Levine, B.B. (1965B). The nature of the antigen-antibody complexes which initiate anaphylactic reactions. II. The effect of molecular size on the abilities of homologous multivalent benzyl penicilloyl haptens to evoke PCA and passive Arthus reactions in guinea pigs. J. Immunol. *94*, 121.

Levine, B.B. (1966). Immunologic mechanisms of penicillin allergy. A haptenic model system for the study of allergic diseases of man. N. England J. Med. *275*, 1115.

Levine, B.B. and Ovary, Z. (1961). Studies on the mechanisms of the formation of the penicillin antigen. III. The N-(D-α-benzyl penicilloyl) group as an antigenic determinant responsible for hypersensitivity to penicillin G. J. Exp. Med. *114*, 875.

Levine, B.B. and Zolov, D.M. (1969). Prediction of penicillin allergy by immunological tests. J. Allergy *43*, 231.

Levine, B.B. and Vaz, N.M. (1970). Effect of combinations of inbred strain, antigen and antigen dose on immune-reproductiveness and reagin production in the mouse. A potential mouse model for immune aspects of human atopic allergy. Int. Arch. Allergy *39*, 156.

Levine, B.B., Chang, H. and Vaz, N.M. (1971). The production of hapten-specific reaginic antibodies in the guinea pig. J. Immunol. *106*, 29.

Levine, P. and Coca, A.F. (1926). Studies in hypersensitiveness. XX. A quantitative study of the interaction of atopic reagin and atopen. XXI. A quantitative study of the atopic reagin in hayfever. The regulation of skin sensitivity to reagin content of serum. J. Immunol. *11*, 411, 435.

Levy, D.A. and Osler, A.G. (1966). Studies on the mechanisms of hypersensitivity phenomena. XIV. Passive sensitisation in vitro of human leucocytes to ragweed pollen antigen. J. Immunol. *97*, 203.

Levy, D.A. and Lichenstein, L.M. (1967). Unpublished observation, quoted in Lichenstein, L.M., Norman, P.S. and Connell, J.T. (1967).

Levy, D.A. and Carlton, J.A. (1969). Influence of temperature on the inhibition by colchicine of allergic histamine release. Proc. Soc. Exp. Biol. Med. *130*, 1333.

Lichenstein, L.M. (1968). Mechanisms of allergic histamine release from human leucocytes. In: C.I.O.M.S. Symp., Biochemistry of the acute allergic reactions, eds. Austen. K.F. and Becker, F.L. (Blackwell) p. 153.

Lichenstein, L.M. and Osler, A.G. (1964). Studies on the mechanisms of hypersensitivity phenomena. IX. Histamine release from human leucocytes by ragweed pollen antigen. J. Exp. Med. *120*, 507.

Lichenstein, L.M. and Osler, A.G. (1966B). Studies on the mechanisms of hypersensitivity phenomena. XI. The effect of normal human serum on the release of histamine from human leucocytes by ragweed pollen antigen. J. Immunol. *96*, 159.

Lichenstein, L.M. and Osler, A.G. (1966A). Studies on the mechanisms of hypersensitivity phenomena. XII. An in vitro study of the reaction between ragweed pollen antigen, allergic human serum and ragweed-sensitive human leucocytes. J. Immunol. *96*, 169.

Lichenstein, L.M., King, T.P. and Osler, A.G. (1966). In vitro assay of allergenic properties of ragweed pollen antigens. J. Allergy *38*, 174.

Lichenstein, L.M. Norman, P.S. and Connell, J.T. (1967). Comparison between skin-sensitising antibody titers and leucocyte sensitivity measurements as an index of severity of ragweed hay fever. J. Allergy *40*, 160.

Lichenstein, L.M. and Margolis, S. (1968). Histamine release in vitro: inhibition by catecholamines and methyl xanthines. Science *161*, 902.

Lidd, D. and Farr, R.S. (1962). Primary interaction between ^{131}I-labelled ragweed pollen and antibodies in the sera of humans and rabbits. J. Allergy *33*, 45.

Lidd, D. and Connell, J.T. (1964). Specific binding of an ^{131}I-labelled ragweed pollen fraction by sera of untreated sensitive humans. J. Allergy *35*, 289.

Lindqvist, K.J. (1968). A unique class of rabbit immunoglobulins eliciting passive cutaneous anaphylaxis in homologous skin. Immunochem. *5*, 525.

Ljaljevic, M., Ljaljevic, J. and Parker, C.W. (1968A). Modification of the amino groups of rabbit γG-globulin. I. The effect on skin sensitizing activity. J. Immunol. *100*, 1041.

Ljaljevic, M., Ljaljevic, J. and Parker, C.W. (1968B). Modification of the amino groups of rabbit γG-globulin. II. Selective effects on Fc function. J. Immunol. *100*, 1051.

Loveless, M.H. (1940). Immunological studies of pollinosis. I. The presence of two antibodies related to the same pollen antigen in the serum of treated hayfever patients. J. Immunol. *38*, 25.

Loveless, M.H. (1964). Reagin production in a healthy male who forms no detectable β_2A immunoglobulins. Federation Proc. *23*, 403 (Abstr.).

Mäkelä, O. (1966). Assay of anti-hapten antibody with the aid of hapten-coupled bacteriophage. Immunol. *10*, 81.

Malley, A. and Dobson, R.L. (1966). Isolation of the allergens of timothy grass pollen. Federation Proc. *25*, 729 (Abstr.).

Malley, A. and Perlman, F. (1966). Isolation of a reaginic antibody fraction with properties of γG-globulin. Proc. Soc. Exp. Biol. Med. *122*, 152.

Mancini, G., Carbonara, A.O., and Heremans, J.F. (1965). Immunochemical quantitation of antigens by single radial immunodiffusion. Immunochem. *2*, 235.

Marsh, D.G., Milner, F.H. and Johnson, P. (1966). The allergenic activity and stability of purified allergens from the pollen of common rye grass (*Lolium perenne*). Int. Arch. Allergy *29*, 521.

Marsh, D.G., Haddad, Z.H. and Campbell, D.H. (1970A). A new method for determining the distribution of allergenic fractions in biological materials: its application to grass pollen extracts. J. Allergy *46*, 107.

Marsh, D.G., Lichenstein, L.M. and Campbell, D.H. (1970B). Studies on 'Allergoids' prepared from naturally occuring antigens. I. Assay of allergenicity and antigenicity of formalinized rye group I component. Immunol. *18*, 705.

Martin, R.R. and White, A. (1969). The in vitro release of leucocyte histamine by staphylococcal antigens. J. Immunol. *102*, 437.

Matthews, N. and Stanworth, D.R. (1972). Further studies on the nature of the reactivity of rheumatoid factor with human immunoglobulin G. In preparation.

May, C.D., Lyman, M., Alberto, R. and Cheng, J. (1970). Procedures for immunochemical study of histamine release from leucocytes with small volume of blood. J. Allergy *46*, 12.

McEwen, C.R., Stallard, R.W. and Juhos, E.Th. (1968). Separation of biological particles by centrifugal elutriation. Anal. Biochem. *23*, 369.

McLaughlan, P. (1971). The development of radio-immunoassays for the study of skin sensitising antibodies (IgE). Birmingham M.Sc Thesis (Unpublished).

McLaughlan, P., Stanworth, D.R., Kennedy, J.F., and Cho Tun, H. (1971). Use of antibody-coupled cellulose as immunosorbent in the estimation of human immunoglobulin IgE. Nature (New Biol.) *232*, 245.

McLaughlan, P. and Stanworth, D.R. (1972). Studies of the fate of radio-labelled myeloma IgE following injection into baboons. In preparation.

Middleton, E. (1960). Passive transfer of atopic hypersensitivity. Proc. Soc. Exp. Biol. and Med. *104*, 245.

Middleton, E. and Sherman, W.B. (1960). Relationship of complement to allergic histamine release in blood of ragweed-sensitive subjects. J. Allergy *31*, 441.

Miescher, P. and Cooper, N. (1960). The fixation of soluble antigen-antibody complexes upon thrombocytes. Vox Sang. *5*, 138.

Miller, J.J. and Cole, L.J. (1968). Proliferation of mast cells after antigenic stimulation in adult rats. Nature *217*, 263.

Minden, P., Reid, R.T. and Farr, R.S. (1966). A comparison of some commonly used methods for detecting antibodies to bovine albumin in human serum. J. Immunol. *96*, 180.

Mongar, J.L. (1965). Mechanism of passive sensitisation. Arch. exp. path. U. Pharmakol. *250*, 124.

Mongar, J.L. and Schild, H.O. (1953). Quantitative measurement of the histamine releasing activity of a series of monoalkyl amines using minced guinea pig lung. Brit. J. Pharmacol. *8*, 103.

Mongar, J.L. and Schild, H.O. (1957). Inhibition of the anaphylactic reaction. J. Physiol. *135*, 301.

Mongar, J. and Schild, H.O. (1958). The effect of calcium and *p*H on the anaphylactic reaction. J. Physiol. *140*, 272.

Mongar, J.L. and Schild, O. (1962). Cellular mechanisms in anaphylaxis. Physiol. Revs. *42*, 226.

Mongar, J.L. and Winne, D. (1966). Further studies of the mechanism of passive sensitization. J. Physiol. *182*, 79.

Moran, N.C., Uvnäs, B. and Westerholm, B. (1962). Release of 5-hydroxytryptamine and histamine from rat mast cells. Acta Physiol. Scand. *56*, 26 .

Morse, H.C., Austen, K.F. and Bloch, K.J. (1969). Biologic properties of rat antibodies. III. Histamine release mediated by two classes of antibodies. J. Immunol. *102*, 327.

Morse, S.J. and Bray, K.K. (1969). The occurrence and properties of leucocytosis and lymphocytosis-stimulating material in the supernatant fluids of *Bordetella pertussis* cultures. J. Exp. Med. *129*, 523.

Mortelmans, J. (1969). Tranquillization and anaesthesia. In: *Primates in medicine*,Vol. 2, p. 113, ed. W.I.B. Beveridge (Karger).

Mota, I. (1959). Effect of antigen and octylamine on mast cells and histamine content of sensitised guinea pig tissues. J. Physiol. (Lond.) *147*, 425.

Mota, I. (1964). The mechanism of anaphylaxis. I. Production and biological properties of mast cell sensitising antibody. Immunol. *7*, 681.

Moussatché, H. and Danon, A.P. (1957). The effect of succinate and malonate upon the histamine released during the anaphylactic reaction in vitro. Naturwissenschaften *44*, 637.

Movat, H.J., Di Lorenzo, N.L., Taichman, N.S., Berger, S. and Stein, H. (1967). Suppression by antihistamines of passive cutaneous anaphylaxis produced with anaphylactic antibody in the guinea pig. J. Immunol. *98*, 230.

Mulligan, W., Urquhart, G.M., Jennings, F.W. and Neilson, J.T.M. (1965). Immunological studies on *Nippostrongylus brasiliensis* infection in the rat: the 'self-cure' phenomenom. Exp. Parasit. *16*, 341.

Murray, M., Miller, H.R.P. and Jarrett, W.F.H., (1968). The globule leucocyte and its derivation from the subepithelial mast cell. Lab. Invest. *19*, 222.

Murray, M., Jarrett, W.F.H. and Jennings, F.W. (1971). Mast cells and macromolecular leak reactions. The influence of sex of rats infected with *Nippotrongylus brasiliensis*. Immunol. *21*, 17.

Murray, M., Miller, H.R.P., Sanford, J. and Jarrett, W.F.H. (1971). 5-Hydroxytryptamine in intestinal immunological reactions. Its relationship to mast cell activity and worm expulsion in rats infected with *Nippostrongylus brasiliensis.* Int. Arch. Allergy *40*, 236.

Murray, M., Smith, W.D., Wadell, A.H. and Jarrett, W.F.H. (1971). The effect of inhibitors of histamine and 5-hydroxytryptamine on intestinal immunological reactions. Exp. Parasit. *30*, 58.

Newcomb, R.W. and Ishizaka, K. (1967). Human diphtheria antitoxin in immunoglobulin classes IgG and IgA. J. Immunol. *99*, 40.

Newcomb, R.W. and Ishizaka, K. (1969). Skin reactions to anti-γE antibody in atopic, non-atopic and immunologically deficient children and adults. J. Allergy *43*, 292.

Nicholson, G.L. Masouredis, S.P. and Singer, S.J. (1971). Quantitative two-dimensional ultrastructural distribution of Rh_0(D) antigenic sites on human erythrocyte membranes. Proc. Nat. Acad. Sci. *68*, 1416.

Nilsson, W.K. (1971). Synthesis and secretion of IgE by an established human myeloma cell line. Clin. Exp. Immunol. *9*, 785.

Nisonoff, A. and Mandy, W.J. (1962). Quantitative estimation of the hybridisation of rabbit antibodies. Nature *194*, 355.

Noah, J. (1954). Release of histamine in the blood of ragweed-sensitive individuals. J. Allergy *25*, 210.

Noah, J. and Brand, A. (1955). Correlation of blood histamine release and skin test response to multiple antigens. J. Allergy *26*, 385.

Noah, J.W. and Brand, A. (1961). A fluorimetric method to determine levels of histamine in human plasma. J. Allergy *32*, 236.

Noelken, M.E., Nelson, C.A., Buckley, C.E. and Tanford, C. (1965). Gross conformation of rabbit *7S* γ-immunoglobulin and its papain cleaved fragments. J. Biol. Chem. *240*, 218.

Norman, P.S., (1969). A rational approach to desensitization. J. Allergy *44*, 129.

Norman, P.S., Winkenwerder, W.L. and Lichenstein, L.M. (1971). Maintenance immunotherapy in radweed hay fever booster injections at six week intervals. J. Allergy *47*, 273.

Nosal, R., Slorach, S.A. and Uvnäs, B. (1970). Quantitative correlation between degranulation and histamine release following exposure of rat mast cells to compound 48/40 in vitro. Acta Physiol. Scand. *80*, 215.

Nussenzweig, R.S., Merryman, C. and Benacerraf, B. (1964). Electrophoretic separation and properties of mouse anti-hapten antibodies involved in passive cutaneous anaphylaxis and passive hemolysis. J. Exp. Med. *120*, 315.

Nussenzweig, V., Benaceraff, B., Ovary, Z. (1969). Further evidence of the role of γ_1 guinea pig antibodies in mediating passive cutaneous anaphylaxis (PCA). J. Immunol. *103*, 1152.

Nussenzweig, V. and Green, I. (1971). Lack of correlation between the net charge of antigen and antibodies in guinea pigs immunized with some charged antigens. J. Immunol. *106*, 1089.

Ogawa, M., Kochwa, S., Smith, C., Ishizaka, K. and McIntyre, O.R. (1969). Clinical aspects of IgE immunoglobulin. New England J. Med. *281*, 1217.

Ogawa, M., Berger, P.A., McIntyre, O.R., Glendenning, W.E. and Ishizaka, K. (1971). IgE in atopic dermatitis. Arch. Dermatol. *103*, 575.

Ogilvie, B.M. (1967). Reagin-like antibodies in rats infected with the nematode parasite *Nippostrongylus brasiliensis.* Immunol. *12*, 113.

Opit, L.J., Potter, H. and Charnock, J.S. (1966). The effect of anions on (N^+ + K^+) activated ATP-ase. Biochim. Biophys. Acta *120*, 159.

Orange, R.P., Valentine, M.D. and Austen, K.F. (1968). Antigen-induced release of slow reacting substance of anaphylaxis (SRS-A rat) in rats prepared with homologous antibody. J. Exp. Med. *127*, 767.

Orange, R.P., Stechschulte, D.J. and Austen, K.F. (1970). Immunochemical and biologic properties of rat IgE. II. Capacity to mediate the immunologic release of histamine and slow reacting substance of anaphylaxis (SRS-A). J. Immunol. *105*, 1087.

Orr, T.S.C. and Blair, A.M.J.N. (1969). Potentiated reagin response to egg albumin and conalbumin in *Nippostrongylus brasiliensis* infected rats. Life Sciences *8*, 1073.

Orr, T.S.C. and Cox, J.S.G. (1969). Disodium cromoglycate, an inhibitor of mast cell degranulation and histamine release induced by phospholipase A. Nature *223*, 197.

Orr, T.S.C., Pollard, M.C., Gwilliam, J. and Cox, J.S.G. (1970). Mode of action of disodium cromoglycate; studies on immediate-type hypersensitivity reaction using double sensitisation with two antigenically distinct rat reagins. Clin. Exp. Immunol. *7*, 745.

Orr, T.S.C., Hall, D.F., Gwilliam, J.M. and Cox, J.S.G. (1971). The effect of disodium cromoglycate on the release of histamine and degranulation of rat mast cells induced by compound 48/80. Life Sciences *10*, 805.

Orr, T.S.C., Riley, P. and Doe, J.E. (1971). Potentiated reagin response to egg albumin in *Nippostrongylus brasiliensis* infected rats. II. Time course of the reagin response. Immunol. *20*, 185.

Osler, A.G. (1961). Functions of the complement system. Advan. Immunol. *1*, 131.

Osler, A.G., Lichenstein, L.M. and Levy, D.A. (1968). In vitro studies of human reaginic antibodies. Adv. Immunol. *8*, 183.

Ovary, Z. (1958). Immediate reactions in the skin of experimental animals provoked by antibody-antigen interaction. Prog. Allergy *5*, 549.

Ovary, Z. (1965). PCA reaction and its elicitation by species specific immunoglobulin and fragments. Federation Proc. *24*, 94.

Ovary, Z. and Karush, F. (1961). Studies on the immunologic mechanisms of anaphylaxis. II. Sensitising and combining capacity in vitro of fractions separated from papain digests of antihapten antibody. J. Immunol. *86*, 146.

Ovary, Z., Benacerraf, B. and Bloch, K.J. (1963). Properties of guinea pig 7S antibodies. II. Identification of antibodies involved in passive cutaneous and systemic anaphylaxis. J. Exp. Med. *117*, 951.

Ovary, Z. and Taranta, A. (1963). Passive cutaneous anaphylaxis with antibody fragment. Science *140*, 193.

Ovary, Z., Bloch, K.J. and Benacerraf, B. (1964). Identification of rabbit, monkey and dog antibodies with PCA activity for guinea pigs. Proc. Soc. Exp. Biol. N.Y. *116*, 840.

Ovary, Z., Vaz, N.M. and Warner, N.L. (1972). Immunol. In press. Cited in Tigelaar, R.E., Vaz, N.M. and Ovary, Z. (1971).

Padawar, J. (1970). The reaction of rat mast cells with poly-lysine. J. Cell. Biol. *47*, 352.

Paraskevas, F. and Goodman, J.W. (1965). Components of fraction III and pepsin-digested fraction III from papain-digested rabbit γ-globulin. Immunochem. *2*, 391.

Parish, W.E. (1967). Release of histamine and slow reacting substance with mast cell changes after challenge of human lung sensitised passively with reagin in vitro. Nature (Lond.) *215*, 738.

Parish, W.E. (1969). Detection of reagins, IgG, IgA and IgM antibodies in human sera. Int. Arch. Allergy *36*, 245.

Parish, W.E. (1970). Absorption of reagin by human tissues in vitro. Int. Arch. Allergy *37*, 184.

Parish, W.E. (1970). Short-term anaphylactic IgG antibodies in human sera. Lancet ii, 591.

Parker, C.W., Kern, M. and Eisen, H.N. (1962A). Polyfunctional dinitrophenyl haptens as reagents for elicitation of immediate type allergic skin responses. J. Exp. Med. *115*, 789.

Parker, C.W., De Weck, A.L., Kern, M. and Eisen, H.N. (1962B). The preparation and some properties of penicillenic acid derivatives relevant to penicillin hypersensitivity. J. Exp. Med. *115*, 803.

Parker, C.W., Shapiro, T., Kern, M. and Eisen, H.N. (1962C). Hypersensitivity to penicillenic acid derivatives in human beings with penicillin allergy. J. Exp. Med. *115*, 821.

Paton, W.D.M. (1958). The release of histamine. Prog. Allergy *5*, 79.

Patterson, R. (1969). Laboratory models of reaginic allergy. Prog. Allergy *13*, 332.

Patterson, R. and Correa, J. (1959). The demonstration of a quantitiative relationship between the skin-sensitising antibody and antigen. Int. Arch. Allergy *15*, 335.

Patterson, R. and Sparks, D.B. (1962). The passive transfer to normal dogs of skin reactivity, asthma and anaphylaxis from a dog with spontaneous ragweed pollen hypersensitivity. J. Immunol. *88*, 262.

Patterson, R., Fink, J.N., Nishimura, E.T. and Pruzansky, J.J. (1965). The passive transfer of immediate type hypersensitivity from man to other primates. J. Clin. Invest. *44*, 140.

Patterson, R., Miyamato, T., Reynolds, L. and Pruzansky, J.J. (1967). Comparative studies of two models of allergic respiratory disease. Int. Arch. Allergy *32*, 31.

Patterson, R. and Pruzansky, J.J. (1968). Inhibition of reagin-induced passive cutaneous anaphylaxis. Lancet ii, 1395.

Paul, W. and Weir, D.M. (1969). Histamine release from human lung by specific antisera. Clin. Exp. Immunol. *5*, 311.

Paul, C., Shimizu, A., Kohler, H. and Putnam, F.W. (1971). Structure of the hinge region of the μ chain of human IgM immunoglobulins. Science *172*, 69.

Pedersen-Bjergaard, J. (1969). Skin sensitising antibodies in serum from patients with penicillin allergy studied by passive transfer to monkey skin and compared with results obtained on human skin (Prausnitz-Küstner technique). Acta Allergol. *24*, 57.

Pepys, J., Hargreave, F.E., Longbottom, J.L. and Faux, J. (1969). Allergic reactions of the lungs to enzymes of *Bacillus subtilis*. Lancet ii, 1181.

Perelmutter, L. Rose, B. and Goodfriend, L. (1969). The relationship between the skin-sensitising antibody and γA in the sera of ragweed-allergic individuals. J. Allergy *37*, 236.

Perelmutter, L. and Khera, K., (1970). A study on the detection of human reagins with rat peritoneal mast cells. Int. Arch. Allergy *39*, 27.

Perera, B.A.V. and Mongar, J.L. (1965). Effect of anoxia, glucose and thioglycollate on anaphylactic and compound 48/80 induced histamine release in isolated rat mast cells. Immunol. *8*, 519.

Perlman, F. and Layton, L.L. (1967). Stability and behaviour of reaginic antibodies: effects of freezing, thawing and lyophilizing on skin sensitising activity of reaginic sera. J. Allergy *39*, 205.

Perlman, P. and Holm, G. (1970). Cytotoxic effects of lymphoid cells in vitro. Adv. Immunol. *11*, 117.

Pernis, B.; Forni, L. and Amante, L. (1970). Immunoglobulin spots on the surface of rabbit lymphocytes. J. Exp. Med. *132*, 1001.

Perry, W.L.M. (1956). Skin histamine. In: Ciba Symposium on Histamine, eds. G.E.W. Wolstenholme and C.M. O'Connoy, (J. and A. Churchill) p. 242.

Perutz, M.F. (1970). Stereochemistry of cooperative effects in haemoglobin. Nature *228*, 726.

Pike, B.L. and Robinson, W.A. (1970). Human bone marrow colony growth in agar-gel. J. Cell. Physiol. *76*, 77.

Pondman, K. (1971). Personal communication.

Poole, A.R., Howell, J.I. and Lucy, J.A. (1970). Lysolecithin and cell fusion. Nature (Lond.) *227*, 810.

Porter, R.R. (1959). The hydrolysis of rabbit γ-globulin and antibodies with crystalline papain. Biochem. J. *73*, 119.

Portier, P. and Richet, C. (1902). De l'action anaphylactique de certains venims. Compt. Rend. Soc. Biol. *54*, 170.

Prahl, J.W. (1967). Enzymatic degradation of the Fc fragment of rabbit immunoglobulin IgG. Biochem. J. *104*, 647.

Prausnitz, C. and Küstner, H. (1921). Studien über die Überempfindlichkeit. Zbl. Bakt. I. Abt. Orig. *86*, 160.

Prouvost-Danon, A., Stiffel, O., Moulton, D. and Biozzi, G. (1971). Anaphylactic antibodies in mice genetically selected for antibody production. Immunol. *20*, 25.

Pruzansky, J.J., Patterson, R. and Feinberg, S.M. (1962). Binding of ragweed allergen labelled with iodine-131 by sera of untreated allergic subjects. Nature *195*, 1113.

Pruzansky, J.J., Patterson, R. and Feinberg, S.M. (1962). Studies on reactions of human allergic serum with serum protein antigens. II. Method of quantitative demonstration by a coprecipitation technique. J. Allergy *33*, 381.

Pruzansky, J.J. and Patterson, R. (1964). Binding of I^{131}-labelled ragweed antigen by sera of ragweed-sensitive individuals. J. Allergy *35*, 1.

Pruzansky, J.J. and Paterson, R. (1966). The interaction of antigen with leucocytes of allergic individuals. J. Immunol. *97*, 854.

Pruzansky, J.J., and Patterson, R. (1967). Histamine release from leucocytes of hypersensitive individuals. II. Reduced sensitivity of leucocytes after injection therapy. J. Allergy *39*, 44.

Pruzansky, J.J. and Patterson, R. (1970). Decrease in basophils after incubation with specific antigen of leucocytes from allergic donors. Int. Arch. Allergy *38*, 522.

Radermecker, M. (1969). Presence of human reagin in immunochemically pure IgG serum fractions. Acta Allergologica *24*, 1.

Rademecker, M. and Goodfriend, L. (1968). Inhibition of reagin-induced passive cutaneous anaphylaxis. Lancet ii, 1086.

Rappaport, B.Z. and Becker, E.L. (1949). Quantitative studies in skin testing. IV. The volume-response relationship. J. Allergy *20*, 358.

Reid, R.T., Minden, P. and Farr, R.S. (1966). Reaginic activity associated with IgG immunoglobulin. J. Exp. Med. *123*, 845.

Reid, R.T., Minden, P. and Farr, R.S. (1968). Biological and chemical differences among proteins having reaginic activity. J. Allergy *41*, 326.

Reisman, R.E., Arbesman, C.E. and Yagi, Y. (1965). Radioimmunoelectrophoretic studies of ragweed-binding antibodies in allergic sera. J. Allergy *36*, 362.

Revoltella, R. and Ovary, Z. (1969). Preferential production of rabbit reaginic antibodies. Int. Arch. Allergy *36*, 282.

Richerson, H., Cheng, H. and Sebohm, P. (1968). Heterogeneity of rabbit anti-ovalbumin antibodies sensitising human, guinea pig and rabbit skin. J. Immunol. *101*, 1291.

Richter, W. (1970). Absence of immunogenic impurities in clinical dextran tested by passive cutaneous anaphylaxis. Int. Arch. Allergy *39*, 469.

Richter, W. (1971). Hapten inhibition of passive anaphylaxis in the antidextran system. Role of molecular size in anaphylacto-genicity and precipitability of dextran fractions. Int. Arch. Allergy *41*, 826.

Ritzen, M. (1966). Quantitative fluorescence microspectrophotometry of 5-hydroxytryptamine formaldehyde products in models and in mast cells. Exp. Cell. Res. *45*, 178.

Rixon, R.H., Whitfield, J.F. and MacManus, J.P. (1970). Stimulation of mitototic activity in rat bone marrow and thymus by exogenous adenosine 3′5′-monophosphate (cyclic AMP). Exp. Cell. Res. *63*, 110.

Robbins, K.C., Wu, H. and Hsein, B. (1966). Physical, chemical and immunochemical studies on a low ragweed pollen antigen. Immunochem. *3*, 71.

Robert, B. and Grabar, P. (1957). Dosage des groupements thiol protéiniques dans des réactions immunochimiques. Ann. Inst. Pasteur *92*, 56.

Roberts, A. (1966). Cellular localization and quantitation of tritiated antigen in mouse lymph nodes during early primary immune response. Amer. J. Path. *49*, 889.

Roberts, A. (1970). Early mast cell responses in mouse popliteal lymph nodes to localised primary antigenic stimulus. J. Immunol. *105*, 187.

Robison, G.A., Butcher, R.W. and Sutherland, E.W. (1967). Adenyl cyclase as an adrenergic receptor. Ann. N.Y. Acad. Sci. *139*, 703.

Robison, G.A. Butcher, R.W. and Sutherland, E.W. (1968). Cyclic AMP. Ann. Rev. Biochem. *37*, 149.

Rockey, J.H. and Kunkel, H.G. (1962). Unusual sedimentation and sulphydryl sensitivity of certain isohemagglutinins and skin sensitising antibody. Proc. Soc. Exp. Biol. *110*, 101.

Rodkey, L.S. and Freeman, M.J. (1969). Occurrence and properties of rabbit IgG1 antibody. J. Immunol. *102*, 713.

Rose, N.R., Kent, J.H., Reisman, R.E. and Arbesman, C.E. (1964). Passive sensitisation of monkey skin with sera of untreated atopic patients. J. Allergy *35*, 520.

Rothschild, A.M. (1966). Histamine release by basic compounds. In: *Handbook of Experimental Pharmacology*, eds. D. Eichler and A. Farah, Vol. 18, Part 1 (Histamines and antihistaminics), eds. M. Rocha and E. Silva (Springer-Verlag, New York) p. 386.

Rowe, D.S. (1968). Personal communication to S.G.O. Johansson quoted in Acta Universitatis Upsaliensis no. 52 (1968).

Rowe, D.S. (1969). Radioactive single radial diffusion: a method for increasing the sensitivity of immunochemical quantification of proteins in agar gel. Bull. Wld. Hlth. Org. *40*, 613.

Rowe, D.S. and Fahey, J.L. (1965). A new class of immunoglobulins. I. A unique myeloma protein. II. Normal serum IgD. J. Exp. Med. *121*; 171, 185.

Rowe, D.S., Tackett, L., Bennich, H., Ishizaka, K., Johansson, S.G.O. and Anderson, S.G. (1970). A research standard for human serum immunoglobulin E. Bull. Wld. Hlth. Org. *43*, 609.

Russo, J. and Lichenstein, L.M. (1967). Unpublished observations quoted in Lichenstein, L.M. (1968). In: C.I.O.M.S. Symp., Biochemistry of the acute allergic reactions, eds. Austen, K.F. and Becker, E.L. (Blackwell), p.153.

Salmon, S.E., Mackey, G. and Fudenberg, H.H. (1969). Sandwich solid phase radioimmunoassay for the quantitative determination of human immunoglobulins. J. Immunol. *103*, 129.

Salvaggio, J., Cavanaugh, J., Lowell, F.C. and Leskowitz, S. (1964). A comparison of the immunologic responses of normal and atopic individuals to intranasally administered antigen. J. Allergy *35*, 62.

Sampson, D. and Archer, G.T. (1967). Release of histamine from human basophils. Blood *29*, 722.

Schild, H.O. (1968). Mechanism of anaphylactic histamine release. In: C.I.O.M.S. Symp., Biochemistry of the acute allergic reactions, eds. Austen, K.F. and Becker, E.L. (Blackwell) p. 99.

Schild, H.O., Hawkins, D.F., Mongar, J.L. and Herxheimer, H. (1951). Reactions of isolated human asthmatic lung and bronchial tissue to a specific antigen. Histamine release and muscular contraction. Lancet ii, 376.

Schimmer, B.P., Veda, K. and Sato, G.H. (1968), Site of action of adrenocorticotropic hormone (ACTH) in adrenal cell cultures. Biochem. Biophys. Res. Commun. *32*, 806.

Schneider, C.H. and De Weck, A.L. (1965). A new chemical aspect of penicillin allergy: the direct reaction of penicillin with ϵ-amino groups. Nature (Lond.) *208*, 57.

Schneider, C.H. and De Weck, A.L. (1966). Chemische aspekte der penicillin allergie: die direkte penicilloylierung von ϵ-amino gruppen durch penicilline bei *p*H 7·4. Helv. Chim. Acta *49*, 1695.

Schwartz, A. (1965). A sodium and potassium-stimulated adenosine triphosphatase from cardiac tissues. IV. Localization and further studies of a basic protein inhibitory factor. Biochim. Biophys. Acta *100*, 202.

Schwartz, J., Klopstock, A. and Vardinon, N. (1965A). The role of the complement in the basophile cell test. Int. Arch. Allergy *26*, 142.

Schwartz, J., Klopstock, A., Zikert-Dudevani, P. and Hönig, S. (1965B). Detection of hypersensitivity by indirect rat mast cells degranulation. Int. Arch. Allergy *26*, 333.

Schwartzman, R.M., Rockey, J.H. and Halliwell, R.E. (1971). Immune reaginic antibody: characterisation of the spontaneous anti-ragweed and induced anti-DNP reaginic antibodies of the atopic dog. Clin. Exp. Immunol. *9*, 549.

Seegers, W. and Janoff, A. (1966). Mediators of inflammation in leukocyte lysosomes. VI. Partial purification and characterisation of a mast cell rupturing component J. Exp. Med. *124*, 833.

Sehon, A.H., Fyles, T.W., and Rose, B. (1955). Electrophoretic separation of skin sensitising antibody from the sera of ragweed-sensitive patients. J. Allergy *26*, 329.

Sela, M. and Mozes, E. (1966). Dependence of the chemical nature of antibodies on the net electrical charge of antigens. Proc. Nat. Acad. Sci. (Wash.) *55*, 445.

Sessa, G., Freer, J.H., Colacicco, G. and Weissmann, G. (1969). Interaction of a lytic polypeptide, melittin, with lipid membrane systems. J. Biol. Chem. *244*, 3575.

Shaw, G. and Yeadon, A. (1966). Chemical studies on the constitution of some pollen and spore membranes. J. Chem. Soc. (C) Org. *1*, 16.

Sheard, P., Killingback, P.G. and Blair, A.M.J.N. (1967). Antigen induced release of histamine and sera from human lung passively sensitised with reaginic serum. Nature *216*, 283.

Sheard, P. and Blair, A.M.J.N. (1970). Disodium cromoglycate. Activity in three in vitro models of the immediate hypersensitivity reaction in lung. Int. Arch. Allergy *38*, 217.

Shelley, W.B. (1962). New serological test for allergy in man. Nature (Lond.) *195*, 1181.

Shelley, W.B. (1965). Further experiences with the indirect basophil test. Arch. Dermatol. *91*, 165.

Shelley, W.B. and Juhlin, L. (1961). A new test for detecting anaphylactic sensitivity: the basophil reaction. Nature (Lond.) *191*, 1056.

Shelley, W.B. and Juhlin, L. (1962). Functional cytology of the human basophil in allergic and physiologic reactions: technic and atlas. Blood *19*, 208.

Sehon, A.H., Hollinger, H.Z., Harter, J.G., Schweitzer, A.E. and Rose, B. (1957). Localization of blocking antibody in sera of ragweed-sensitive individuals by starch electrophoresis. J. Allergy *28*, 229.

Shore, P.A., Bukhacter, A. and Cohn, V.H. (1959). A method for the fluorimetric assay of histamine in tissues. J. Pharmacol. Expt. Therap. *127*, 182.

Siqueria, M. and Nelson, R.A. (1961). Platelet agglutination by immune complexes and its possible role in hypersensitivity. J. Immunol. *86*, 516.

Siraganian, R.P. and Oliveira, B. (1968). The allergic response of rabbit platelets and leukocytes. Federation Proc. *27*, 315 (Abstr. 562).

Sjöquist (1971). Personal communication.

Skom, J.H. and Talmage, D.W. (1958). The role of non-precipitating insulin antibodies in diabetes. J. Clin. Invest. *37*, 783.

Skou, J.C. (1965). Enzymatic basis for active transport of Na^+ and K^+ across cell membrane. Physiol. Rev. *45*, 596.

Skou, J.C. and Hilberg, C. (1969). The effect of cations, g-strophanthin and oligomycin on the labelling from (^{32}P) ATP of the ($Na^+ - K^+$) activated enzyme system and the effect of cations and g-strophanthin on the labelling from (^{32}P) ITP and $^{32}P_i$. Biochim. Biophys. Acta *185*, 198.

Slavin, R.G. and Lewis, C.R. (1971). Enzyme asthma: an occupational disease of laundry detergent workers. J. Allergy *47* (Abstr. 26).

Smyth, D.G. and Utsumi, S. (1967). Structure at the hinge region in rabbit immunoglobulin G. Nature (Lond.) *216*, 332.

Sparks, D.B., Feinberg, S.M. and Becker, R.J. (1962). Immediate skin reactivity induced in atopics and non-atopic persons following injection of emulsified pollen extracts. J. Allergy *33*, 245.

Spieksma, F.ThM. (1970). Biological aspects of the house dust mite (*Dermatophagoides pteronyssinus*) in relation to house dust atopy. Clin. Exp. Immunol. *6*, 61.

Spieksma, F.ThM. and Voorhorst, R. (1969). Comparison of skin reactions to extracts of house dust, mites, and human skin scales. Acta Allergol. (kbk) *24*, 124.

Spies, J.R., Stevan, M.A. Stein, W.J. and Coulson, E.J. (1969). The Chemistry of Allergens. XX. New antigens generated by pepsin hydrolysis of bovine milk proteins. J. Allergy *45*, 208.

Squire, J.R. (1950). The relationship between horse dander and horse serum antigens in asthma. Clin. Sci. *9*, 127.

Stanley, R.G. and Linskens, H.F. (1965). Protein diffusion from germinating pollen. Physiol. Plant *18*, 47.

Stanworth, D.R. (1957A). The isolation and identification of horse dandruff allergen. Biochem. J. *65*, 582.

Stanworth, D.R. (1957B). The use of the gel-precipitation technique in the identification of horse dandruff allergen, and in the study of the serological relationship between horse dandruff and horse serum proteins. Int. Arch. Allergy *11*, 170.

Stanworth, D.R. (1959). Studies on the physico-chemical properties of reagin to horse dandruff. Immunol. *2*, 384.

Stanworth, D.R. (1963). Reaginic antibodies. Adv. in Immunol. *3*, 181.

Stanworth, D.R. (1964). Immunological relationships between human serum, horse serum and horse dandruff proteins. Protides of Biol. Fluids, 12th Bruges Colloq. ed. H. Peeters, p. 265.

Stanworth, D.R. (1965A). The structure of reagins. Int. Arch. Allergy *28*, 71.

Stanworth, D.R. (1965B). The characterisation of antigens and antibodies involved in immediate-type hypersensitivity. Trans. World Asthma Conf. (Eastbourne), p.56.

Stanworth, D.R. (1965C). Measurement of histamine release in vitro as an alternative to the P-K test in the assay of skin sensitising antibodies. Acta. Allergologica *20*, 221 (Abstr.).

Stanworth, D.R. (1967). Ultracentrifugation of Immunoglobulins. In: *Handbook of Experimental Immunology,* ed. D.M. Weir, (Blackwell) p. 44.

Stanworth, D.R. (1967). Tissue sensitising antibodies. Paper presented at a British Soc. for Immunology symposium on The Biological Effects of Different Immunoglobulin Classes (London).

Stanworth, D.R. (1969). The mechanism of the reagin reaction. Proc. VIIth European Congress of Allergology, Berlin, October 1968. Published in La Revue Francais D'Allergie *9*, 240.

Stanworth, D.R. (1970). Immunochemical mechanisms of immediate-type hypersensitivity reactions. Clin. Exp. Immunol. *6*, 1.

Stanworth, D.R. (1971). Immunoglobulin E (reagin) and allergy. Nature *233*, 310.

Stanworth, D.R. (1971). The experimental inhibition of reagin-mediated reactions. Clin. Allergy *1*, 25.

Stanworth, D.R. (1971). Unpublished data.

Stanworth, D.R. (1972). IgE and hypersensitivity in man. In: Scientific basis of medicine. 1971 Lecture series.

Stanworth, D.R., James, K. and Squire, J.R. (1961). Application of zone-centrifugation to the study of normal and pathological human sera. Anal. Biochem. *2*, 324.

Stanworth, D.R. and Kuhns, W.J. (1965). Quantitative studies on the assay of human skin sensitising antibodies (Reagins). I. An examination of factors affecting the accuracy of the Prausnitz-Küstner (P-K) test. Immunol. *8*, 323.

Stanworth, D.R. and Henney, C.S. (1967). Some biological activities associated with the 10S form of human γG-globulin. Immunol. *12*, 267.

Stanworth, D.R., Humphrey, J., Bennich, H. and Johansson, S.G.O. (1967). Specific inhibition of the Prausnitz-Küstner reaction by an atypical human myeloma protein. Lancet ii, 330.

Stanworth, D.R., Humphrey, J.H., Bennich, H. and Johansson, S.G.O. (1968). Inhibition of Prausnitz-Küstner reaction by proteolytic-cleavage fragments of a human myeloma protein of immunoglobulin class E. Lancet ii, 17.

Stanworth, D.R., Housley, J., Bennich, H. and Johansson, S.G.O. (1969A). Inhibition of reagin-induced passive anaphylaxis in baboons by myeloma IgE and certain of its proteolytic cleavage fragments. To be published (quoted in Stanworth, D.R. (1971). Clin. Allergy *1* 25).

Stanworth, D.R., Housley J., Bennich, H. and Johansson, S.G.O. (1969B). Effect of reduction upon the tissue-binding activity of immunoglobulin E. Immunochem. *7*, 32.

Stanworth, D.R., Housley, J., Bennich, H. and Johansson, S.G.O. (1969C). Studies of the skin reactivity of aggregated IgE in baboons. To be published (quoted in Stanworth, D.R. (1971). Nature *233*, 310).

Stanworth, D.R. and Johansson, S.G.O. (1973). Studies on the stability of γE antibodies during storage under various conditions. In preparation.

Stanworth, D.R., Smith, A.K. and Matthews, N. (1971). Demonstration of aggregate-specific determinants of heated human IgG by in vitro anaphylaxis in guinea pig ileum. In preparation.

Stanworth, D.R., Johns, P. and Jasani, B. (1972). Investigation of the possible application of microcalorimetry to the study of immediate hypersensitivity reactions in vitro. Science Tools *19*, 6.

Stechschulte, D.J., Austen, K.F. and Bloch, K.J. (1967). Antibodies involved in antigen-induced release of slow reacting substance of anaphylaxis (SRS-A) in the guinea pig. J. Exp. Med. *125*, 127.

Steele, A.S.V. and Coombs, R.R.A. (1964). The red cell-linked antigen test for incomplete antibodies to soluble proteins. Int. Arch. Allergy *25*, 11.

Stenius, B. and Wide, L. (1969). Reaginic antibody (IgE), skin, and provocation tests to *Dermatophagoides culinae* and house dust in respiratory allergy. Lancet ii, 455.

Stewart, D.F. (1955). Self-cure in nematode infestation of sheep. Nature *176*, 1273.

Stewart, G., Smith, A.K. and Stanworth, D.R. (1972). Studies of the biological properties of Facb fragments from rabbit IgG. In preparation.

Stewart, G.T. (1967). Allergenic residues in penicillins. Lancet i, 1177.

Storck, H., Hoigné, R. and Koller, F. (1955). Thrombocytes in allergic reactions. Int. Arch. Allergy *6*, 372.

Strannegård, Ö. (1971). Regulatory effects of antigen and antibody on the reagin response in rabbits. Clin. Exp. Immunol. *8*, 963.

Strannegård, Ö. and Yurchison, A. (1969). Formation of agglutinating and reaginic antibodies in rabbits following oral administration of soluble and particulate antigens. Int. Arch. Allergy *35*, 579.

Strannegård, Ö. and Yurchison, A. (1969A). Formation of rabbit reaginic antibodies to protein conjugates. Immunol. *16*, 387.

Strannegård, Ö. and Yurchison, A. (1969B). Formation of agglutinating and reaginic antibodies in rabbits following oral administration of soluble and particulate antigens. Int. Arch. Allergy *35*, 579.

Strannegård, Ö. and Belin, L. (1970). Suppression of reagin synthesis in rabbits by passively administered antibody. Immunol. *18*, 775.

Strannegård, Ö. and Belin, L. (1971). Enhancement of reagin formation in rabbits by passively administered 19S antibody. Immunol. *20*, 427.

Straus, H.W. (1937). Studies in experimental hypersensitiveness in the rhesus monkey. II. Passive local cutaneous sensitisation with human reaginic sera. J. Immunol. *32*, 251.

Strejan, G. and Campbell, D.H. (1967). Hypersensitivity to Ascaris antigens. II. The skin sensitising properties of 7S γ_2 antibody from sensitised guinea pigs as tested in guinea pigs. J. Immunol. *99*, 347.

Strejan, G. and Campbell, D.H. (1968). Skin sensitising properties of guinea pig antibodies to keyhole limpet hemocyanin. J. Immunol. *100*, 1245.

Strejan, G. and Campbell, D.H. (1970). Hypersensitivity to Ascaris antigens, V. Production of homocytotropic antibodies in the rabbit. J. Immunol. *105*, 1264.

Strejan, G. and Campbell, D.H. (1971). Hypersensitivity to Ascaris antigens. VI. Physico-chemical, immunochemical and biologic properties of rabbit homocytotropic antibodies produced to crude extracts. J. Immunol. *106*, 1363.

Swain, H.H. and Becker, E.L. (1952). Quantitative studies in skin testing, V. The whealing reactions of histamine and ragweed pollen extract. J. Allergy *23*, 441.

Tada, T. and Ishizaka, K. (1970). Distribution of E forming cells in lymphoid tissues of the human and monkey. J. Immunol. *104*, 377.

Tada, T. and Okumura, K. (1971A). Regulation of homocytotropic antibody formation in the rat. I. Feed-back regulation by passively administered antibody. J. Immunol. *106*, 1002.

Tada, T. and Okumura, K. (1971B). Regulation of homocytotropic antibody formation in the rat. II. Effect of X-irradiation. J. Immunol. *106*, 1012.

Tada, T. and Okumura, K. (1971C). Regulation of homocytotropic antibody formation in the rat. III. Effect of thymectomy and splenectomy. J. Immunol. *106*, 1019.

Tada, T. and Okumura, K. (1971D). Regulation of homocytotropic antibody formation in the rat. IV. Cell cooperation in the anti-hapten homocytotropic antibody response. J. Immunol. *107*, 1137.

Tanaka, R. and Strickland, K.P. (1965). Role of phospholipid in the activation of Na^+, K^+-activated adenosine triphosphatase of beef brain. Arch. Biochem. *111*, 583.

Taylor, A.B., Hayward, B.J. and Augustin, R. (1958). An investigation of Hoigné's light scattering method for the diagnosis of allergies. Int. Arch Allergy *12*, 365.

Taylor, S.H. and Thorp, J.M. (1959). Properties and biological behaviour of Coomassie Blue. Brit. Heart. J. *21*, 492.

Terr, A.I. and Bentz, J.D. (1964). Gel-filtration of human skin-sensitising antibody and β_2A-globulin. J. Allergy *35*, 206.

Terry, W.D. (1965). Skin sensitising activity related to γ-polypeptide chains characteristic of human IgG. J. Immunol. *95*, 1041.

Terry, W., Ogawa, M. and Kochwa, S. (1970). Structural studies of immunoglobulin E. II. Amino terminal sequence of the heavy chain. J. Immunol. *105*, 783.

Thon, I.L. and Uvnäs, B. (1967). Degranulation and histamine release, two consecutive steps in the response of rat mast cells to compound 48/80. Acta Physiol. Scand. *71*, 303.

Tigelaar, R.E., Vaz, N.M. and Ovary, Z. (1971). Immunoglobulin receptors on mouse mast cells. J. Immunol. *106*, 661.

Todorov, D.M., Wilkinson, P.C. and White, R.G. (1968). Affinity of immunoglobulin for heterologous tissue mast cells. A study with the fluorescent antibody method. Immunol. *15*, 51.

Tollackson, K.A. and Frick, U.L. (1966). Response of human smooth muscle in Schultz-Dale experiment. J. Allergy *37*, 195.

Turner, M.W., Johansson, S.G.O., Barratt, T.M. and Bennich, H. (1970). Studies on the levels of immunoglobulins in normal human urine with particular reference to IgE. Int. Arch. Allergy *37*, 409.

Underdown, B.J. and Goodfriend, L. (1969). Isolation and characterisation of an allergen from short ragweed pollen. Biochem. *8*, 980.

Underdown, B.J. and Goodfriend, L. (1970). Correlation of charge properties of human reaginic antibodies with charge of the corresponding allergens. J. Immunol. *104*, 530.

Urquhart, G.M., Mulligan, W., Eadie, R.M. and Jennings, F.W. (1965). Immunological studies on *Nippostrongylus brasiliensis* infection in the rat: the role of local anaphylaxis. Exp. Parasit. *17*, 210.

Utsumi, S. (1969). Stepwise cleavage of rabbit immunoglobulin G by papain and isolation of four types of biologically active Fc fragment. Biochem. J. *112*, 343.

Uvnäs, B. (1967). Mode of binding and release of histamine in mast cell granules. Federation Proc. *26*, 219.

Uvnäs, B. (1968). Metabolic and non-metabolic processes in the mechanism of histamine release from mast cells. In: C.I.O.M.S. Symp., Biochemistry of the acute allergic reactions, eds. K.F. Austen and E.L. Becker (Blackwell) p. 131.

Vaerman, J.P., Epstein, W., Fudenburg, H. and Ishizaka, K. (1964). Direct demonstration of reagin activity in purified γ_1A-globulin. Nature *203*, 1046.

Vaerman, J.P. and Heremans, J.F. (1969). Distribution of various immunoglobulin containing cells in canine lymphoid tissue. Immunol. *17*, 627.

Vaerman, J.P. and Heremans, J.F. (1970). Origin and molecular size of immunoglobulin-A in the mesenteric lymph of the dog. Immunol. *18*, 27.

Van Arsdel, P. (1962). Effects of humoral factors on antigenic histamine released from human leucocytes. J. Clin. Invest. *41*, 1407.

Van Arsdel, P.P. (1965). Effect of specific hyposensitisation on antigenic histamine release from human leucocytes. Federation Proc. *24*, 632.

Van Arsdel, P., Wack, S., Middleton, E., Sherman, W.B. and Buchwald, H. (1958). A quantitative study on the in vitro release of histamine from leukocytes of atopic persons. J. Allergy *29*, 429.

Van Arsdel, P.P. and Sells, C.J. (1963). Antigenic histamine release from passively sensitised human leukocytes. Science *141*, 1190.

Van Es, L., Den Harink, H. and Pondman, K.W. (1970). The specificity of skin sensitising antibody in the guinea pig. Clin. Exp. Immunol. *6*, 741.

Vaughan, J.H. and Kabat, E.A. (1953). Studies on the antibodies in rabbit antisera responsible for sensitization of human skin. I. The role of impurities in crystalline egg albumin in stimulating the production of skin-sensitising antibody. J. Exp. Med. *97*, 821.

Vaughan, W.T. and Black, J.H. (1954). Practice of Allergy. 3rd Ed., ch. XVIII (Henry Kimpton, London).

Vaz, E.M., Vaz, N.M. and Levine, B.B. (1971). Persistent formation of reagins in mice injected with low doses of ovalbumin. Immunol. *21*, 11.

Vaz, N.M. and Prouvost-Danon, A. (1969). Behaviour of mouse mast cells during anaphylaxis in vitro. Prog. Allergy *13*, 111.

Vaz, N.M. and Levine, B.B. (1970). Immune responses of inbred mice to repeated low doses of antigen: relationship to histocompatibility (H-2) type. Science *168*, 852.

Vaz, N.M., Vaz, E.M. and Levine, B.B. (1970). Relationship between histocompatibility (H-2) genotype and immune responsiveness to low doses of ovalbumin in the mouse. J. Immunol. *104*, 1572.

Versie, R. and Brocteur, J. (1967). Identification de proteines humaines dans les extracts allergeniques de poussieres de maison. Acta Allergologica *22*, 11.

Von Pirquet, C. (1906). Allergy. Münch. med. Wochschr *53*, 1457.

Voorhorst, R., Spieksma, F. ThM., Varekamp, H., Leupen, M.J. and Lyklema, A.W. (1967). The house-dust mite (*Dermatophagoides pteronyssinus*) and the allergens it produces. Identity with the house-dust allergen. J. Allergy *39*, 325.

Waldmann, T.A. (1969). Disorders of immunoglobulin metabolism. New Eng. J. Med. *281*, 1170.

Walzer, M. and Bowman, K.L. (1960). Leucocytic transfer of immediate-type hypersensitiveness in man. V. Transfer of experimental sensitivity to Ascaris antigen. Proc. Soc. Exp. Biol. Med. *105*, 246.

Ward, P.A. and Becker, E.L. (1970). Biochemical demonstration of the activatable esterase of the rabbit neutrophil involved in the chemotactic response. J. Immunol. *105*, 1057.

Weiszer, I., Patterson, R. and Pruzansky, J.J. (1968). Ascaris hypersensitivity in the rhesus monkey. A model for the study of immediate hypersensitivity in the primate. J. Allergy *41*, 14.

Weissmann, G., Dukor, P. and Zurier, R.B. (1971). Effect of cyclic AMP on release of lysosomal enzymes from phagocytes. Nature (New Biol.) *231*, 131.

Whittam, R. (1962). The asymmetrical stimulation of a membrane adenosine triphosphatase in relation to active action transport. Biochem. J. *84*, 110.

W.H.O. Technical Report Series No. 448 (1970). Factors regulating the immune response.

Wicher, V. and Dolovich, J. (1971). Non-immunologic inhibition of *B.* subtilis alkaline proteinases by human serum components. J. Allergy *47*, 98 (Abstract 27B)

Wide, L. and Porath, J. (1966). Radio-immunoassay of proteins with use of Sephadex-coupled antibodies. Biochim. Biophys. Acta *130*, 257.

Wide, L., Bennich, H. and Johansson, S.G.O. (1967). Diagnosis of allergy by an in vitro test for allergen antibodies. Lancet ii, 1105.

Wide, L. and Juhlin, L. (1971). Detection of penicillin allergy of the immediate type by radioimmunoassay of reagins (IgE) to penicilloyl conjugates. Clin. Allergy *1*, 171.

Wilkins, D.J., Ottewill, R.H. and Bangham, A.D. (1962). On the flocculation of sheep leucocytes. I. Electrophoretic studies. II. Stability studies. J. Theoret. Biol. *2*; 165, 176.

Wilson, A.B., Marchand, R. and Coombs, R.R.A. (1971). Passive allergisation in vitro of human basophils with serum containing IgE reaginic antibodies to castor allergen, demonstrated by rosette formation. Lancet ii, 1325.

Wilson, A.F., Novey, H.S., Surpenant, E.L. and Bennett, L.R. (1971). Fate of inhaled whole pollen in asthmatics. J. Allergy *47*, 107 (Abstr. 46).

Wilson, R.J.M. and Bloch, K.J. (1967). Homocytotropic antibody response in the rat infected with the nematode, *Nippostrongylus brasiliensis*: II. Characteristics of the immune response. III. Characteristics of the antibody. J. Immunol. *100*; 622, 629.

Yagi, Y., Maier, P., Pressman, D., Arbesman, C.E. and Reisman, R.E. (1963). The presence of ragweed-binding antibodies in the β_2A-, β_2M- and γ-globulins of sensitive individuals. J. Immunol. *91*, 83.

Yoshida, H., Fujisawa, H. and Ohi, Y. (1965). Influences of protamine on the Na^+, K^+-dependent ATP-ase and on the active transport processes of potassium and L-dopa in brain slices. Canad. J. Biochem. *43*, 841.

Yount, W.J., Dorner, M.M., Kunkel, H.G. and Kabat, E.A. (1968). Studies on human antibodies. VI. Selective variations in sub group composition and genetic markers. J. Exp. Med. *127*, 633.

Zeitz, S.J., Van Arsdel, P.P. and McClure, D.K. (1966). Specific response of human lymphocytes to pollen antigen in tissue culture. J. Allergy *38*, 321.

Zvaifler, N.J. and Becker, E.L. (1966). Rabbit anaphylactic antibody. J. Exp. Med. *123*, 935.

Zvaifler, N.J. and Robinson, J.O. (1969). Rabbit homocytotropic antibody. A unique rabbit immunoglobulin analogous to human IgE. J. Exp. Med. *130*, 907.

Subject index